Lung Transplantation

Editors

LUIS F. ANGEL
STEPHANIE M. LEVINE

CLINICS IN CHEST MEDICINE

www.chestmed.theclinics.com

March 2023 • Volume 44 • Number 1

ELSEVIER

1600 John F. Kennedy Boulevard • Suite 1800 • Philadelphia, Pennsylvania, 19103-2899

http://www.theclinics.com

CLINICS IN CHEST MEDICINE Volume 44, Number 1
March 2023 ISSN 0272-5231, ISBN-13: 978-0-323-96071-7

Editor: Joanna Gascoine
Developmental Editor: Karen Justine S. Dino

Clinics in Chest Medicine (ISSN 0272-5231) is published quarterly by Elsevier Inc., 360 Park Avenue South, New York, NY 10010-1710. Months of issue are March, June, September, and December. Periodicals postage paid at New York, NY and additional mailing offices. Subscription prices are $420.00 per year (domestic individuals), $895.00 per year (domestic institutions), $100.00 per year (domestic students/residents), $449.00 per year (Canadian individuals), $1112.00 per year (Canadian institutions), $514.00 per year (international individuals), $1112.00 per year (international institutions), $100.00 per year (Canadian Students), and $230.00 per year (International Students). International air speed delivery is included in all Clinics subscription prices. All prices are subject to change without notice. **POSTMASTER:** Send address changes to Clinics in Chest Medicine, Elsevier Health Sciences Division, Subscription Customer Service, 3251 Riverport Lane, Maryland Heights, MO 63043. **Customer Service: Telephone: 1-800-654-2452** (U.S. and Canada); **1-314-447-8871** (outside U.S. and Canada). **Fax: 1-314-447-8029. E-mail: journalscustomerservice-usa@elsevier.com (for print support); journalsonlinesupport-usa@elsevier.com (for online support).**

Reprints. For copies of 100 or more of articles in this publication, please contact the Commercial Reprints Department, Elsevier Inc., 360 Park Avenue South, New York, NY 10010-1710. Tel.: 212-633-3874; Fax: 212-633-3820; E-mail: reprints@elsevier.com.

Clinics in Chest Medicine is covered in *MEDLINE/PubMed (Index Medicus), Current Contents/Clinical Medicine, EMBASE/ Excerpta Medica, Science Citation Index,* and *ISI/BIOMED.*

Contributors

EDITORS

LUIS F. ANGEL, MD
Director of Lung Transplantation, Professor of Medicine and Cardiothoracic Surgery, NYU Langone Medical Center, Transplant Institute, New York University, New York, New York, USA

STEPHANIE M. LEVINE, MD
Vice-Chair of Medical Education, Department of Medicine, Professor of Medicine, Division of Pulmonary Diseases and Critical Care Medicine, University of Texas Health San Antonio, Staff Physicians South Texas Veterans Healthcare System, San Antonio, Texas, USA

AUTHORS

LUIS F. ANGEL, MD
Director of Lung Transplantation, Professor of Medicine and Cardiothoracic Surgery, NYU Langone Medical Center, Transplant Institute, New York University, New York, New York, USA

SELIM M. ARCASOY, MD, MPH
Lung Transplant Program, Columbia University Irving Medical Center, New York, New York, USA

CARL ATKINSON, PhD
Professor of Medicine, University of Florida, Gainesville, Florida, USA

DIEGO AVELLA, MD
Thoracic Surgery, Department of Surgery, Feinberg School of Medicine, Northwestern University, Chicago, Illinois, USA

MEGHAN AVERSA, MD, MS
Assistant Professor, Division of Respirology, Department of Medicine, University Health Network and University of Toronto, Toronto, Ontario, Canada

HANNE BEECKMANS, MD
Department of Chronic Diseases and Metabolism, KU Leuven, Laboratory of Respiratory Diseases and Thoracic Surgery (BREATHE), Leuven, Belgium

ANKIT BHARAT, MD
Thoracic Surgery, Department of Surgery, Feinberg School of Medicine, Northwestern University, Chicago, Illinois, USA

SASKIA BOS, MD
Department of Respiratory Diseases, University Hospitals Leuven, Leuven, Belgium; Newcastle University, Translational and Clinical Research Institute, Newcastle upon Tyne, United Kingdom

MARIE M. BUDEV, DO, MPH, FCCP
Professor, Lerner College of Medicine, Respiratory Institute, Cleveland Clinic, Cleveland, Ohio, USA

FAY BURROWS, BPharm (Hons)
Department of Pharmacy, St Vincent's Hospital, Sydney, New South Wales, Australia

RYAN CHABAN, MD
Department of Surgery, Center for Transplantation Sciences, Massachusetts General Hospital, Harvard Medical School, Boston, Massachusetts, USA; Department of Cardiovascular Surgery, University Hospital of Johannes Gutenberg University, Mainz, Germany

JUSTIN C.Y. CHAN, MD, MPhil
Assistant Professor of Cardiothoracic Surgery, Division of Thoracic Surgery, Department of

Cardiothoracic Surgery, NYU Transplant Institute, New York University, NYU Langone Health, New York, New York, USA

STEPHANIE H. CHANG, MD
Assistant Professor of Cardiothoracic Surgery, Surgical Director of Lung Transplant, Division of Thoracic Surgery, Department of Cardiothoracic Surgery, NYU Transplant Institute, New York University, NYU Langone Health, New York City, New York, USA

EMILY S. CLAUSEN, MD
Assistant Professor of Clinical Medicine, Division of Pulmonary, Allergy, and Critical Care, Department of Medicine, Perelman School of Medicine, University of Pennsylvania, Philadelphia, Pennsylvania, USA

ANDREW COURTWRIGHT, MD, PhD
Assistant Professor of Medicine, Hospital of University of Pennsylvania, Philadelphia, Pennsylvania, USA

MARCELO CYPEL, MD, MSC
Professor of Surgery, Toronto Lung Transplant Program, Toronto General Hospital, Toronto, Ontario, Canada

ALLAN R. GLANVILLE, MD
Lung Transplant Unit, St. Vincent's Hospital, Sydney, Australia

HILARY J. GOLDBERG, MD, MPH
Brigham and Women's Hospital, Harvard Medical School, Boston, Massachusetts, USA

HARPREET SINGH GREWAL, MD
Lung Transplant Program, Columbia University Irving Medical Center, New York, New York, USA

RAMSEY R. HACHEM, MD
Division of Pulmonary and Critical Care, Washington University School of Medicine, St Louis, Missouri, USA

LAURA P. HALVERSON, MD
Division of Pulmonary and Critical Care, Washington University School of Medicine, St Louis, Missouri, USA

ELAINE C. JOLLY, MBChB, BSc, PhD
Division of Renal Medicine, Department of Medicine, University of Cambridge, Cambridge, United Kingdom

SIDDHARTHA G. KAPNADAK, MD
Associate Professor, Division of Pulmonary, Critical Care, and Sleep Medicine, Department of Medicine, University of Washington School of Medicine

THOMAS KELLER, MD
Clinical Instructor, Division of Pulmonary, Critical Care, and Sleep Medicine, Department of Medicine, University of Washington School of Medicine

ERIKA D. LEASE, MD, FCCP
Associate Professor of Medicine, Division of Pulmonary, Critical Care, and Sleep Medicine, University of Washington, Seattle, Washington, USA

MELISSA B. LESKO, DO
Assistant Professor of Medicine, Assistant Program Director, Pulmonary and Critical Care Fellowship, Division of Pulmonary and Critical Care Medicine, NYU Langone Medical Center, New York, New York, USA

HAIFA LYSTER, MSc, FRPharmS, FFRPS
Cardiothoracic Transplant Unit, Royal Brompton and Harefield Hospitals, Part of Guy's & St Thomas' NHS Foundation Trust, Kings College, London, United Kingdom

GABRIELA MAGDA, MD
Assistant Professor of Medicine, Columbia University Lung Transplant Program, Division of Pulmonary, Allergy, and Critical Care Medicine, Columbia University Irving Medical Center, Columbia University Vagelos College of Physicians and Surgeons, New York, New York, USA

HANNAH MANNEM, MD
Associate Professor, Division of Pulmonary and Critical Care Medicine, University of Virginia School of Medicine

BRYAN F. MEYERS, MD, MPH
Washington University School of Medicine, Barnes-Jewish Hospital, St Louis, Missouri, USA

ROBERT A. MONTGOMERY, MD, DPhil
NYU Transplant Institute, New York University, New York, New York, USA

JAKE G. NATALINI, MD, MSCE
Assistant Professor of Medicine, Division of Pulmonary and Critical Care Medicine, New

York University, NYU Langone Health, New York, New York, USA

HENRY NEUMANN, MD
Transplant Infectious Diseases, Division of Infectious Diseases, Assistant Professor, Department of Medicine, NYU School of Medicine

CAROLINE M. PATTERSON, BMBS, BMedSci, MD
Transplant Continuing Care Unit, Royal Papworth Hospital NHS Foundation Trust, Cambridge, United Kingdom

G. ALEXANDER PATTERSON, MD
Joseph C. Bancroft Professor of Surgery, Editor-in-Chief AATS Journals, Division of Cardiothoracic Surgery, Department of Surgery, Washington University School of Medicine, St Louis, Missouri, USA

ANDRES PELAEZ, MD
Associate Professor of Medicine, Jackson Health System, University of Miami Miller School of Medicine, Miami Transplant Institute, Miami, Florida, USA

RICHARD N. PIERSON III, MD
Department of Surgery, Center for Transplantation Sciences, Massachusetts General Hospital, Harvard Medical School, Boston, Massachusetts, USA

NICOLA J. RONAN, MbBCh, PhD
Transplant Continuing Care Unit, Royal Papworth Hospital NHS Foundation Trust, Cambridge, United Kingdom

DARYA RUDYM, MD
Assistant Professor of Medicine, Division of Pulmonary and Critical Care Medicine, New York University, NYU Langone Health, New York, New York, USA

SAHAR A. SADDOUGHI, MD, PhD
Assistant Professor of Surgery, Division of Thoracic Surgery, Department of Cardiovascular Surgery, Mayo Clinic, Rochester, Minnesota, USA

MELANIE SUBRAMANIAN, MD
Washington University School of Medicine, Barnes-Jewish Hospital, St Louis, Missouri, USA

TANY THANIYAVARN, MD
Brigham and Women's Hospital, Harvard Medical School, Boston, Massachusetts, USA

ANIL J. TRINDADE, MD
Assistant Professor of Medicine, Division of Allergy, Pulmonary, and Critical Care Medicine, Vanderbilt University Medical Center, Nashville, Tennessee, USA

WAYNE M. TSUANG, MD, MHS
Assistant Professor of Medicine, Lerner College of Medicine, Respiratory Institute, Cleveland Clinic, Cleveland, Ohio, USA

ROBIN VOS, MD, PhD
Department of Chronic Diseases and Metabolism, KU Leuven, Laboratory of Respiratory Diseases and Thoracic Surgery (BREATHE), Department of Respiratory Diseases, University Hospitals Leuven, Leuven, Belgium

Contents

> Lung transplantation remains the only available therapy for many patients with end-stage lung disease. The number of lung transplants performed has increased significantly, but development of the field was slow compared with other solid-organ transplants. This delayed growth was secondary to the increased complexity of transplanting lungs; the continuous needs for surgical, anesthetics, and critical care improvements; changes in immunosuppression and infection prophylaxis; and donor management and patient selection. The future of lung transplant remains promising: expansion of donor after cardiac death donors, improved outcomes, new immunosuppressants targeted to cellular and antibody-mediated rejection, and use of xenotransplantation or artificial lungs.

> Lung transplantation can be lifesaving for patients with advanced lung disease. Demographics are evolving with recipients now sicker but determining candidacy remains predicated on one's underlying lung disease prognosis, along with the likelihood of posttransplant success. Determining optimal timing can be challenging, and most programs favor initiating the process early and proactively to allow time for patient education, informed decision-making, and preparation. A comprehensive, multidisciplinary evaluation is used to elucidate disease progrnosis and identify risk factors for poor posttransplant outcomes. Candidacy criteria vary significantly by center, and close communication between referring and transplant providers is necessary to improve access to transplant and outcomes.

> Selection of lung transplant candidates is an evolving field that pushes the boundaries of what is considered the norm. Given the continually changing demographics of the typical lung transplant recipient as well as the growing list of risk factors that predispose patients to poor posttransplant outcomes, we explore the dilemmas in lung transplant candidate selections pertaining to older age, frailty, low and high body mass index, preexisting cancers, and systemic autoimmune rheumatic diseases.

> This article examines the existing literature regarding single (SLT) and bilateral lung transplantation (BLT) to help answer the question of which approach is preferable.

Specifically, this review highlights the following subjects: disease-specific indications for SLT versus BLT; the impact of procedure type on posttransplantation functional status; the impact of procedure type on posttransplantation quality of life; chronic rejection after lung transplantation; ethical challenges facing the choice between single and bilateral transplants; and, novel strategies in this arena.

The first official donor lung allocation system in the United States was initiated by the United Network of Organ Sharing in 1990. The initial policy for lung allocation was simple with donor lungs allocated based on ABO match and the amount of time the candidates accrued on the waiting list. Donor offers were first given to candidates' donor service area. In March 2005, the implementation of the lung allocation score (LAS) was the major change in organ allocation. International adoption of the LAS-based allocation system can be seen worldwide.

Rates of lung donation have increased over the past several years. This has been accomplished through the utilization of donors with extended criteria, the creation of donor hospitals or centers, and the optimization of lungs through the implementation of donor management protocols. These measures have resulted in augmenting the pool of available donors thereby decreasing the wait time for lung transplantation candidates. Although transplant programs vary significantly in their acceptance rates of these organs, studies have not shown any difference in the incidence of primary graft dysfunction or overall mortality for the recipient when higher match-run sequence organs are accepted. Yet, the level of comfort in accepting these donors varies among transplant programs. This deviation in practice results in these organs going to lower-priority candidates thereby increasing the waitlist time of other recipients and ultimately has a deleterious effect on an institution's waitlist mortality.

Organ shortage remains a limiting factor in lung transplantation. Traditionally, donation after brain death has been the main source of lungs used for transplantation; however, to meet the demand of patients requiring lung transplantation it is crucial to find innovative methods for organ donation. The implementation of extended donors, lung donation after circulatory death (DCD), the use of ex-vivo lung perfusion (EVLP) systems, and more recently the acceptance of hepatitis C donors have started to close the gap between organ donors and recipients in need of lung transplantation. This article focuses on the expansion of donor lungs for transplantation after DCD, the use of EVLP in evaluating extended criteria lungs, and the use of lung grafts from donors with hepatitis C.

Justin C.Y. Chan, Ryan Chaban, Stephanie H. Chang, Luis F. Angel, Robert A. Montgomery, and Richard N. Pierson III

Xenotransplantation promises to alleviate the issue of donor organ shortages and to decrease waiting times for transplantation. Recent advances in genetic engineering have allowed for the creation of pigs with up to 16 genetic modifications. Several combinations of genetic modifications have been associated with extended graft survival and life-supporting function in experimental heart and kidney xenotransplants. Lung xenotransplantation carries specific challenges related to the large surface area of the lung vascular bed, its innate immune system's intrinsic hyperreactivity to perceived 'danger', and its anatomic vulnerability to airway flooding after even localized loss of alveolocapillary barrier function. This article discusses the current status of lung xenotransplantation, and challenges related to immunology, physiology, anatomy, and infection. Tissue engineering as a feasible alternative to develop a viable lung replacement solution is discussed.

CLINICS IN CHEST MEDICINE

SERIES OF RELATED INTEREST

Critical Care Clinics
Available at: https://www.criticalcare.theclinics.com/

THE CLINICS ARE AVAILABLE ONLINE!
Access your subscription at:
www.theclinics.com

Preface

40 Years in the Making: Lung Transplantation Past, Present, and Future

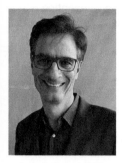
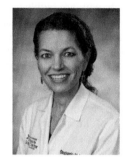

Luis F. Angel, MD   Stephanie M. Levine, MD
Editors

The year 2023 has marked historic milestones in the evolution of lung transplantation. Sixty years ago, on June 11, 1963, Dr James Hardy performed the first human lung transplant at the University of Mississippi. It was not until November 7, 1983 that the current modern era of lung transplantation began after a successful single-lung transplantation performed by Dr Joel D. Cooper at the Toronto Lung Transplant Program. Today, 40 years later and with nearly ninety thousand transplant procedures performed worldwide, we confidently feel that lung transplantation has evolved—becoming an excellent alternative for thousands of patients with advanced lung diseases. Due to lung transplantation's challenging nature, perhaps being the most complex of solid organ transplants, these improvements have been incremental—feeling sometimes painfully slow for patients and transplant teams alike.

In this commemorative issue of *Clinics in Chest Medicine*, we highlight some of the major advancements in lung transplantation. To properly recount the history of lung transplantation, Dr Alexander Paterson shared his memories of 40 years of lung transplantation, starting with the very first transplant in Toronto. In addition to looking at the past and present, we also look into the future of lung transplantation, including an article on Xenotransplantation and Lung Bioengineering, seeing recent major advancements in both early human heart and kidney xenotransplantation. This article provides an updated review on the current state of lung xenotransplantation as we work toward eventually allowing this to be a workable possibility for patients in need of lung transplantation.

Another article focuses on the lung-transplant candidates themselves, describing the major advances that have allowed us to transplant older and sicker patients as well as recommendations for best timing for referral. We also include a more detailed article of some of the most frequent dilemmas faced when listing, including older age, low and high body weight, frailty, preexisting cancers, and systemic diseases. The critical care management of the pre–lung-transplant and post–lung-transplant patients is then reviewed, providing an overview of the intensive management of patients requiring mechanical ventilation and extracorporeal membrane oxygenation (ECMO) support.

Once a patient is approved as a candidate for lung transplantation, the next decision is on what would be the ideal type of transplant procedure

Clin Chest Med 44 (2023) xiii–xv
https://doi.org/10.1016/j.ccm.2022.12.001

followed by the proper placement on the transplant list. We include an article that elaborates on, in a comprehensive manner, the options of either a single- or a bilateral lung-transplant procedure. The authors support what has become the most widespread practice worldwide of performing bilateral lung transplantation in 80% of the lung-transplant candidates. The discussion about the type of procedure (single-lung transplant vs bilateral lung transplant) now needs to move from the focus on short-term survival to a broader discussion that focuses on the quality of life in patients who are now living longer, and the benefits of having an "extra lung" to provide higher lung capacity and better handling of many of the potential complications of this procedure. In the article on donor management review, the authors share our view that listing for bilateral lungs offers more opportunities to use "not perfect" bilateral lungs for patients who otherwise will be waiting for the ideal single organ while also decreasing the number of discarded organs.

Led in part by the efforts made in the United States, the allocation systems around the world have evolved, now providing more fair distribution of organs. This year a new allocation system based on a continuous distribution of organs was implemented in the United States based on medical urgency, outcomes, efficiency, and patient access. This new allocation system, like other systems around the world, is reviewed in detail. Lung donation has always been considered to be one of the main limitations to the process of lung transplantation; however, the article on donor management and the use of donors after cardiac death, ex vivo lung perfusion, and hepatitis C donors shows how despite the increasing number of lung transplants, the implementation of donor management protocols, and the use of other types of donors offer a hope to close the gap between the number of donors and transplant candidates waiting for transplantation. This gap is now much smaller and could be further closed with a unity in practices among donor procurement organizations and transplant programs. A better understanding of the patient arriving at the donor hospital with no history of lung diseases, normal lung images, and lung mechanics can, despite the common presence of single-lobar pneumonia, atelectasis, and fluid overload, become a "nonperfect" lung donor while still providing comparable results for transplant recipients with the rarely available "perfect" donor lungs.

Major progress has been made in the understanding of both antibody-mediated and T-cell immunity in lung transplantation. This is unfortunately not yet reflected as a standardized way to prevent and treat both acute and chronic lung allograft dysfunction, but it has established a more solid basis for new and promising therapies for lung-transplant recipients, as reviewed in an article devoted to this topic. The advancements to this approach are more commonly seen in patients who are highly sensitized, presenting alternatives for the diagnosis, listing, and potential management, while also providing a better alternative to allow a successful transplant (now included in the new continuous distribution system for allocation of organs discussed above) and are reviewed in another article. The presence of newly formed or preformed antibodies in the role of acute and chronic rejection is now a routine part of the monitoring of our patients, and these new therapeutic targets are further discussed in an accompanying article. Also, the classic definitions of lung rejection are discussed in a detailed article with a provocative and helpful renaming of acute rejection based more on the actual immunologic mechanisms in the two groups, the antibody-mediated rejection, as discussed above, and the new classification of T-cell–mediated rejection. We also believe that with our better understanding of immunology, better diagnostic tools, and new therapeutic agents, this classification will become the standard in the near future.

The evolution of lung transplantation has now provided a longer survival rate for most patients, in particular, bilateral lung recipients, who are now commonly surviving 8 to 10 years. This improved survival is also related to the better understanding and management of infectious and noninfectious complications for our patients (also reviewed in detail in two articles). Finally, in these unprecedented years of a global pandemic with SARS-CoV-2, we have faced further challenges in both preventing and treating this infection in our lung-transplant patients, as well as a new indication for lung transplantation for severely acute patients with COVID-19 acute respiratory distress syndrome, most on ECMO support. This experience is reviewed in detail in the COVID-19 and lung-transplantation article.

Ultimately, as reviewed in this issue of the *Clinics in Chest Medicine*, we have seen considerable progress in multiple areas. Surviving a lung-transplant surgery and the acute postoperative period is no longer a major limitation, yet we will continue to face challenges for long-term survival in transplant recipients, and this will continue for the near future as we advance our knowledge about the immune and nonimmune mechanisms associated with chronic lung allograft dysfunction. In the meantime, after these past 40 years of successful lung transplantation, we will focus on better use of our potential lung donors, aiming to perform the best type of procedure, and striving to have more similar practices among donor procurement organizations and lung-transplant programs worldwide, allowing recipients the opportunity of a successful lung transplant regardless of location. We want to sincerely thank all the authors who contributed to writing these excellent reviews, which will, it is hoped, make this issue of the *Clinics in Chest Medicine* a source of information for the hundreds of health care workers currently taking part in this exciting field.

Luis F. Angel, MD
SurgeryNYU Langone Health - NYU Grossman
School of Medicine
New York, NY 10530, USA

Stephanie M. Levine, MD
Division of Pulmonary Diseases and
Critical Care Medicine
University of Texas Health San Antonio
South Texas Veterans Healthcare System
San Antonio, TX 78229, USA

E-mail addresses:
luis.angel@nyulangone.org (L.F. Angel)
levines@uthscsa.edu (S.M. Levine)

History of Lung Transplantation

Stephanie H. Chang, MD[a],*, Justin Chan, MD[a], G. Alexander Patterson, MD[b]

KEYWORDS

• Lung transplantation • History • Single lung transplant • Double lung transplant

KEY POINTS

- Initial lung transplants in the 1960s and 1970s were unsuccessful because of issues with surgical techniques and lack of effective immunosuppression.
- The first successful single lung transplant was performed in 1983 and the first successful double lung transplant was performed in 1986, by Dr Joel Cooper at the University of Toronto.
- Standardization of surgical technique, organ preservation, prophylaxis, and treatment of opportunistic infections and immunosuppression led to a rapid worldwide expansion of lung transplantation in the 1990s.
- Recent developments with the frequent use of extended donors, increased donation after circulatory death, and use of hepatitis C–positive donors has contributed to the increased number of patients receiving lung transplants.

INTRODUCTION

Lung transplantation remains the only available therapy for many patients with end-stage lung disease, increasing their quality of life along with prolonging survival. The number of lung transplants performed has increased significantly over the recent decades,[1] but the development of the field was slow compared with other solid-organ transplants. This delayed growth was secondary to the increased complexity of transplanting lungs; the continuous needs for surgical, anesthetics, and critical care improvements; changes in immunosuppression and infection prophylaxis; and donor management and patient selection, among many other developments.

EARLY EXPERIENCE: THE 1960S TO 1970S

The first human lung transplant was performed on June 11, 1963, by Dr James Hardy (**Fig. 1**) at the University of Mississippi.[2] The recipient was a 58-year-old male prisoner with emphysema who presented to the hospital with increased shortness of breath. He had a central left lung carcinoma with nodal metastases, postobstructive pneumonia, and severe emphysema in the right lung. Because of his poor baseline lung function, a left pneumonectomy would have led to respiratory failure. Thus, a single left lung transplant was performed. Without a definition at that time for brain death and organ donation, the lung allograft was harvested from a donor after cardiac death (DCD). Perioperative immunosuppression included azathioprine, cortisone, and radiation of the thymic region.[2] The patient initially survived 18 days but died of renal failure and advanced lung cancer with no respiratory failure. At the time of autopsy, no rejection was present, although there was a small defect on the membranous aspect of the bronchial anastomosis that had been sealed by surrounding inflammatory reaction.[3]

Over the subsequent two decades, approximately 40 lung or heart-lung transplants were attempted with minimal success.[4] Those patients

[a] Division of Thoracic Surgery, Department of Cardiothoracic Surgery, New York University Langone Health, New York City, NY, USA; [b] Division of Cardiothoracic Surgery, Department of Surgery, Washington University School of Medicine, St Louis, MO, USA
* Corresponding author. Department of Cardiothoracic Surgery, New York University Langone Health, 530 First Avenue, Suite 9V, New York City, NY 10016.
E-mail address: stephanie.chang@nyulangone.org

Clin Chest Med 44 (2023) 1–13
https://doi.org/10.1016/j.ccm.2022.11.004
0272-5231/23/© 2022 Elsevier Inc. All rights reserved.

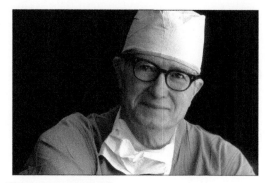

Fig. 1. Dr James Hardy.

died of rejection, pneumonia, pulmonary insuffi-ciency, and often bronchial dehiscence, as was seen in a single right lung transplant performed in 1978 at the University in Toronto.[4] The recipient was a 19-year-old man with inhalational injury from a fire, requiring preoperative extracorporeal membrane oxygenator (ECMO) support. He initially did well with methylprednisolone and azathioprine immunosuppression. He was able to ambulate and was weaned off ventilator support, but he died in the third postoperative week from a bronchial anastomotic breakdown.

Initial Advances in Immunosuppression

As a result of their own experience and improve-ments in immunosuppression with other solid or-gans, the group in Toronto performed experiments in animal models to evaluate the role of immunosup-pression and ischemia on bronchial anastomoses. Autotransplantation was performed in animals, comparing no immunosuppression with the stan-dard immunosuppression at the time, prednisone and azathioprine.[5] In these studies, the animals with no immunosuppression had good primary heal-ing, but the group with prednisone and azathioprine had a higher rate of bronchial complications. Further studies comparing prednisone and azathioprine noted that prednisone alone was associated with poor bronchial healing.

During this time, another key immunosuppres-sive agent was developed. In the 1970s, cyclo-sporine was discovered and found to be a "novel antilymphocyte agent."[6] Clinical trials were per-formed for kidney transplants, which showed improved graft survival and function.[7] Dr Joel Coo-per's laboratory next performed lung transplanta-tion in animal models evaluating (1) no immunosuppression, (2) prednisone and azathio-prine, and (3) cyclosporine A.[8] They demonstrated normal bronchial wound healing in the no immuno-suppression group and cyclosporine A group, with no difference in bronchial strength between those two groups.

Initial Advances in Surgical Technique

Another concern was ischemia of the bronchus, because the bronchial arterial blood supply is not reattached during lung transplant. Abdominal omentum is well recognized as an excellent source of collateral circulation. Dr Cooper's laboratory group studied the use of an omental pedicle flap in animal models using a bronchial stump graft. They found that all the animals without omental wraps had necrosis of the bronchus within 5 days, whereas the group with omental wraps had viable bronchial grafts with full revasculariza-tion on Day 23.[9] Comparable results were found with omental wraps for animal lung transplanta-tion.[10,11] A follow-up animal study evaluated the use of cyclosporine in combination with pedicled omental flaps, which showed good bronchial heal-ing with no stenosis after the lung transplant.[12]

During this time, Dr Bruce Reitz and Dr Norman Shumway (**Fig. 2**) were modifying the technique used for heart-lung transplantation. Previously, animal models evaluating heart-lung transplanta-tion were performed using a lateral thoracotomy, with anastomosis of the trachea, aorta, superior vena cava, and inferior vena cava. Because of the small size of the primates, this technique resulted in stenosis of the inferior vena cava.[13] Reitz and colleagues[14] thus modified their tech-nique using a median sternotomy and retaining part of the right atrium for inflow anastomosis, which had superior results in combination with cyclosporine immunosuppression.

BEGINNING OF SUCCESSFUL LUNG TRANSPLANTATION: THE 1980S
Heart-Lung Transplant

Based on the advances in immunosuppression and surgical models, Dr Reitz and Dr Shumway per-formed a heart-lung transplant on March 9, 1981, at Stanford Hospital (**Fig. 3**). The recipient was a 45-year-old woman with primary pulmonary hyper-tension with progressive right heart failure.[15] Her immunosuppression regimen consisted of cyclo-sporine, methylprednisolone, and azathioprine. Although she had two early initial episodes of rejec-tion, she overall did well and was discharged home with good lung function, heralding the first suc-cessful heart-lung transplant. This technique used an en bloc allograft of the heart and both lungs, which included anastomoses of the distal tracheal, ascending aortic and right atrium. An added benefit was preservation of collateral blood flow from the coronary to bronchial arteries. Combined heart-lung transplant was indicated for patients with elevated pulmonary vascular resistance and

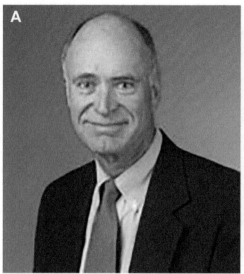
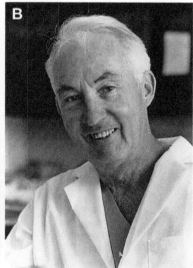

Fig. 2. (A) Dr Bruce Reitz. (B) Dr Norman Shumway.

associated heart failure,[16] and for patients with septic lung disease.

Single Lung Transplant for Pulmonary Fibrosis

Isolated lung transplants continued to have difficulty with long-term survival. In 1982, the group in Toronto General Hospital performed a right lung transplant in a 31-year-old man with paraquat poisoning requiring preoperative ECMO support.[17] However, the right allograft was damaged postoperatively by continued paraquat entering the bloodstream. The patient was placed on a charcoal dialysis system to clear the paraquat from the bloodstream, then underwent left lung transplant 3 weeks after his initial right lung transplant. Despite these efforts, the patient eventually died of myopathy and a cerebrovascular accident. This incident led to further scrutiny regarding selection criteria for appropriate recipients, as many transplants

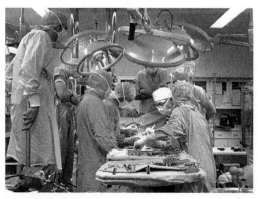

Fig. 3. The operating room during the first long-term surviving heart-lung transplant.

were performed for acutely ill patients with multiorgan failure or who were ventilator dependent.

Based on their prior experience, the group in Toronto determined that patients with pulmonary fibrosis were ideal candidates for single lung transplant. They stated that "the poor compliance and increased pulmonary vascular resistance of the native lung would ensure that ventilation and perfusion will be directed preferentially toward the transplanted lung, then avoiding a ventilation-perfusion imbalance."[18] Additionally, patients who were ventilator dependent or could not be weaned from long-term corticosteroid use were not considered eligible lung transplant candidates at the time.

On November 7, 1983, a 58-year-old man with pulmonary fibrosis underwent a laparotomy with omental mobilization, followed by a right lung transplant with the pedicled omental flap[18] at the Toronto General Hospital (**Fig. 4**). Perioperative immunosuppression was cyclosporine and azathioprine. Although he had two initial rejection episodes, the patient did well and survived for years after his transplant. A second single lung transplant was performed on November 30, 1984, in a 42-year-old woman with idiopathic pulmonary fibrosis. She underwent a single left lung transplant, with similar perioperative immunosuppression. Although she also had an early rejection episode, she was also discharged home with a good clinical outcome.[18] These two patients marked the first successful isolated lung transplants, ushering in a new era for lung transplantation.

Bilateral Lung Transplant

Despite the advances in single lung transplant, bilateral lung transplant without the heart was still

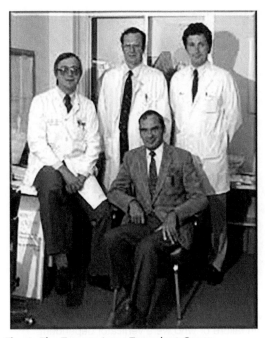

Fig. 4. The Toronto Lung Transplant Group.

not feasible in the early 1980s. Moreover, single lung transplant was not considered an appropriate option for patients with chronic obstructive pulmonary disease, because of concern that the native lung would overinflate and shift the mediastinum toward the transplanted lung. Animal models were used to create a technique for en bloc double lung transplant, which involved circulatory arrest with anastomoses at the distal trachea, posterior left atrium, and main pulmonary artery (PA).[19]

Based on their research, Dr G. Alexander Patterson and Dr Cooper (**Fig. 5**) performed a successful en bloc double lung transplant on November 26, 1986, for a 42-year-old woman with end-stage emphysema from α_1-antitrypsin deficiency.[20] This surgery was performed using cardiopulmonary bypass with cardioplegia arrest through a median sternotomy. The tracheal anastomosis was wrapped with omentum, the donor atrial cuff was sewn to the back of the recipient's left atrium, and the main PA was anastomosed.[21] The patient did well and survived for many years, as did the subsequent two recipients who underwent the same procedure. However, the fourth recipient developed ischemic necrosis of the donor trachea and died 3 weeks after transplantation.

In the mid-1980s, patients with septic lung disease were treated with a heart-lung transplant because of their ineligibility for single lung transplant, because the remaining native lung would remain as an infectious source after transplantation. However, many patients with end-stage lung disease did not require a heart-lung transplant because of normal cardiac function. Dr Magdi Yacoub (**Fig. 6**) developed domino transplants, using the heart from the heart-lung recipient as an allograft for transplantation in another recipient.[22] This domino transplant strategy was used in a few other centers but never gained wide acceptance.[23] Furthermore, heart-lung transplantation still had a high operative mortality with poor 1-year survival.[24] Given these limitations, en bloc double lung transplant was next expanded to patients with cystic fibrosis and bronchiectasis.[25]

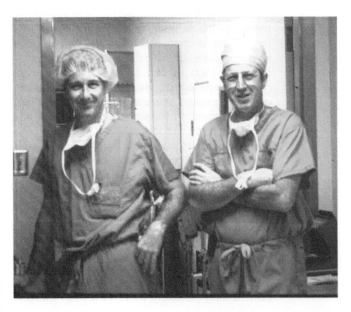

Fig. 5. Dr G. Alexander Patterson and Dr. Joel Cooper.

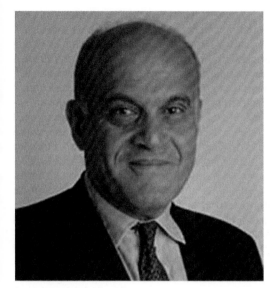

Fig. 6. Dr Magdi Yacoub.

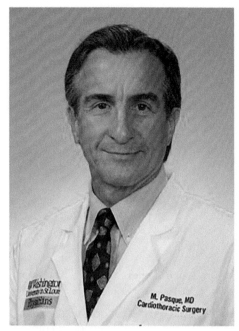

Fig. 7. Dr Michael Pasque.

Despite the success of en bloc double lung transplant, this technique was still complex[21] and had increased airway complications compared to heart-lung transplantation,[26] with a 25% mortality rate from airway ischemia.[27] Because of the issues with the tracheal anastomosis, surgeons adopted a bilateral bronchial anastomoses strategy, although that technique continued to have issues with necrosis and dehiscence.[26,28] The proposed solution was to evaluate if bronchial artery revascularization was feasible.[29] En bloc bilateral lung transplant with tracheal and bronchial revascularization was proposed. The en bloc double lung allograft was harvested with a cuff of donor aorta containing a bronchial artery orifice. The aortic cuff was then anastomosed to the recipient left internal mammary artery[30] or right intercostobrachial artery.[31] This strategy did result in reliable bronchial revascularization. However, the technique was associated with significant perioperative blood loss, cardiac complications from prolonged cardiopulmonary bypass, and cardioplegic arrest times.[27] As a result, the technique was never widely adopted.

Further technical improvements in bilateral lung transplant were described by Dr Michael Pasque (Fig. 7) and his colleagues at Washington University in St. Louis in 1990.[32] To eliminate the need for cardiopulmonary bypass and cardioplegic arrest, they performed sequential bilateral lung transplants through bilateral anterior thoracotomies with a transverse sternotomy (otherwise known as a clamshell incision).[32] Using this technique, if the patient can tolerate single lung ventilation, the sequential transplant does not require bypass to complete the bilateral lung transplant.[33]

Early outcomes in these initial patients showed excellent exposure, rare use of cardiopulmonary bypass, and improved mortality compared with en bloc bilateral lung transplant. Furthermore, four recipients who were ventilator dependent underwent successful bilateral lung transplant using this new technique.[33] The sequential bilateral lung transplant described by the group in Washington University in St. Louis (minus an omental patch to buttress the bronchus) is still used today and has become worldwide the most offered lung transplant for all indications.

Living Donor Lung and Lobar Transplant

The next evolution in lung transplant was to expand the donor pool from deceased donors to living donors. A lobar transplant was technically feasible, as demonstrated by Dr Kingo Shinoi and his team in 1966.[34] A 44-year-old man with severe bronchiectasis who suffered from persistent hemoptysis from the lingula and left lower lobe underwent a left lower lobe transplant. The donor was a 49-year-old man with a central left lung cancer who underwent a left pneumonectomy, with the left lower lobe uninvolved with tumor. This left lower lobe was then implanted into the recipient, with initial good function. However, on postoperative day 18, the transplanted lobe was necrotic and removed, likely from venous congestion.

In 1990, Dr Vaughn Starnes (Fig. 8) performed a successful living related lobar transplant. The recipient was a 12-year-old girl with pulmonary fibrosis,

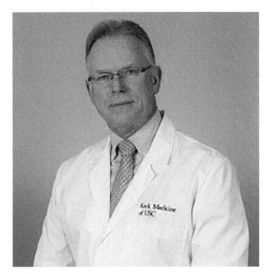

Fig. 8. Dr Vaughn Starnes.

with her 44-year-old mother donating her right upper lobe.[35] During this initial period, one other child received a living related lobar transplant, and a neonate received a lobar transplant from a 2-year-old deceased donor.[35] This success stimulated the adoption of living lobar transplantation in a few transplant centers. It was used for recipients (usually children) who were critically ill and not likely to survive the usually prolonged wait time for a suitable donor. At that time, in the United States, recipient waiting time priority was only dependent on time on the waiting list, not disease severity. However, in 2005 with the adoption of the lung allocation score (LAS) in the United States, recipient priority on the waiting list was determined by severity of disease and probability of posttransplant survival. This change eliminated the need for living lobar transplantation in the United States. However, the living lobar strategy has been successfully used in Japan where, because of cultural and religious reasons, there is a significant donor shortage.[36]

Preservation Solutions

Another significant advancement that contributed to progressive success in lung transplant was improved preservation techniques and solutions. During the early lung transplant experience, allografts were preserved by topical hypothermic immersion.[25] By 1990, most programs shifted to using PA and retrograde pulmonary vein flush with cold crystalloid solution.[25] Preservation solutions were slowly being developed along with organ transplantation. One of the first solutions was the Collins solution, which was created in the 1960s and was used for kidney transplants.[37] This solution was modified by the Eurotransplant Organization, with Euro-Collins removing magnesium from the solution.[38] Euro-Collins has an intracellular electrolyte composition with a strong phosphate buffer.[39] Euro-Collins was the preservation solution most commonly used[32]; however, there was no consensus on the ideal approach.[40]

In the late 1980s, Fujimura and colleagues[41] reported prolonged lung preservation in animal models using extracellular low-potassium dextran solution. This new solution, known at the "Fujimura solution," fostered further investigation by Keshavjee and coworkers,[42] leading to commercial development of Perfadex,[43] which is used worldwide as the preferred lung preservation solution. Prostaglandin E_1, a potent pulmonary vasodilator when bolus injected into the PA before flushing the allograft with perfusate, was reported as safe and improved preservation, by improving the distribution of the cold perfusate.[32,44]

EXPANSION OF LUNG TRANSPLANT: THE 1990S

At the start of 1990, few programs had a meaningful clinical experience. In the United States, only six programs performed more than two transplants in 1989, and Washington University in St. Louis was the only one to perform greater than 20 that year.[45] There were five centers in Europe with reasonable volume, and the University of Toronto in Canada. There were no lung transplant programs in Asia, South America, or Oceania at that time.

Standardized Lung Transplant Technique

In the early 1990s, the technique for single lung transplant[46] and sequential bilateral lung transplant[32] became standardized. The initial technique for single lung transplant was slightly different when initially described in 1987. The omentum was first mobilized via a laparotomy.[46] Afterward, a posterolateral thoracotomy was performed, and the lung was removed with extrapericardial division of the superior and inferior pulmonary veins, division of the PA, and transection of the distal mainstem bronchus. The donor lung was prepared from en bloc lungs by dividing the bronchus at the level of the trachea and left mainstem bronchus, dividing the PA at the origin of the left and right PAs, and dividing the left atrium with a good donor cuff. The donor bronchus was trimmed to two rings above the secondary carina. Implantation first occurred with performing the left atrial anastomosis with Prolene suture followed by the PA anastomosis with running Prolene. Before finishing the front wall of the PA, the atrial clamp was released for back bleeding. Then the PA clamp was transiently opened to flush the PA, before completing the PA anastomosis. After restoration of blood flow, the bronchial anastomosis was performed, with the omental pedicle wrapped around the bronchus.

In 1990, the technique was modified for a sequential bilateral lung transplant. The thoracotomy, pneumonectomy, and preparation of the donor remained similar. However, the order of the anastomoses was changed[32] because of the exposure from bilateral anterior thoracotomies or a clamshell incision. The membranous wall was sewn with running 4–0 absorbable monofilament suture, with interrupted 4–0 absorbable suture for the cartilaginous portion. Next, the PA was clamped centrally, and the PA anastomosis was performed with 5–0 Prolene. Finally, a clamp was placed on the left atrium with creation of a recipient left atrial cuff and the anastomosis was performed with running 4–0 Prolene. Before tying the anastomosis, the PA clamp was transiently released until blood is flushed through the lung and out the atrial anastomosis. Then, the left atrial clamp was removed to allow for backbleeding, before tying the final suture. An omental patch was placed around the bronchial anastomosis. Once that lung was reinflated, the lung transplant on the other side was performed with similar steps. This order of anastomoses allowed for decreased incidence of severe hypoxia after reperfusion of the lung. When the lung allograft is reperfused before the bronchial anastomosis, the patient can have a significant ventilation-perfusion mismatch leading to profound hypoxia. However, if the bronchial anastomosis is already complete, the new lung is reinflated to mitigate that mismatch.

After these seminal papers describing surgical technique for lung transplant, surgeons continued to tweak and perfect their surgical approach. For bronchial anastomoses, various techniques emerged, including running the cartilaginous portion of the bronchus,[47] telescoping the smaller airway into the larger airway,[48] and eliminating the use of omental wrap or any wrap around the bronchial anastomosis.[48,49] As experience increased, bronchial anastomotic complications decreased, with one group showing a decrease from 14% to 4% of lung transplant patients.[50] In the left atrial/pulmonary venous anastomosis, the pulmonary venous cuff was trimmed more, to exclude donor atrial muscle.[49] The suture line was also changed to a continuous vertical mattress suture for good endothelial contact with exclusion of atrial muscle or fat.[49]

Donor and Recipient Selection

Alongside the technical advances in surgery, donor and recipient selection criteria for lung transplant also evolved. Additionally, sicker patients, such as those requiring mechanical ventilation, were also candidates for lung transplant, with good survival.[33] The guidelines for donor selection were also slowly refined through this time frame. The early reports on donor quality emphasized normal chest radiograph, no active infection, and minimal ventilation/perfusion mismatch.[51] As experience with lung transplantation grew, standard criteria for ideal donor selection were defined as age less than 55 years, smoking history less than 20 pack-years, arterial oxygen level greater than 300 mm Hg (with 100% inspired oxygen and positive end-expiratory pressure of 5 cm H_2O), and normal chest radiograph.[52] Because of the shortage of donors, centers started expanding to extended who did not meet the ideal criteria.[53] Despite not meeting the standard requirements, lungs from extended donors used in well-selected recipients resulted in good outcomes with similar survival as ideal donors. These advancements in allograft selection helped increase the pool of potential donors for lung transplantation.

Improved Immunosuppression and Monitoring

During this time, immunosuppression and understanding of rejection also made significant advances. Chronic lung rejection was first described by a working group in St. Louis, which described bronchiolitis obliterans syndrome, a term to describe the clinical manifestations of chronic lung allograft rejection.[54] The guidelines for bronchiolitis obliterans syndrome were important for classifying post–lung transplant allograft disease that did not require histologic findings, instead using pulmonary function tests. Given that chronic rejection is the leading cause of post-1-year lung transplant mortality, further research went into improving immunosuppression and improving surveillance.

Other major advancements occurred during that period to help with detection and prevention of rejection. Donor-specific cytotoxicity testing was introduced in animal models in 1990,[55] building the foundation for evaluating donor-specific antibodies and antibody-mediated rejection in posttransplant patients. Additionally, the use of transbronchial lung biopsy to diagnose rejection without a surgical biopsy[56] was developed as a standard technique. Tacrolimus was also introduced as an immunosuppressive agent, with Food and Drug Administration approval in 1994.[57] All these developments are still used in the management of lung transplant recipients.

Worldwide Growth of Lung Transplant

With the standardization of surgical technique, donor and recipient selection, and allograft preservation, the rate of lung transplantation rapidly grew through the 1990s in North America and Europe.[58] In the United States, 82 more lung transplant programs were opened throughout the 1990s, compared with the six programs at the beginning of the decade.[45] In 1990, an isolated lung transplant was performed at St. Vincent's hospital in Sydney, heralding the first program in Australia.[59] Although two prior lung transplants in China had been attempted in 1979, lung transplantation was halted until a left lung transplant was performed in 1995, marking the start of lung transplant in China.[60] With programs in Turkey, South Africa, Brazil, Argentina, Colombia, and multiple other countries, lung transplants are now performed worldwide.

IMPROVEMENTS IN ALLOCATION AND GUIDELINES: THE 2000S

Lung transplantation in the 2000s continued to improve via a multitude of factors. The most notable improvements were regarding lung allocation and the publication of consensus documents using data from the International Society for Heart and Lung Transplantation (ISHLT). These consensus documents used the ISHLT registry to help expand knowledge in various aspects of lung transplant, including primary graft dysfunction (PGD).

In the United States, the donor lung allocation system was initially based on ABO match and overall time on the waitlist.[61] The result of waitlist time prioritization was many deaths on the waitlist, because it did not account for severity of illness. To address this problem, the LAS was implemented in 2005. The goal of the change was to "(1) reduce the number of deaths on the lung transplant list; (2) increase transplant benefit for lung recipients; and (3) ensure the efficient and equitable allocation of lungs to active transplant recipients."[62] The LAS was created to address this by creating a score from 0 to 100 that is an aggregate of the weighted components: the expected survival during the following year on the waitlist and the expected survival during the first year after lung transplant.[61] There was a notable reduction in waitlist mortality after the LAS, with a 40% decrease compared with pre-LAS waitlist mortality.[63] Recipients also experienced a decrease in waitlist time,[63,64] with an improvement in 1-year survival[65] after the LAS was instituted. The system is currently updated to a continuous distribution allocation system that considers multiple patient and donor attributes all at once with an overall score. This overall score includes medical urgency, patient outcomes, biologic make-up, other candidate factors, and efficiency of organ placement, without hard geographic boundaries.[66]

With the global increase in transplants (**Fig. 9**), a significant volume of data regarding all aspects of lung transplantation was available. The ISHLT was established in 1981 as an organization committed to research and education. The ISHLT was a major repository of recipient and donor data, allowing development of guidelines for recipient and donor criteria, and allograft dysfunction and rejection.[65,67–77]

THE CURRENT ERA: THE 2010S ONWARD
Increased Donor Lung Recovery

Before the implementation of the LAS in 2005, one of the most limiting factors to the number of lung transplants was the lack of donor lungs, with only 43% of the patients on the waiting list being transplanted annually. Since then, the increase in overall organ donation and lung allocation from ideal and more frequent extended donors has significantly closed the gap with nearly 85% of the listed patients transplanted within a year. Numerous new developments have been implemented to help expand the donor pool.

Extended Donor Recovery

A major area of expansion has been regarding the use of extended donors. Based on the characteristics of ideal, standard, and extended donors for lung transplant, more than 91% of donors from 2006 to 2019 were considered extended donors, with 77.6% of transplanted lungs from extended donors.[78] Over time, extended donor use increased: they accounted for 63.9% of lung transplants in 2006 to 2009, and 83.3% of lung transplants in 2015 to 2019.[79] Multiple studies have shown no difference in postoperative outcomes, such as PGD,[78] duration of ventilation,[78,80] in-hospital mortality,[78] and long-term survival.[78,80–82]

Donor Recovery Centers

Traditional donor management and organ procurement is managed by the organ procurement organizations, with donors at the facility where brain death occurs. In this model, small hospitals with minimal experience managing donors are responsible for most donors. However, a different model arose using specialized donor care facilities (SDCF) or donor recovery centers. The concept of SDCF was established in 2001 with Mid-America Transplant.[83] Studies have demonstrated improved donor management at an SCDF is

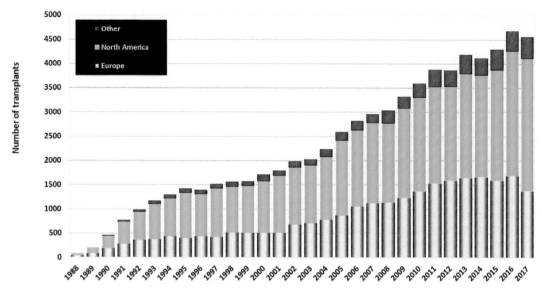

Fig. 9. Number of adult and pediatric lung transplants by year and location. (*Adapted from* Hayes D Jr, Cherikh WS, Chambers DC, et al. The International Thoracic Organ Transplant Registry of the International Society for Heart and Lung Transplantation: Twenty-second pediatric lung and heart-lung transplantation report-2019; Focus theme: Donor and recipient size match. J Heart Lung Transplant. 2019;38(10):1015-1027 and Khush KK, Cherikh WS, Chambers DC, et al. The International Thoracic Organ Transplant Registry of the International Society for Heart and Lung Transplantation: Thirty-sixth adult heart transplantation report - 2019; focus theme: Donor and recipient size match [published correction appears in J Heart Lung Transplant. 2020 Jan;39(1):91]. J Heart Lung Transplant. 2019;38(10):1056-1066.)

associated with increased organ yield compared with local hospital yield with decreased cost and increased efficiency.[79,84] When donor management protocols are implemented in conjunction with an SCDF,[85] lung utilization rates increase, with one SDCF showing an increase from 19.8% to 33.9%.[83] Based on the improved organ yield with decreased costs, SDCFs are slowly expanding, with 13 freestanding centers in 2020, and more organ procurement organizations using designated hospitals as donor recovery centers.

Hepatitis C Positive Donors

Before the development of direct-acting antivirals against hepatitis C virus (HCV), organ transplants from HCV-positive donor resulted in HCV transmission in most recipients.[86] However, the advent of direct-acting antivirals that could eradicate HCV led to heart and lung transplants from HCV-positive donors to negative recipients.[87,88] These early trials demonstrated 95% to 100% 6-month recipient survival with 0% having detectable HCV viral loads.[87,88] Additional data have demonstrated no difference in acute cellular rejection or infection requiring treatment at 1 year after transplant.[89] As HCV donor usage has increased, the ISHLT has since released a consensus statement to help with use of these donors.[90]

Ex Vivo Lung Perfusion

Another method to increase organ utilization is the use of ex vivo lung perfusion (EVLP). For donors with marginal lungs that would otherwise not be accepted for transplantation, the lungs can be retrieved and evaluated using EVLP. Early data demonstrated no difference in PGD, early mortality, bronchial complications, length of mechanical ventilation, or length of stay.[91] Long-term outcomes comparing EVLP with non-EVLP lung transplant recipients show no difference in lung allograft dysfunction or 3-year, 5-year, and 9-year survival.[92] As experience with EVLP grows, its use is increasing, accounting for 25% of the lung transplants performed in the University of Toronto between 2008 and 2017.[92]

Donor After Circulatory Death

Traditional lung transplant donors are donors after brain death, with few DCD.[1] Although use of DCD lungs was initially described in 1995,[93] DCD lungs only accounted for 0.1% (n = 1) of lung transplants in 2001.[1] However, studies evaluating the ISHLT registry[94] and the United Network for Organ Sharing registry[95] have shown equivalent outcomes between DCD and donors after brain death. The advent of EVLP has also allowed for centers to evaluate DCD allografts before implantation, helping to increase the DCD to 10% (n = 264) in 2021[1] in the United States.

Extracorporeal Membrane Oxygenation

Previously, patients with severe hypoxemia/hypercarbia or severe pulmonary hypertension that required intraoperative cardiopulmonary support would be placed on cardiopulmonary bypass during lung transplantation. However, the use of ECMO has significantly increased over the last decade. Use of intraoperative ECMO has been associated with decreased blood utilization, decreased mechanical ventilation time, and improved short-term survival when compared with cardiopulmonary bypass.[96] Based on these outcomes, ECMO is the current preferred method for intraoperative support.

SUMMARY

In the 60-year history of the first lung transplant by Dr Hardy in Mississippi and 40-year history of the first successful lung transplant by Dr Cooper in Toronto, there has been a slow but continuous evolution in lung transplantation that has resulted in a significant increase in the number of patients benefiting from this procedure worldwide with improvement in survival and quality of life. Current 1-year post transplant survival is around 90%, despite the increased severity of disease and age of recipients, with improving long-term outcomes. The future of lung transplant remains promising with the expansion of DCD, new immunosuppressants targeted to cellular and antibody-mediated rejection, better diagnosis, prophylaxis for opportunistic infections and, in the not-too-distant future, the possible use of xenotransplant and artificial lungs.

DISCLOSURES

S.H. Chang, J. Chan, and G.A. Patterson have no relevant conflicts of interest.

REFERENCES

1. Transplants by donor type: lung national data. US transplants performed: January 1, 1988-May 31, 2022. Organ procurement and transplantation network. Available at: https://optn.transplant.hrsa.gov/data/view-data-reports/national-data/#. Accessed June 8, 2022.
2. Hardy JD, Webb WR, Dalton ML, et al. Lung homo-transplantations in man. JAMA 1963;186:1065–74.
3. Hardy JD, Araslan S, Webb WR. Transplantation of the lung. Ann Surg 1964;160:440–8.
4. Nelems JM, Rebuck AS, Cooper JD, et al. Human lung transplantation. Chest 1980;78:569–73.
5. Lima O, Cooper JD, Peters WJ, et al. Effects of methylprednisolone and azathioprine on bronchial healing following lung autotransplantation. J Thorac Cardiovasc Surg 1981;82:211–5.
6. Borel JF, Feurer C, Gubler HU, et al. Biological effects of cyclosporine A: a new antilymphocytic agent. Agents Actions 1976;6:468.
7. The Canadian Multicentre Transplant Study Group. A randomized clinical trial of cyclosporine in cadaveric renal transplantation. N Engl J Med 1983;309:809–15.
8. Goldberg M, Lima O, Morgan E, et al. A comparison between cyclosporine A and methylprednisolone plus azathioprine on bronchial healing following canine lung allotransplantation. J Thorac Cardiovasc Surg 1983;85:821–6.
9. Morgan E, Lima O, Goldber M, et al. Successful revascularization of totally ischemic bronchial autografts with omental pedicle flaps in dogs. J Thorac Cardiovasc Surg 1982;94:204–10.
10. Dubois P, Choiniere L, Cooper JD. Bronchial omentopexy in canine lung allotransplantation. Ann Thorac Surg 1984;38:211–4.
11. Lima O, Goldberg M, Peters WJ, et al. Bronchial omentopexy in canine lung transplantation. J Thorac Cardiovasc Surg 1982;83:418–21.
12. Saunders NR, Egan TM, Chamberlain D, et al. Cyclosporine and bronchial healing in canine lung transplantation. J Thorac Cardiovasc Surg 1984;88:993–9.
13. Rietz BA, Burtion NA, Jamieson SW, et al. Heart and lung transplantation: autotransplantation and allotransplantation with extended survival. J Thorac Cardiovasc Surg 1980;80:360.
14. Reitz BA, Pennock JL, Shumway NE. Simplified operative method for heart and lung transplantation. J Surg Res 1981;31:1–5.
15. Reitz BA, Wallwork JL, Hunt SA, et al. Heart-lung transplantation: successful therapy for patients with pulmonary vascular disease. N Engl J Med 1982;306:557–64.
16. Reitz BA, Hunt SA, Gaudiani V, et al. Clinical heart-lung transplantation. Transplant Proc 1983;15:1256–9.
17. Toronto Lung Transplant Group. Sequential bilateral lung transplantation for paraquat poisoning. A case report. J Thorac Cardiovasc Surg 1985;89:734–42.
18. Toronto Lung Transplant Group. Unilateral lung transplantation for pulmonary fibrosis. N Engl J Med 1986;314:1140–5.
19. Dark JH, Patterson GA, Al-Jilaihawi AN, et al. Experimental en bloc double-lung transplantation. Ann Thorac Surg 1986;42:394–8.
20. Patterson GA, Cooper JD, Dark JH, et al. Experimental and clinical double lung transplantation. J Thorac Cardiovasc Surg 1988;95:70–4.

21. Patterson GA, Cooper JD, Goldman B, et al. Technique of successful clinical double-lung transplantation. Ann Thorac Surg 1988;45(6):626–33.

22. Yacoub MH, Khagani A, Fitzgerald M, et al. Cardiac transplantation from live donors (abstract). J Am Coll Cardiol 1988;11:102A.

23. Cooper JD. Dominoes: pragmatism or piracy? Transpl Int 1991;4:1–2.

24. Griffith BP, Hardesty RL, Trento A, et al. Heart-lung transplantation: lessons learned and future hopes. Ann Thorac Surg 1987;43:6–16.

25. Ramirez J, Patterson GA, Winton TL, et al. Bilateral lung transplantation for cystic fibrosis. J Thorac Cardiovasc Surg 1992;103:287–94.

26. Patterson GA, Todd TR, Cooper JD, et al. Airway complications after double lung transplantation. J Thorac Cardiovasc Surg 1990;99:14–20.

27. Cooper DJ. The evolution of techniques and indications for lung transplantation. Ann Surg 1990;212:249–56.

28. Noirclerc MJ, Metras D, Vaillant A, et al. Bilateral bronchial anastomosis in double lung and heart-lung transplantations. Eur J Cardiothorac Surg 1990;4:314–7.

29. Schreinemakers H, Weder W, Miyoshi S, et al. Direct revascularization of bronchial arteries for lung transplantation: an anatomical study. Ann Thorac Surg 1990;49:44–54.

30. Pettersson G, Arendrup H, Mortensen SA. Early experience of double-lung transplantation with bronchial artery revascularization using mammary artery. Eur J Cardiothorac Surg 1994;8(10):520–4.

31. Couraud L, Baudet E, Nashef SAM, et al. Lung transplantation with bronchial revascularization. Eur J Cardiothorac Surg 1992;6:490–5.

32. Pasque MK, Cooper JD, Kaiser LR, et al. Improved technique for bilateral lung transplantation: rationale and initial clinical experience. Ann Thorac Surg 1990;49:785–91.

33. Kaiser LR, Pasque MK, Trulock EP, et al. Bilateral sequential lung transplantation: the procedure of choice for double lung replacement. J Thorac Cardiovasc Surg 1991;52:438–46.

34. Shinoi K, Hayata Y, Aoki H, et al. Pulmonary lobe homotransplantations in human subjects. Am J Surg 1966;111:617–28.

35. Starnes VA, Lewiston NJ, Luikart H, et al. Current trends in lung transplantation. Lobar transplantation and expanded use of single lungs. J Thorac Cardiovasc Surg 1992;104(4):1060–5.

36. Date H. Current status and problems of lung transplantation in Japan. J Thorac Dis 2016;8:S631–6.

37. Collins GM, Bravo-Shugarman M, Terasaki P. Kidney preservation for transplantation. Initial perfusion and 30 hour's ice storage. The. Lancet 1969;294:1219–22.

38. Cohen B, Persjin G, De Meester J. Eurotransplant foundation annual report 1994. Leiden: Niederlande); 1994.

39. Egan TM, Kaiser LR, Cooper JD. Lung transplantation. Curr Probl Surg 1989;26:675–751.

40. Muhlbacher F, Langer F, Mittermayer C. Preservation solutions for transplantation. Transplant Proc 1999;31:2069–70.

41. Fujimura S, Handa M, Kondo T, et al. Successful 48-hour simple hypothermic preservation of canine lung transplant. Transplant Proc 1987;19:1334–6.

42. Keshavjee SH, Yamazaki F, Cardoso PF, et al. A method for safe twelve-hour pulmonary preservation. J Thorac Cardiovasc Surg 1989;98:529–34.

43. Perfadex plus. Xvivo. Available at: https://www.xvivoperfusion.com/products/perfadex-plus/. Accessed June 8, 2022.

44. Wallwork J, Jones K, Cavarocchi N, et al. Distant procurement of organs for clinical heart-lung preservation. J Heart Transplant 1986;5:89–98.

45. Center data. Organ Procurement and Transplantation Network. Available at: https://optn.transplant.hrsa.gov/data/view-data-reports/center-data/. Accessed June 8, 2022.

46. Cooper JD, Pearson FG, Patterson GA, et al. Technique of successful lung transplantation in humans. J Thorac Cardiovasc Surg 1987;93:173–81.

47. Puri V, Patterson GA. Adult lung transplantation: technical considerations. Semin Thorac Cardiovasc Surg 2008;20:152–64.

48. Calhoon JH, Grover FL, Gibbons WJ, et al. Single lung transplantation. Alternative indications and techniques. J Thorac Cardiovasc Surg 1991;101(5):816–24.

49. Griffith BP, Magee MJ, Gonzalez IF, et al. Anastomosis pitfalls in lung transplantation. J Thorac Cardiovasc Surg 1994;107:743–54.

50. Date H, Trulock EP, Arcidi JM, et al. Improved airway healing after lung transplantation. An analysis of 348 bronchial anastomoses. J Thorac Cardiovasc Surg 1995;110:1424–32.

51. Griffith BP, Zenati M. The pulmonary donor. Clin Chest Med 1990;11:217–26.

52. Sundaresan S, Trachiotis GD, Aoe M, et al. Donor lung procurement: assessment and operative technique. Ann Thorac Surg 1993;56:1409–13.

53. Sundaresan S, Semenkovich J, Ochoa L, et al. Successful outcome of lung transplantation is not compromised by the use of marginal donor lungs. J Thorac Cardiovasc Surg 1995;109(6):1075–9.

54. Cooper JD, Billingham M, Egan T, et al. A working formulation for the standardization of nomenclature and for clinical staging of chronic dysfunction in lung allografts. J Heart Lung Transplant 1993;12:713–6.

55. Dal Col RH, Zeevi A, Rabinowich H, et al. Donor-specific cytotoxicity testing: an advance in detecting pulmonary allograft rejection. Ann Thorac Surg 1990;49:754–8.

56. Higenbottam T, Stewart S, Penketh A, et al. Transbronchial lung biopsy for the diagnosis of rejection

in heart-lung transplant patients. Transplantation 1988;46:532–9.

57. Hausen B, Morris RE. Review of immunosuppression for lung transplantation. Novel drugs, new uses for conventional immunosuppressants, and alternative strategies. Clin Chest Med 1997;18:353–66.

58. Chambers DC, Perch MP, Zuckermann A, et al. The International Thoracic Organ Transplant Registry of the International Society for Heart and Lung Transplantation: Thirty-eighth adult lung transplantation report – 2021; Focus on recipient characteristics. J Heart Lung Transplant 2021;40:1060–72.

59. Tait BD. More than a footnote: the story of organ transplantation in Australia and New Zealand. Melbourne: Australian Scholarly; 2012.

60. Wu B, Hu C, Chen W, et al. China lung transplantation developing: past, present, and future. Ann Transl Med 2020;8:41.

61. Egan TM, Murray S, Bustami RT, et al. Development of the new lung allocation system in the United States. Am J Transplant 2006;6:1212–27.

62. Report of the OPTN thoracic organ transplantation committee to the board of directors. Exhibit A; 2004.

63. Egan TM, Edwards LB. Effects of the lung allocation score on lung transplantation in the United States. J Heart Lung Transplant 2016;35:433–9.

64. Hachem RR, Trulock EP. The new lung allocation system and its impact on waitlist characteristics and post-transplant outcomes. Semin Thorac Cardiovasc Surg 2008;20:1399-42.

65. Ross DJ, Marchevsky A, Kramer M, et al. Refractoriness of airflow obstruction associated with isolated lymphocytic bronchiolitis in pulmonary allografts. J Heart Lung Transplant 1997;16:832–8.

66. Continuous distribution format provides a single, composite score for each match. UNOS. Available at: https://unos.org/news/new-lung-allocation-policy-approved/. Accessed September 14, 2022..

67. Estenne M, Maurer JR, Boehler A, et al. Bronchiolitis obliterans syndrome 2001: an update of the diagnostic criteria. J Heart Lung Transplant 2002;21:297–310.

68. Patterson GM, Wilson S, Whang JL, et al. Physiologic definitions of obliterative bronchiolitis in heart-lung and double lung transplantation a comparison of the forced expiratory flow between 25% and 75% of the forced vital capacity and forced expiratory volume in one second. J Heart Lung Transplant 1996;15:175–81.

69. Girgis RE, Tu I, Berry GJ. Risk factors for the development of obliterative bronchiolitis after lung transplantation. J Heart Lung Transplant 1996;12:1200–8.

70. Orens JB, Boehler A, de Perrot M, et al. A review of lung transplant donor acceptability criteria. J Heart Lung Transplant 2003;22:1183–200.

71. Christie JD, Van Raemdonck D, de Perrot M, et al. Report of the ISHLT working group on primary lung graft dysfunction part I: introduction and methods. J Heart Lung Transplant 2005;24:1451–3.

72. Christie JD, Carby M, Bag R, et al. Report of the ISHLT working group on primary lung graft dysfunction part II: definition. A consensus statement of the International Society for Heart and Lung Transplantation. J Heart Lung Transplant 2005;24:1454-49.

73. Arcasoy SM, Fisher A, Hachem RR, et al. Report of the ISHLT working group on primary lung graft dysfunction part V: predictors and outcomes. J Heart Lung Transplant 2005;24:1483–8.

74. de Perrot M, Bonser RS, Dark J, et al. Report of the ISHLT working group on primary lung graft dysfunction part III: donor-related risk factors and markers. J Heart Lung Transplant 2005;24:1460–7.

75. Barr ML, Kawut SM, Whelan TP, et al. Report of the ISHLT working group on primary lung graft dysfunction part IV: recipient-related risk factors and markers. J Heart Lung Transplant 2005;24:468–82.

76. Shargall Y, Guenther G, Ahya VN, et al. Report of the ISHLT working group on primary lung graft dysfunction part VI: treatment. J Heart Lung Transplant 2005;24:1489–500.

77. Orens JB, Estenne M, Arcasoy S, et al. International guidelines for the selection of lung transplant candidates: 2006 update – a consensus report from the Pulmonary Scientific Council of the International Society for Heart and Lung Transplantation. J Heart Lung Transplant 2006;25:745–55.

78. Wadowski B, Chang SH, Carillo J, et al. Assessing donor organ quality according to recipient characteristics in lung transplantation. J Thorac Cardiovasc Surg 2022. https://doi.org/10.1016/j.jtcvs.2022.03.014.

79. Doyle M, Subramanian V, Vachharajani N, et al. Organ donor recovery performed at an organ procurement organization-based facility is an effective way to minimize organ costs and increase organ yield. J Am Coll Surg 2016;11:591–600.

80. Zych B, Garcia Saez D, Sabashnikov A, et al. Lung transplantation from donors outside standard acceptability criteria: are they really marginal? Transpl Int 2014;1024(27):1183–91.

81. Loor G, Radosevich DM, Kelly RF, et al. The University of Minnesota Donor Lung Quality Index: a consensus-based scoring application improved donor lung use. Ann Thorac Surg 2016;102:1156–65.

82. Singh E, Schecter M, Towe C, et al. Sequence of refusals for donor quality, organ utilization, and survival after lung transplantation. J Heart Lung Transplant 2019;38:35–42.

83. Chang SH, Kreisel D, Marklin GF, et al. Lung focused resuscitation at a specialized donor care facility improves lung procurement rates. Ann Thorac Surg 2018;105:1531–56.

84. Doyle MB, Vachharajani N, Wellen JR, et al. A novel organ donor facility: a decade of experience with liver donors. Am J Transplant 2014;14:615–20.

85. Angel LF, Levine DJ, Restrepo MI, et al. Impact of a lung transplantation donor-management protocol on lung donation and recipient outcomes. Am J Respir Crit Care Med 2006;174:710–6.

86. Pereira BJG, Milford EL, Kirkman RL, et al. Transmission of hepatitis C virus by organ transplantation. N Engl J Med 1991;325:454–60.

87. Wooley AE, Singh SK, Goldberg HJ, et al. Heart and lung transplant from HCV-infected donors to uninfected recipients. N Engl J Med 2019;380:1606–17.

88. Cypel M, Feld JJ, Galasso M, et al. Prevention of viral transmission during lung transplantation with hepatitis C-viraemic donors: an open-label, single-centre, pilot trial. Lancet Resp Med 2020;8: 192–201.

89. Lewis TC, Lesko M, Rudym D, et al. One-year immunologic outcomes of lung transplantation utilizing hepatitis C-viremic donors. Clin Transplant 2022; 36(8):e14749.

90. Aslam S, Grossi P, Schlendorf KH, et al. Utilization of hepatitis C virus-infected organ donors in cardiothoracic transplantation: an ISHLT expert consensus statement. J Heart Lung Transplant 2020;39: 418–32.

91. Cypel M, Yeung JC, Liu M, et al. Normothermic ex vivo lung perfusion in clinical transplantation. N Engl J Med 2011;364:1431–40.

92. Divithotawela C, Cyper M, Martinu T, et al. Long-term outcomes of lung transplant with ex vivo lung perfusion. JAMA Surg 2019;154:1143–50.

93. Love RB, Stringham JC, Chomiak PN, et al. Successful lung transplantation using a non-heart beating donor. J Heart Lung Transplant 1995;14:S88.

94. Van Raemdonck D, Keshavjee S, Levvey B, et al. Donation after circulatory death in lung transplantation: five-year follow-up from ISHLT registry. J Heart Lung Transplant 2019;38:1235–45.

95. Villavicencio MA, Axtell AL, Spencer PJ, et al. Lung transplantation from donation after circulatory death: United States and single-center experience. Ann Thorac Surg 2018;106:1619–27.

96. Machuca TN, Collaud S, Mercier O, et al. Outcomes of intraoperative extracorporeal membrane oxygenation versus cardiopulmonary bypass for lung transplantation. J Thorac Cardiovasc Surg 2015;149: 1152–7.

The Lung Transplant Candidate, Indications, Timing, and Selection Criteria

Hannah Mannem, MD[a], Meghan Aversa, MD, MS[b], Thomas Keller, MD[c], Siddhartha G. Kapnadak, MD[c],*

KEYWORDS

- Lung transplantation • Advanced lung disease • Candidacy • Prognosis
- Idiopathic pulmonary fibrosis • Chronic obstructive lung disease • Cystic fibrosis
- Pulmonary hypertension

KEY POINTS

- Candidacy for lung transplantation is determined by assessing a patient with advanced lung disease's risk of death and quality of life without transplant, as well as the likelihood of success with transplantation.
- Important, often overlapping steps leading up to lung transplant include pulmonary risk assessment, early referral if able, optimization of modifiable barriers to transplant, planning and education, multidisciplinary evaluation by the transplant team, and listing.
- Lung transplant selection criteria have evolved considerably but still vary significantly by center, and adequate, transparent communication between referring and transplant providers is needed to optimize patient care and provide equity to the overall population in need.

INTRODUCTION

Lung transplantation (LTx) is one of the most important treatment options for patients with advanced lung disease. The field of LTx is growing, and if excluding the recent negative impact of the COVID-19 pandemic, the International Society for Heart and Lung Transplantation (ISHLT) has reported a gradual increase in worldwide transplant volume during the past 3 decades to approximately 4500 per year in the most recent registry report.[1,2] This trend is noticeable globally, and the increase in volume has been most pronounced *outside* of North America and Europe, with other nations now accounting for 8.5% of total lung transplants performed.[2] Additionally, recipients are surviving long after LTx, and with a growing population of pretransplant and posttransplant patients around the world there is a need for not only transplant pulmonologists but also other subspecialists to understand transplant candidacy and selection. In this article, we review LTx candidacy along with important considerations for transplant and nontransplant providers during the selection and listing processes.

[a] Division of Pulmonary and Critical Care Medicine, University of Virginia School of Medicine, PO Box 800546, Clinical Department Wing, 1 Hospital Drive, Charlottesville, VA 22908, USA; [b] Division of Respirology, Department of Medicine, University Health Network and University of Toronto, C. David Naylor Building, 6 Queen's Park Crescent West, Third Floor, Toronto, ON M5S 3H2, Canada; [c] Division of Pulmonary, Critical Care, and Sleep Medicine, Department of Medicine, University of Washington School of Medicine, 1959 Northeast Pacific Street, Campus Box 356522, Seattle, WA 98195, USA
* Corresponding author. Division of Pulmonary, Critical Care, and Sleep Medicine, Department of Medicine, University of Washington School of Medicine, 1959 Northeast Pacific Street, Campus Box 356122, Seattle, WA 98195.
E-mail address: skap@uw.edu

Clin Chest Med 44 (2023) 15–33
https://doi.org/10.1016/j.ccm.2022.10.001
0272-5231/23/© 2022 Elsevier Inc. All rights reserved.

Table 1
Most common indications for lung transplantation by era[a] (% of worldwide transplants reported to the ISHLT registry)

Indication	2005–2009 N = 13,934	2010–6/2018 N = 33,657
COPD[b]	34.7%	29.6%
ILD[c]	30.7%	38.0%
CF and other bronchiectasis	18.6%	16.7%
Retransplant	4.9%	4.1%
Sarcoidosis	2.8%	2.3%
IPAH	2.3%	2.8%

Abbreviations: CF, cystic fibrosis; COPD, chronic obstructive lung disease; ILD, interstitial lung disease; IPAH, idiopathic pulmonary arterial hypertension; ISHLT, international society for heart and lung transplantation.

[a] Data from Chambers DC, et al. The International Thoracic Organ Transplant Registry of the International Society for Heart and Lung Transplantation: Thirty-sixth adult lung and heart-lung transplantation Report-2019; Focus theme: Donor and recipient size match; J Heart Lung Transplant 2019. Oct;38(10):1042-1055.

[b] Includes alpha-one antitrypsin deficiency.

[c] Includes idiopathic pulmonary fibrosis.

DEMOGRAPHICS AND OVERVIEW OF LUNG TRANSPLANT CANDIDACY

Along with increasing transplant volumes, there has also been significant evolution in demographics including the indications for LTx (**Table 1**). Interstitial lung disease (ILD) surpassed chronic obstructive pulmonary disease (COPD) as the most common indication in 2009, with the former accounting for 40.5% of total worldwide transplants in 2017, including 32.4% for idiopathic pulmonary fibrosis (IPF).[1]

The trend toward transplanting more patients with ILD is most pronounced in North America. In fact, the United States Organ Procurement and Transplantation Network Registry reported that candidates with restrictive lung disease accounted for 60.2% of the total wait list in 2020, compared with 26.5% for obstructive lung disease, and only 4.1% for cystic fibrosis (CF).[3]

The average age of transplant recipients is also increasing internationally to now 57 years,[2–4] and candidates are sicker, with higher lung allocation scores, and such that more than 20% are now hospitalized at the time of LTx.[2,5,6] In combination, the changes in LTx demographics reflect several factors including an aging of the population, survival-improving treatments for some diagnoses including CF, and perhaps most importantly, a move in the community toward transplanting patients who are at highest risk of short-term mortality from their underlying disease.[7]

Although volumes and experience with higher risk candidates are increasing, the basic tenets of LTx candidate selection remain similar, incorporating the fact that donor lungs remain a scarce resource. In fact, mortality on the LTx waiting list is approximately 15 to 20 deaths per 100 waitlist-years,[3] and there is a large subset of the overall population with advanced lung disease in whom access to transplant is impeded by various medical and nonmedical factors.[5,8,9] With access limited, programs carry an important obligation to avoid futile transplants, offering the potentially life-saving intervention to only those who are considered to have a reasonable likelihood of an adequate outcome.[10,11] In keeping with this concept, the most recent ISHLT guidelines support consideration of LTx in patients who have a[10]

1. High (>50%) risk of death from lung disease within 2 years if LTx is not performed and
2. High (>80%) likelihood of 5-year posttransplant survival from a general medical perspective provided that there is adequate graft function.

Implementing these criteria requires providers to estimate prognosis without, as well as likelihood of success with LTx. Especially given the imprecise nature of prognostic predictions, most consider there to be an "optimal window" period for both referral and listing, during which initiation of the process allows for a lower risk of death before LTx, as well as for transplant to occur at a stage where the perioperative risks are lower. Although lung allocation mechanisms including the lung allocation score (LAS) prioritize donor lungs to the sickest wait-listed patients, it is important to recognize that a strategy of earlier referral also allows candidates time to learn about and consider their options, fully prepare, and modify any potential barriers or risk factors to improve candidacy and the likelihood of successful post-transplant outcomes (**Fig. 1**).[10,12–15]

DISEASE-SPECIFIC INDICATIONS AND TIMING

In addition to the general considerations above, the recent ISHLT consensus statement provides updated, disease-specific recommendations to general pulmonologists on the timing of referral for LTx, as well as to transplant pulmonologists on the timing of both referral and listing (**Table 2**).[10] Although intended to provide a general, prognosis-based framework on transplant timing for advanced lung disease, it is important to recognize that patient, provider, and program-specific

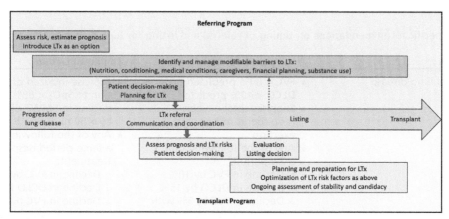

Fig. 1. Optimal approach to lung transplant referral, listing, and pretransplant management, emphasizing the overlapping roles of the referring and lung transplant programs. The suggested approach also highlights the importance of initiating the pretransplant process proactively to allow for important steps in preparation, planning, and intervening on potential barriers to transplantation. LTx, lung transplantation.

practices by necessity affect decisions on an individual basis.

Interstitial Lung Diseases

With epidemiologic data suggesting a median survival of 3 to 5 years among patients with IPF,[16,17] guidelines have traditionally recommended clinicians refer for LTx at the time of diagnosis. More recently, clinical trials have demonstrated that antifibrotic therapy (eg, nintedanib and pirfenidone) can slow the rate of decline in forced vital capacity (FVC), slow radiographic progression, and decrease the incidence of acute exacerbations among patients with IPF.[18–20] In addition, subsequent registry studies and pooled post hoc analyses suggest antifibrotic therapy may also confer a mortality benefit in some individuals, with only 25.9% of patients who received full-dose nintedanib dying during a 3-year period.[19,21–23] Despite these treatment options, long-term prognosis in the overall IPF population remains guarded, with a high risk of 2-year mortality persisting in the modern era particularly in those with risk factors including poor functional status, desaturation on 6-minute walk testing, low diffusing capacity for carbon monoxide (DLCO), pulmonary hypertension, and progressive fibrosis on computed tomography (CT) scan (with high fibrosis score).[24–27] Prediction models have been validated but are not widely used in practice,[24,25] and the ISHLT continues to recommend a conservative philosophy of early referral for patients with IPF given the unpredictable nature of disease progression and high mortality associated with acute exacerbations (referral and listing criteria in **Table 2**).[10]

Survival among patients with other fibrotic ILDs is highly variable. Although some experience a rapidly progressive course, the 5-year survival among this heterogenous group may be as high as 72%.[28–30] Moreover, recent studies indicate that antifibrotic therapy can also benefit patients with fibrotic lung diseases other than IPF (eg, connective tissue disease [CTD]-related ILD, chronic hypersensitivity pneumonitis, and idiopathic nonspecific interstitial pneumonitis), particularly those who progress despite standard management.[31–34] Consequently, determining the optimal timing for LTx referral and listing among this diverse group is challenging. Worsening symptoms despite treatment, declining FVC or DLCO, supplemental oxygen need, lower exercise capacity (as measured by 6-minute walk testing), prior hospitalization, and secondary pulmonary hypertension predict poor outcomes in fibrotic ILD and inform the current recommendations (see **Table 2**).[10,24,35–41] Recognizing the unpredictable nature of these diseases,[3] the ISHLT recommendations largely adopt a conservative philosophy of grouping IPF with other forms of ILD, again emphasizing the concept of early referral.[10]

Chronic Obstructive Lung Disease

Determining LTx need among patients with COPD is notoriously difficult because, even in the presence of severe obstructive impairment with functional limitations, many patients will demonstrate prolonged survival. The BODE index, a composite score incorporating body mass index (BMI), severity of airflow obstruction based on the forced expiratory volume in 1 second (FEV$_1$), dyspnea

Table 2
Disease-specific recommendations on timing of referral and listing for lung transplantation[a]

Diagnosis	Timing of Referral	Timing of Listing

Interstitial lung disease	• FVC < 80% predicted or DLCO < 40% predicted
	• Supplemental oxygen required at rest or with exertion
	• Any of the following during a 2-y period:
	  ○ Decline in FVC by 10%
	  ○ Decline in DLCO by 15%
	  ○ Decline in FVC by 5% with radiographic or symptomatic progression
	• Consider referral at:
	  ○ Time of diagnosis of IPF
	  ○ Time of diagnosis of connective tissue disease related ILD
	  ○ Radiographic progression among patients with inflammatory ILD
		• Exercise-induced desaturation to SpO_2 < 88% or decline in 6MWT distance by > 50 m during 6 mo
		• Any of the following during a 6-mo period despite treatment:
		  ○ Decline in FVC by 10%
		  ○ Decline in DCLO by 15%
		  ○ Decline in FVC by >5% with radiographic progression of disease
		• Evidence of pulmonary hypertension
		• Hospitalization for acute exacerbation of ILD

Chronic obstructive pulmonary disease[b]	• BODE score of 5–6 and any of the following:
	  ○ Frequent exacerbations
	  ○ FEV_1 20%–25% predicted
	  ○ Increase in BODE score >1 point during 24 mo
	  ○ Radiographic evidence of pulmonary hypertension
	• Consider referral if:
	  ○ Clinical decline despite optimized treatment
	  ○ Unacceptable quality of life
		• BODE score of 7–10
		• Consider when:
		  ○ FEV_1 < 20% predicted
		  ○ History of recurrent hospitalization
		  ○ Moderate-to-severe pulmonary hypertension

Cystic fibrosis	• Any of the following despite optimal medical management (including CFTR modulator therapy)
	  ○ FEV_1 < 30% predicted
	  ○ FEV_1 < 40% predicted and
	    ■ 6MWT distance <400 m
	    ■ $Paco_2$ > 50
	    ■ Supplemental oxygen requirement at rest or with exertion
	    ■ Pulmonary hypertension
	    ■ Ongoing weight loss
	    ■ History of massive hemoptysis requiring embolization
	    ■ Pneumothorax
	    ■ 2+ exacerbations per year requiring IV therapy
		• Among patients meeting referral criteria, any of the following:
		  ○ FEV_1 < 25% predicted
		  ○ Frequent hospitalizations (>28 d in past year)
		  ○ >30% relative decline in FEV_1 during 12 mo
		  ○ Exacerbation requiring mechanical ventilation
		  ○ Pulmonary hypertension with estimated or measured pulmonary artery systolic pressure >50 mm Hg
		  ○ BMI < 18 kg/m^2 despite nutritional optimization
		  ○ Recurrent hemoptysis despite embolization

(continued on next page)

Table 2 (continued)		
Diagnosis	**Timing of Referral**	**Timing of Listing**
	○ FEV$_1$ < 50% predicted with rapidly declining trajectory ○ Any exacerbation requiring positive pressure ventilation	
Pulmonary arterial hypertension	• Any of the following despite IV therapy: ○ ESC/ERS intermediate or high risk ○ Significant RV dysfunction ○ Progression of disease or hospitalization • Suspected PCH/PVOD or scleroderma • Evidence of secondary liver of kidney injury • Consider when initiating IV or SQ prostacyclin therapy	• ESC/ERS high risk (REVEAL score >10) despite appropriate therapy (including IV) • Progressive hypoxemia • Progressive liver or kidney injury • Life-threatening hemoptysis

Abbreviations: 6MWT; 6-minute walk test; CFTR, cystic fibrosis transmembrane conductance regulator; DLCO, diffusing capacity for carbon monoxide; ERS, European Respiratory Society; ESC, European Society of Cardiology; FEV$_1$, forced expiratory volume in 1 second; FVC, forced vital capacity; IPF, idiopathic pulmonary fibrosis; IV, intravenous; Paco$_2$, arterial partial pressure of carbon dioxide; PCH/PVOD, Pulmonary capillary hemangiomatosis/pulmonary veno-occlusive disease; RV; right ventricle, SpO$_2$; oxygen saturation via pulse oximetry.

[a] Adapted from Leard LE, et al. Consensus document for the selection of lung transplant candidates: An update from the International Society for Heart and Lung Transplantation. J Heart Lung Transplant 2021. Nov;40(11):1349-1379.

[b] Includes alpha-1-antitrypsin deficiency.

severity, and 6-minute walk distance, remains one of the best validated prognostic models.[42,43] In the original validation cohort, patients with BODE scores of 7 or higher had an estimated 4-year survival of 57%,[42] suggesting a survival benefit with LTx for this subset of the overall COPD population. Subsequent studies have demonstrated that the BODE index overestimates mortality among patients with COPD and without contraindications to transplantation, likely reflecting a younger subgroup with fewer medical comorbidities.[44,45] Nonetheless, the ISHLT continues to recommend use of the BODE Index to inform the timing of referral (BODE scores of 5–6) and listing (BODE scores ≥7) for LTx (see **Table 2**).[10]

In addition to the absolute BODE Index, progression of BODE scores despite optimal treatment, FEV$_1$ less than 20% predicted pulmonary hypertension, and history of frequent exacerbations have all been associated with higher mortality in COPD and should thus be considered in the timing of referral and listing for LTx.[46–50] Acute exacerbations requiring intensive care unit admission for invasive or noninvasive ventilatory support are of particular prognostic importance,[51,52] and "severe" exacerbations are thus

designated as an ISHLT listing criterion among patients with advanced COPD (see **Table 2**).[10] Importantly, the ISHLT also recommends that clinicians incorporate quality[a] of life in LTx decisions, recognizing that although many patients with advanced COPD are unlikely to live longer with transplant, they may have severe symptoms and functional limitations without alternate treatment options.[10]

Cystic Fibrosis and Non-Cystic Fibrosis Bronchiectasis

For many patients with CF, the advent of highly effective CF transmembrane conductance regulator (CFTR) modulator therapy (eg, elexecaftor/tezacaftor/ivacaftor) has revolutionized management and led to significant improvements in lung function, exacerbation frequency, nutritional status, and quality of life.[53–58] It is generally accepted that highly effective modulators will improve long-term survival in CF and obviate or significantly delay the need for LTx. Despite this, LTx will continue to remain an important option for those who currently have advanced CF lung disease, those who progress despite modulators, as well as for whom this therapy is unavailable.[12,59,60]

Although the median survival among patients with CF and an FEV_1 < 30% predicted has improved substantially during the past 3 decades, this subgroup as a whole was shown in a 2017 study to experience a 10% annual risk of death.[61–63] Additional risk factors for disease progression and early mortality include a rapid decline in FEV_1 and/or a value < 25% predicted, frequent exacerbations and hospitalization, hypercapnia ($Paco_2$ > 50), supplemental oxygen requirement, pulmonary hypertension, low exercise capacity, malnutrition (BMI < 18 kg/m^2), and massive hemoptysis requiring bronchial artery embolization.[62,64–71] These data inform the current recommendations for LTx referral and listing (see Table 2).[10] One recent study confirmed FEV_1 as the most important prognostic marker in CF patients with the G551D genotype who had been treated since 2012 with ivacaftor, considered the first available highly effective CFTR modulator.[72] The specific indications for LTx among patients with CF will evolve further as more data become available on the long-term impact of CFTR modulators including elexecaftor/tezacaftor/ivacaftor.

In general, the criteria for LTx referral and listing among patients with non-CF bronchiectasis are similar to those with CF. These recommendations are based on older studies demonstrating higher mortality among patients with an FEV_1 < 30% predicted, frequent exacerbations or hospitalization, lower BMI, and worsening dyspnea.[73] Importantly, a 2015 study demonstrated that patients with non-CF bronchiectasis listed for LTx had a 44% lower risk of death than those with CF,[64] with only 25% dying during 5 years despite having a mean FEV_1 of 25% predicted. These findings may reflect the heterogenous nature of non-CF bronchiectasis. It is thus recommended that clinicians should consider the underlying cause and risk for progression in their decisions to refer and list patients with non-CF bronchiectasis for LTx.[10,73]

Pulmonary Arterial Hypertension

The ISHLT, European Society of Cardiology (ESC), and European Respiratory Society (ERS) currently emphasize the use of either the 2015 ESC/ERS model or the second iteration of the Registry to Evaluate Early and Long-term Pulmonary Arterial Hypertension Disease Management (REVEAL 2.0) score to guide decisions on referral and listing for LTx among patients with PAH (World Health Organization [WHO] Group I disease).[10,74] The 2015 ESC/ERS model, which incorporates functional status, exercise capacity (6WMT distance), and laboratory, echocardiographic, and right heart catheterization parameters, suggest patients who have intermediate-risk and high-risk disease experience a 5% to 10%, and >10% annual mortality, respectively.[74,75] Although not prospectively validated, registry studies suggest patients with REVEAL 2.0 scores >8 experience similar risk of short-term mortality.[76,77] Thus, the ISHLT recommends clinicians refer patients who remain at least ESC/ERS intermediate-risk (REVEAL 2.0 scores >8) despite 6 months of optimal therapy for LTx, whereas ERS/ESC high-risk patients (REVEAL scores >10) warrant listing (see Table 2).[10]

Apart from these predictive models, data suggest worsening RV dysfunction on imaging and low peak oxygen consumption on cardiopulmonary exercise testing are associated with higher short-term mortality and can further inform the timing of LTx referral.[78,79] In addition, patients with certain underlying diagnoses such as familial PAH, pulmonary capillary hemangiomatosis/pulmonary veno-occlusive disease, and CTD-related PAH tend to experience more rapid progression and may warrant earlier referral and listing.[80–82] Finally, it is important to note that current LAS systems likely underestimate mortality risk for patients with PAH.[83–85] Although some, including the US system, have adopted mechanisms to account for this increased risk (by granting score exceptions for patients with right atrial pressure >15 mm Hg, and/or cardiac index <1.8 $L/min/m^2$),[86] in nations using the LAS, the ISHLT recommends a lower threshold for LTx referral when considering the potential for longer waiting times.[10]

Despite improved understanding of prognosis in PAH, it is important to recognize that this remains a particularly challenging disease for transplant and referring providers. On one hand, with considerable evolution in medical treatments, the survival has improved,[87] such that many patients remain stable for years without LTx, with functional status often relatively preserved in the context of a comparatively young age compared with candidates with ILD or COPD. On the other hand, disease destabilization can be acute, often presenting with right ventricular failure that remains associated with poor prognosis and may require urgent LTx.[88–90] In fact, in the United States, the median LAS at the time of transplant in 2020 was highest among patients with pulmonary vascular disease, with a value of 46.6 compared with an overall median of 40.7.[3] Acute decompensation in PAH should be reviewed in multidisciplinary fashion when possible, including the role for inotropic and/or mechanical support, along with urgent transplant evaluation/listing when relevant.

Other Lung Diseases

Lymphangioleiomyomatosis

Given the effectiveness of mammalian target of rapamycin (mTOR) inhibitor therapy (eg, sirolimus) at slowing the rate of decline in FEV_1,[91–93] median transplant-free survival among patients with lymphangioleiomyomatosis (LAM) is currently estimated at greater than 20 years from time of diagnosis.[94] However, survival is significantly worse among patients with FEV_1 or DLCO less than 50% predicted, severe dyspnea as the presenting symptom, and those requiring supplemental oxygen.[94,95] Considering these risk factors, the ISHLT currently recommends referring LAM patients for LTx if they develop any of the following despite mTOR inhibitor therapy: FEV_1 less than 30% predicted New York Heart Association Class III or IV dyspnea, supplemental oxygen requirement at rest, pulmonary hypertension, or refractory pneumothorax.[10]

Sarcoidosis

Although observational studies suggest 90% of patients with sarcoidosis will survive greater than 10 years after diagnosis, LTx may still be indicated for those with progressive disease including advanced radiographic fibrosis, WHO Group V pulmonary hypertension, or advanced bronchiectasis with frequent exacerbations.[96] The timing of LTx referral and listing should follow the disease-specific recommendations for each patient's predominant manifestation (eg, ILD or pulmonary hypertension).[10,97] Although patients with advanced pulmonary sarcoidosis experience favorable outcomes with LTx, transplant clinicians should carefully evaluate for cardiac involvement because the presence of sarcoid cardiomyopathy may represent a contraindication to isolated LTx.[10,98] These patients, with severe mediastinal lymphadenopathy and calcifications, present a significant surgical risk and challenge for listing.

Combined pulmonary fibrosis and emphysema

In general, recommendations for LTx in combined pulmonary fibrosis and emphysema (CPFE) follow those for other ILDs. However, FVC is a less reliable predictor of disease progression and outcomes among patients with CPFE.[99,100] Consequently, the ISHLT emphasizes the use of other parameters (eg, decline in DLCO, radiographic progression, or development of pulmonary hypertension) to inform the timing of LTx in this subset of the ILD population.[10]

Acute respiratory distress syndrome

Historically, LTx has been rarely feasible among patients with acute respiratory distress syndrome (ARDS) given the associated risks including high likelihood of concomitant organ failure.[101] Additionally, the "optimal window" for LTx for ARDS can be challenging to define given that a subset of patients may ultimately demonstrate late recovery. However, there has been momentum in the LTx community toward transplanting in sicker patients, and particularly during the COVID-19 pandemic, more transplantations are being performed in the setting of acute respiratory failure (also see "Special considerations" section and a later article in this issue). The ISHLT guidelines propose that it is reasonable to consider LTx for young patients with isolated respiratory failure despite 4 to 6 weeks of supportive care, recognizing that this population does carry significant risks, and that recovery from ARDS may be possible even after prolonged life support.[102–104]

Chronic lung allograft dysfunction and retransplantation

Lung retransplantation remains somewhat controversial and not universally performed. Survival is worse than after the initial transplantation, particularly among patients who underwent retransplantation for primary graft dysfunction or restrictive CLAD (restrictive allograft syndrome; RAS).[1,2,105–109] Outcomes among patients who underwent retransplantation for bronchiolitis obliterans syndrome (BOS) have been shown to be more favorable than for RAS, with one study demonstrating a 5-year survival of 51% versus 23%, respectively.[107] Additional factors associated with improved survival include age younger than 50 years, time since initial transplant greater than 2 years, absence of renal dysfunction, and outpatient status at the time of retransplantation.[105,108] Thus, consideration of retransplantation may be reasonable in carefully selected candidates.

EVALUATION PROCESS

After a patient with advanced lung disease is referred for LTx, evaluation on the part of the transplant team involves a detailed multistage assessment (see **Fig. 1**). First, on reviewing the patient's underlying diagnosis, it is imperative to confirm that no other treatment options are available that could provide disease stabilization or improvement. For example, some transplant programs engage in a combined evaluation for COPD, where a patient referred with advanced disease is evaluated not only for LTx but also for bronchoscopic or surgical lung volume reduction surgery. If treatment options are available to improve morbidity and/or mortality before or in lieu of LTx, coordination of care between transplantation and referring teams must ensue to ensure that these steps take place in the context of the overall evaluation process including expected timeline. As discussed above, earlier referral for LTx will help facilitate this process in a coordinated manner that allows more flexibility for the patient and providers.

Second, the transplant team will evaluate a patient's current pulmonary status including symptoms, clinical trajectory, and objective testing to confirm that prognosis is limited and determine the most appropriate timing of further evaluation and listing. Depending on clinical status, the subsequent timeline can range from a fully elective workup over the course of months, to a prescheduled workup over weeks, to an expedited inpatient evaluation over days.

Arguably most challenging is an assessment of a patient's cumulative risk for adverse outcomes with LTx. Due to the scarcity of viable donor lungs, the ISHLT suggests that transplant programs have an ethical and societal responsibility to ration transplantation to the candidates who have a relatively high probability of overall success.[10] However, most risk factors for poorer posttransplant outcomes have been identified in isolation using retrospective analyses, and prediction can be exceedingly difficult on an individual basis. Diagnostic testing during the evaluation process is intended to identify risk factors, including those that may be modifiable in the pretransplant period to improve the likelihood of a successful outcome (see "Selection criteria" section).

Although significant variability exists, most LTx centers have similar core diagnostics that include not only assessment for risk factors but also age-appropriate screening and vaccines, and testing for markers of pulmonary disease severity (Box 1). Laboratory analysis includes hematologic, hepatic, renal, and endocrinologic testing, infectious disease biomarkers, and screening for nicotine and other substances. Pulmonary function and 6-minute walk testing are completed at all centers and repeated at multiple time points to determine the trajectory of disease. Radiographic studies include chest radiograph and CT scan, quantitative ventilation and perfusion scan, bone mineral densitometry, as well as other imaging based on clinical scenario.

Cardiac and gastrointestinal disease in particular may pose significant risk for worse LTx outcomes (Table 3). In patients with moderate-to-severe coronary artery disease, pretransplant percutaneous intervention or simultaneous revascularization at time of LTx may be warranted. Most centers perform routine pretransplant cardiac testing including electrocardiogram, echocardiogram, and right/left (based on risk) heart catheterization, generally keeping a low threshold for consultation with a cardiologist as appropriate. In patients with gastroesophageal reflux and/or esophageal dysmotility, varying evidence exists to suggest an increased risk of posttransplant baseline allograft dysfunction, an acute cellular rejection, and an early onset of CLAD.[110–113] Pretransplant gastrointestinal testing varies by center, and in some cases by patient based on underlying disease and symptomatology. All centers require updated age-appropriate cancer screening and vaccinations, along with dental evaluation. Importantly, the ISHLT, American Society of Transplantation, and American Society for Transplant Surgeons recently released a statement strongly recommending vaccination against SARS-CoV-2, ideally before transplantation.[114]

Finally, consultation with members of the multidisciplinary transplant team is a cornerstone of the LTx evaluation process (Fig. 2). Education of potential candidates and their caregivers is vital, and the pretransplant nurse coordinators, physicians, and other team members need to ensure that patients are aware of the risks, benefits, and expectations of LTx. Incorporating decision aids has been shown to be useful in certain populations.[115] Social work and often neuropsychological evaluation are crucial to evaluate and manage conditions associated with worse posttransplant outcomes including inadequate social support and depression,[116–118] whereas also supporting and assisting patients during a vulnerable time marked by uncertainty about prognosis and LTx candidacy.[119] Mental health conditions, inadequate social support, or limited financial resources may represent barriers to LTx but many times, these are modifiable with time, therapies, and proactive planning. Specialized medical consultation may also be needed to optimize certain conditions including pretransplant diabetes, osteoporosis, or chronic rhinosinusitis.

SELECTION CRITERIA

On completion of the LTx evaluation, the patient is typically presented to a selection committee to determine appropriateness and timing of listing based on disease severity (section III; see Table 2), along with potential risk factors for adverse outcomes (see Table 3). Absolute contraindications are well described in the ISHLT 2021 consensus statement.[10] Importantly, the document also transitioned from the term "relative contraindications,"

Box 1
Testing used during the prelung transplant evaluation[a]

Laboratory

Complete blood count, comprehensive metabolic panel, magnesium, phosphorus, prothrombin time,

Arterial/venous blood gas, ABO (blood type) testing × 2, hemoglobin A1c, lipid panel, vitamin D, parathyroid hormone, TSH/free T4, testosterone (men), immunoglobulins, HLA antibodies, EBV IgM/IgG, CMV IgM/IgG, hepatitis panel (A, B, C), HIV, Quantiferon gold, Treponemal Ig/RPR, Toxoplasma IgM/IgG, HSV IgG, VZV IgG, MMR

Urine studies: Urinalysis, 24-h creatinine clearance/protein, urine drug screen, urine nicotine, urine HcG (women of childbearing age)

Consider: PETH, ANA, RF, ESR, uric acid, BNP, amylase, LDH, CK, iron studies, alpha-1 antitrypsin level, ammonia, telomere testing

Pulmonary

Pulmonary function tests (spirometry, volumes, DLCO), 6-min walk, pulmonary rehabilitation documentation

Consider: Sputum culture (Bacterial/fungal/AFB)

Cardiac

Electrocardiogram, echocardiogram (consider with agitated saline study), right heart catheterization, left heart catheterization (>45–50-year old or coronary artery disease risk factors)

Consider: Cardiac MRI (sarcoidosis)

Gastrointestinal

Consider: Esophagram, pH probe, manometry, gastric emptying study, modified barium swallow

Radiology

Chest radiograph, chest CT, quantitative V/Q scan, abdominal ultrasound/CT, bone mineral density, diaphragmatic fluoroscopy

Consider: Carotid Doppler, lower extremity vascular studies, sinus CT, flexion/extension neck radiographs (rheumatoid arthritis)

Consults

Social work, dietitian, finance, neuropsychology, pharmacy

Consider: Endocrine, otolaryngology, cardiology, physical therapy, infectious diseases

Health-care Maintenance

Age-appropriate cancer screening: Colonoscopy, Pap/pelvic examination (women), mammogram (women), PSA (men)

Dental evaluation

Consider: Fecal occult blood test

Vaccines

Hepatitis A, Hepatitis B, Tetanus, Flu, Prevnar-13, Pneumovax-23, COVID-19

Consider: Shingles, HPV

Abbreviations: AFB, acid fast bacilli; ANA, antinuclear antibodies; BNP, B-type natriuretic peptide; CMV, cytomegalovirus; CPK, creatine phosphokinase; CT, computed tomography; DLCO, diffusing capacity for carbon monoxide; EBV, Ebstein-Barr virus; ESR, erythrocyte sedimentation rate; HcG, human chorionic gonadotropin; HIV, human immunodeficiency virus; HLA, human leukocyte antigen; HPV, human papilloma virus; HSV, herpes simplex virus; LDH, lactate dehydrogenase; MMR, measles, mumps, rubella; MRI, magnetic resonance imaging; PETH, phosphatidylethanol; PSA, prostate specific antigen; Rf, Rheumatoid factor; TSH, thyroid stimulating hormone; V/Q, Ventilation/perfusion (imaging); VZV, varicella zoster virus. [a]Testing protocols were compiled from the following lung transplantation centers: University Health Network-Toronto, University of Washington, Washington University, University of Virginia, University of Pittsburgh Medical Center, University of California San Francisco, University of Florida, St. Joseph's Hospital and Medical Center-Arizona, Duke University, and University of Wisconsin-Madison.

Table 3
Risk factors for adverse posttransplant outcomes in candidates for lung transplantation

Absolute Contraindications	High or Substantially Increased Risk	General
• Lack of patient willingness or acceptance of transplant • Malignancy with high risk of death or recurrence • GFR <40 mL/min/1.73m^2 unless being considered for multiorgan transplant • Acute coronary syndrome within 30 d (excluding demand ischemia) • Stroke within 30 d • Liver cirrhosis with portal hypertension or synthetic dysfunction unless being considered for multiorgan transplant • Acute liver failure • Acute renal failure with rising creatinine or on dialysis and low likelihood of recovery • Active extrapulmonary infection including septic shock • Active tuberculosis infection • HIV infection with detectable viral load • Severely limited functional status with poor rehabilitation potential • Progressive cognitive impairment • Repeated episodes of nonadherence without evidence of improvement • Active substance use or dependence including current tobacco use, vaping, marijuana smoking, or IV drug use • Other severe uncontrolled medical condition expected to limit survival after transplant	• Age >70 y • Severe CAD requiring CABG at transplant • LV ejection fraction <40% • Significant cerebrovascular disease • Severe esophageal dysmotility • Untreatable hematologic disorders (bleeding diathesis, thrombophilia, severe bone marrow dysfunction) • BMI ≥35 kg/m^2 • BMI <16 kg/m^2 • Limited functional status • Psychiatric, psychological or cognitive conditions with potential to interfere with medical adherence • Unreliable support system • Lack of understanding of disease and/or transplant despite teaching • *M abscessus* infection • *Lomentospora prolificans* infection • *Burkholderia cenocepacia* or *Burkholderia gladioli* infection • Hepatitis B or C infection with detectable viral load and liver fibrosis • Chest wall or spinal deformity expected to cause restriction after transplant • Extracorporeal life support • Retransplantation for restrictive CLAD, antibody-mediated rejection, or within 1 y following initial lung transplant	• Age 65–70 y • GFR 40–60 mL/min/1.73m^2 • CAD including prior CABG • LV ejection fraction 40%–50% • Peripheral vascular disease • Connective tissue disease • Severe GERD • Esophageal dysmotility • Bone marrow dysfunction • Osteoporosis • BMI 30–34.9 kg/m^2 • BMI 16–17 kg/m^2 • Frailty • Hypoalbuminemia • Poorly controlled diabetes • Edible marijuana • *Scedosporium apiospermum* infection • HIV with undetectable viral load • Previous thoracic surgery including pleurodesis • Mechanical ventilation • Retransplantation

Abbreviations: BMI, body mass index; CABG, coronary artery bypass graft surgery; CAD, coronary artery disease; CLAD, chronic lung allograft dysfunction; GERD, gastroesophageal reflux disease; GFR, glomerular filtration rate; HIV, human immunodeficiency virus; LV, left ventricular.

Adapted from Leard LE, et al. Consensus document for the selection of lung transplant candidates: An update from the International Society for Heart and Lung Transplantation. J Heart Lung Transplant 2021. Nov;40(11):1349-1379.

to the more descriptive "risk factors," including characterizing some as "high or substantially increased risk," while also recognizing the cumulative nature of multiple smaller risk factors. Finally, the guidelines acknowledge the fact that suitability for transplant is a complex decision, and by nature, centers will have varying levels of risk tolerance based on volumes, specific expertise, and donor availability, all of which will contribute to varying selection criteria.

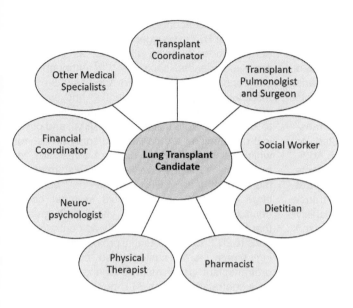

Fig. 2. Multifaceted approach to lung transplantation evaluation.

Absolute contraindications have become fewer as centers gain more experience but still reflect conditions that should preclude LTx at most centers due to the risks being too high in comparison with the potential benefits (see **Table 3**).[10] First and foremost, the patient must be understanding and accepting of the idea of LTx and be able to provide consent. Other contraindications include malignancy with high risk of recurrence, severe extrapulmonary disease not amenable to combined transplantation, some high-risk infections including active septic shock, and active substance abuse or nonadherence.

Factors carrying substantially increased risk have also evolved and become fewer because the field advances (see **Table 3**).[10] For example, LTx is now often possible in patients with severe esophageal dysmotility associated with scleroderma,[120,121] severely reduced BMI in CF,[122,123] age greater than 70 years,[124] and some infections including *Mycobacterium abscessus*,[125,126] but candidates with these conditions should still generally be transplanted in programs having adequate experience, with any modifiable conditions (eg, malnutrition, morbid obesity) optimized as early as possible during the process.[10] For those with prior malignancy, although a 5-year cancer-free survival was historically required, recognizing that this may not be possible in many cases due to pulmonary prognosis, as well as the low risk of recurrence of some cancers, shorter times may be allowable after consultation with oncologic providers.[127,128] Other high-risk medical conditions including severe functional limitations similarly may be considered on a case-by-

case basis while recognizing that certain factors may create additive risk that ultimately leads to a patient being declined at the specific program.

Although psychosocial and behavioral factors are often more challenging to objectively assess, certain problems including severe anxiety or depression, personality disorders, neurocognitive dysfunction, and lack of social support have all been shown to affect postlung transplant outcomes and should be reviewed carefully (see **Table 3**).[119] The habitual nature of high-risk behaviors (eg, substance use) is essential to explore from a psychosocial perspective but LTx is often possible in those who demonstrate prolonged and ongoing compliance (including abstinence from pertinent substances) with a recommended treatment program. It is important to note that the key predictor of poor outcome in the setting of pretransplant psychosocial concerns is the element of true functional impairment that is expected following LTx. Well-controlled psychiatric disease involving the use of psychotropic medications is not considered an absolute contraindication, and some cognitive problems may be allowed if the candidate is well-compensated and previously functional, well-supported, and/or if underlying pulmonary disease or the related treatments are contributing to the limitations. Other problems may be modifiable (eg, social support or financial limitations) with time, careful planning, and fundraising. Mental health therapy, including cognitive behavioral therapy, can also produce favorable results while on the transplant list.[115]

Ultimately, the decision for transplant listing is rarely a straightforward conclusion. Often listing may be deferred until a candidate can optimize certain risk factors, a process that is facilitated by early referral. Even when the decision is made to list a candidate for LTx, attention to optimizable risk factors including conditioning, nutrition, and social support is still required on the part of transplant and referring providers while listed to improve the chance of successful outcome. Additionally, there are contingencies and requirements to remain active on the list, and reevaluation at close intervals while listed is vital to ensure transplant is still in the patient's best interest. Variability in selection criteria by center should be recognized by referring providers, and importantly, the most recent ISHLT guidelines emphasize the importance of transparency regarding LTx candidacy decisions and policies.[10] If a patient is determined to not be a candidate, it is recommended that specific reasons be provided by the center to allow for optimization, or potentially referral to a different center if this is a possibility. Finally, concurrent referral to a palliative care specialist should be considered for all patients that go through the pretransplant process to address symptoms, goals of care, and other means of support, and this should not be viewed as mutually exclusive from curative care including LTx.[59,129–131]

SPECIAL CONSIDERATIONS
Extracorporeal Life Support as Bridge to Transplant

During the last 2 decades, extracorporeal life support (ECLS) as a bridge to transplant (BTT) has been increasingly used when LTx candidates demonstrate refractory hypoxemia, hemodynamic instability, or the inability to participate in physiotherapy despite noninvasive ventilation.[10,132] In the United States, 6.7% of total lung transplants in 2020 occurred following BTT with ECLS, compared with 4.7% in 2015.[3] Increased use of ECLS bridging has occurred in the context of improved outcomes, which correlates with several major practice changes including: (1) increasing use of veno-venous (VV) rather than veno-arterial (VA) ECLS, (2) avoidance of bridging to acute retransplantation, and (3) the transition away from keeping patients sedated on concomitant mechanical ventilation to using ECLS alone in awake patients.[133] In the most recent era, long-term postlung transplant survival among BTT patients is only slightly inferior to non-BTT patients.[133,134]

It is important to recognize that not all LTx candidates can or should be considered BTT candidates. Outcomes have been shown to be better after BTT in younger patients, those who undergo shorter bridging durations, as well as in more experienced centers.[135–139] Although general consensus is that factors such as irreversible extrapulmonary organ dysfunction and systemic infections should be considered contraindications to BTT, other factors, such as age, BMI, and physical conditioning are considered "gray areas" for which centers will have different thresholds for candidacy.[10] Higher volume centers may be more liberal than smaller centers[138,139] but even large transplant centers would in most cases consider age older than 65 years, BMI greater than 30 kg/m^2, and severe frailty as contraindications to BTT. Due to potential prolongation of waiting times, some centers also consider high pretransplant panel reactive antibody values to be a contraindication to BTT; however, this varies widely and depends on centers' management of donor-specific antibodies at the time of transplantation.[140]

Certainly, patients for whom ECLS BTT is initiated require close, ongoing evaluation to determine if survival and rehabilitation after LTx remain reasonably likely. Prioritizing regular physiotherapy is crucial, and when feasible improves transplantation rates, posttransplant recovery time, and survival.[134,137,141] Although historically avoiding femoral cannulation was felt to allow for more effective physiotherapy,[141] more recent literature and experience suggest that adequate rehabilitation can continue with VV, or even VA ECLS via the femoral site(s).[142,143] In summary, the decision to use ECLS BTT should involve a multidisciplinary review by the LTx, critical care, and ECLS physicians and surgeons, ideally before critical illness. The team should discuss risks, expectations, and goals of care with the patient and family when considering ECLS BTT.

Urgent Referrals

Although early and proactive LTx referral is always preferable, as with BTT, urgent referral for a patient in acute or acute-on-chronic respiratory failure has become more common and poses unique challenges. Critical illness often precludes the ability to obtain all the typically required pretransplant testing, fully evaluate the mental status and physical strength of the patient, adequately assess the patient's understanding of LTx and posttransplant care and provide comprehensive education and counseling. Deciding to urgently list a rapidly deteriorating patient within the confines of such limitations requires the center to accept a higher degree of risk compared with electively assessed candidates. Centers have varying levels of comfort in accepting this risk. One large, single center study reported that urgently listed candidates undergo LTx more often than not, and they have similar short-term and long-term outcomes as electively listed candidates.[144] Not surprisingly, urgently listed patients were more likely to die before transplantation if they were older, referred from outside hospitals, required transfusion, required inotropic support, or were in renal failure. Another recent study analyzed outcomes among 43 patients who were urgently evaluated in the intensive care unit and bridged to LTx on mechanical support.[145] Twelve (28%) died before LTx but among the 32 transplanted the 1-year, 5-year, and 10-year survival was 86.8%, 78.4%, and 53.4%, respectively, which did not differ significantly compared with patients who were evaluated and transplanted electively.

Several specific factors must be considered to allow for urgent evaluation and LTx. Younger age is preferable, and absence of extrapulmonary organ dysfunction required. Generally, an inability to participate in physiotherapy is considered an absolute contraindication.[10,137] However, patients who were well before the onset of acute respiratory failure may have greater physical reserve compared with candidates with chronic lung disease. Therefore, a period of immobility may not preclude candidacy if rehabilitation potential is established based on recent history and functional status. The requirement for first-person consent before lung transplant varies among transplant centers. Transplanting a candidate without informed consent is fraught with ethical issues; however, in rare circumstances, centers have obtained consent from the substitute decision maker when a critically ill patient cannot provide consent due to sedation requirements.[146]

THE ROLE OF THE REFERRING PULMONOLOGIST

The referring pulmonologist plays a significant role in the lung transplant process (see **Fig. 1**). The CF community, in particular, has devoted a great deal of attention to educating referring providers on the transplant process through recent and explicit guidelines on advanced lung disease and LTx referral.[10,12,59] Important concepts include early patient education and preparation for LTx well before the need arises, close communication between referring and transplant teams, as well as the concept of modifiable barriers to LTx as reviewed above. CF guidelines also imply that contraindications to LTx should be established by the transplant teams, and not by referring providers,[12] a notion that is particularly important given the continuously evolving landscape of risk tolerance. For example, a perceived barrier to LTx such as malnutrition, obesity, or coronary artery disease, should not necessarily preclude a pulmonologist from contacting or referral to a transplant center, and although the subsequent steps will certainly differ based on the program and specific risk factor(s), it can be argued that this philosophy improves equity for the overall population of patients with advanced lung disease who could benefit from LTx. This is arguably most important for patients with complex psychosocial issues who can benefit from meeting with the transplant team early to establish strong support plans that would be required for LTx candidacy. Ideally, the local LTx team is readily accessible to the referring pulmonologist, and there is a culture of open and frequent communication. In addition to transparency regarding barriers to LTx, communication between transplant and referring pulmonologists should include clearly outlining steps for improving candidacy, relevant timeline, and delineating responsibilities for various aspects of patient management.

Once a patient is listed, the transplant team continues to rely on the referring pulmonologist's ongoing input regarding the patient's clinical status because this may prompt a higher status on the wait list or change in decision regarding candidacy. Following transplant, the referring pulmonologist may continue to participate in the patient's care depending on the respective centers' usual protocols. Local pulmonary follow-up, particularly if the patient is located a far distance from the transplant center, is often encouraged by the transplant team. Patients with CF have been shown to benefit from ongoing involvement from their CF care team,[147] a notion that may be applicable to other diseases although literature is lacking.

SUMMARY

LTx offers the potential to extend and improve quality of life for patients with many forms of advanced lung disease. Volumes are increasing and recipient demographics evolving but the basic tenets of candidate selection remain similar, with LTx best suited for patients with limited life expectancy from their native disease, in whom there is also a reasonable chance of long-term posttransplant success. Predicting outcomes after LTx is extremely challenging and involves estimating the cumulative risks based on previously identified risk factors for posttransplant mortality.

For most candidates, there is an optimal window for referral that allows for the evaluation, education, and listing processes to be performed electively. Specific criteria and processes vary greatly by diagnosis and center but there is general agreement in the transplant and pulmonary communities that early referral is preferable to late referral given the risks of death and rushed evaluation with the latter. In many cases, this may not be possible due to rapid disease progression or acute illnesses including ARDS, where there is an added need for thorough assessment of functional status and extrapulmonary organ dysfunction, as well as close communication between transplant and referring centers to discuss candidacy and bridging options. As the community transitions toward higher-risk, sicker patients, more data are needed on longer term posttransplant outcomes, risk stratification to better determine candidacy, interventions to improve management while approaching LTx, and methods to ensure allocation of donor lungs to those most in need.

CLINICS CARE POINTS

- The demographics of lung transplantation are evolving such that candidates are now older, sicker, and more often have interstitial lung disease than in decades past.

- The 2021 International Society for Heart and Lung Transplantation Consensus Document supports consideration of lung transplantation in patients with a high (>50%) risk of death from their lung disease within two years if transplant is not perfomed, and a high (>80%) likelihood of 5-year post-transplant survival from a general medical perspective provided there is adequate graft function.

- Lung transplant centers conduct a comprehensive, multidisciplinary pre-transplant evaluation in order to assess pulmonary disease severity, extra-pulmonary organ dysfunction, nutrition, conditioning, cancer screening, vaccinations, and psychosocial well-being.

- The referring pulmonolgist plays a crucial role in the pre-lung transplant process including in ensuring timely referral for transplant, working to address modifiable barriers to transplant as soon as possible, and managing the underlying disease in collaboration with the transplant team.

DISCLOSURE

None of the authors has any disclosures relevant to this article.

REFERENCES

1. Chambers DC, Cherikh WS, Harhay MO, et al. The International thoracic organ transplant registry of the international society for heart and lung transplantation: thirty-sixth adult lung and heart-lung transplantation Report-2019; Focus theme: donor and recipient size match. J Heart Lung Transpl 2019;38(10):1042–55.
2. Chambers DC, Perch M, Zuckermann A, et al. The international thoracic organ transplant registry of the international society for heart and lung transplantation: thirty-eighth adult lung transplantation report - 2021; Focus on recipient characteristics. J Heart Lung Transpl 2021;40(10):1060–72.
3. Valapour M, Lehr CJ, Skeans MA, et al. OPTN/SRTR 2020 annual data report: lung. Am J Transpl 2022;22(Suppl 2):438–518.
4. Egan TM, Edwards LB. Effect of the lung allocation score on lung transplantation in the United States. J Heart Lung Transpl 2016;35(4):433–9.
5. Benvenuto LJ, Anderson MR, Aversa M, et al. Geographic disparities in lung transplantation in the United States before and after the November 2017 allocation change. J Heart Lung Transpl 2022;41(3):382–90.
6. Mooney JJ, Bhattacharya J, Dhillon GS. Effect of broader geographic sharing of donor lungs on lung transplant waitlist outcomes. J Heart Lung Transpl 2019;38(2):136–44.
7. Egan TM. How should lungs be allocated for transplant? Semin Respir Crit Care Med 2018;39(2):126–37.
8. Ramos KJ, Quon BS, Psoter KJ, et al. Predictors of non-referral of patients with cystic fibrosis for lung transplant evaluation in the United States. J Cyst Fibros 2016;15(2):196–203.
9. Tague LK, Witt CA, Byers DE, et al. Association between allosensitization and waiting list outcomes among adult lung transplant candidates in the United States. Ann Am Thorac Soc 2019;16(7):846–52.
10. Leard LE, Holm AM, Valapour M, et al. Consensus document for the selection of lung transplant candidates: an update from the International Society for Heart and Lung Transplantation. J Heart Lung Transpl 2021;40(11):1349–79.
11. Network OPaT. Ethical principles in the allocation of human organs. Available at: https://optn.transplant.hrsa.gov/resources/ethics/ethical-principles-in-the-allocation-of-human-organs/.

12. Ramos KJ, Smith PJ, McKone EF, et al. Lung transplant referral for individuals with cystic fibrosis: cystic Fibrosis Foundation consensus guidelines. J Cyst Fibros 2019;18(3):321–33.

13. Clausen ES, Frankel C, Palmer SM, et al. Pre-transplant weight loss and clinical outcomes after lung transplantation. J Heart Lung Transpl 2018;37(12):1443–7.

14. Li M, Mathur S, Chowdhury NA, et al. Pulmonary rehabilitation in lung transplant candidates. J Heart Lung Transpl 2013;32(6):626–32.

15. Wickerson L, Rozenberg D, Janaudis-Ferreira T, et al. Physical rehabilitation for lung transplant candidates and recipients: an evidence-informed clinical approach. Worldj Transpl 2016;6(3):517–31.

16. Fernández Pérez ER, Daniels CE, Schroeder DR, et al. Incidence, prevalence, and clinical course of idiopathic pulmonary fibrosis: a population-based study. Chest 2010;137(1):129–37.

17. Flaherty KR, Toews GB, Travis WD, et al. Clinical significance of histological classification of idiopathic interstitial pneumonia. Eur Respir J 2002;19(2):275–83.

18. King TE Jr, Bradford WZ, Castro-Bernardini S, et al. A phase 3 trial of pirfenidone in patients with idiopathic pulmonary fibrosis. N Engl J Med 2014;370(22):2083–92.

19. Raghu G, Wells AU, Nicholson AG, et al. Effect of nintedanib in subgroups of idiopathic pulmonary fibrosis by diagnostic criteria. Am J Respir Crit Care Med 2017;195(1):78–85.

20. Richeldi L, du Bois RM, Raghu G, et al. Efficacy and safety of nintedanib in idiopathic pulmonary fibrosis. N Engl J Med 2014;370(22):2071–82.

21. Nathan SD, Albera C, Bradford WZ, et al. Effect of pirfenidone on mortality: pooled analyses and meta-analyses of clinical trials in idiopathic pulmonary fibrosis. Lancet Respir Med 2017;5(1):33–41.

22. Lederer DJ, Martinez FJ. Idiopathic pulmonary fibrosis. N Engl J Med 2018;378(19):1811–23.

23. Kapnadak SG, Raghu G. Lung transplantation for interstitial lung disease. Eur Respir Rev 2021;30(161):210017.

24. du Bois RM, Weycker D, Albera C, et al. Ascertainment of individual risk of mortality for patients with idiopathic pulmonary fibrosis. Am J Respir Crit Care Med 2011;184(4):459–66.

25. Ley B, Ryerson CJ, Vittinghoff E, et al. A multidimensional index and staging system for idiopathic pulmonary fibrosis. Ann Intern Med 2012;156(10):684–91.

26. Alhamad EH, Cal JG, Alrajhi NN, et al. Predictors of mortality in patients with interstitial lung disease-associated pulmonary hypertension. J Clin Med 2020;9(12):3828.

27. Chahal A, Sharif R, Watts J, et al. Predicting outcome in idiopathic pulmonary fibrosis: addition of fibrotic score at thin-section ct of the chest to gender, age, and physiology score improves the prediction model. Radiol Cardiothorac Imaging 2019;1(2):e180029.

28. Nasser M, Larrieu S, Si-Mohamed S, et al. Progressive fibrosing interstitial lung disease: a clinical cohort (the PROGRESS study). Eur Respir J 2021;57(2).

29. Park JH, Kim DS, Park IN, et al. Prognosis of fibrotic interstitial pneumonia: idiopathic versus collagen vascular disease-related subtypes. Am J Respir Crit Care Med 2007;175(7):705–11.

30. Cottin V, Hirani NA, Hotchkin DL, et al. Presentation, diagnosis and clinical course of the spectrum of progressive-fibrosing interstitial lung diseases. Eur Respir Rev 2018;27(150):180076.

31. Flaherty KR, Wells AU, Cottin V, et al. Nintedanib in progressive fibrosing interstitial lung diseases. N Engl J Med 2019;381(18):1718–27.

32. Maher TM, Corte TJ, Fischer A, et al. Pirfenidone in patients with unclassifiable progressive fibrosing interstitial lung disease: a double-blind, randomised, placebo-controlled, phase 2 trial. Lancet Respir Med 2020;8(2):147–57.

33. Distler O, Highland KB, Gahlemann M, et al. Nintedanib for systemic sclerosis-associated interstitial lung disease. N Engl J Med 2019;380(26):2518–28.

34. Wells AU, Flaherty KR, Brown KK, et al. Nintedanib in patients with progressive fibrosing interstitial lung diseases-subgroup analyses by interstitial lung disease diagnosis in the INBUILD trial: a randomised, double-blind, placebo-controlled, parallel-group trial. Lancet Respir Med 2020;8(5):453–60.

35. Raghu G, Ley B, Brown KK, et al. Risk factors for disease progression in idiopathic pulmonary fibrosis. Thorax 2020;75(1):78–80.

36. Snyder L, Neely ML, Hellkamp AS, et al. Predictors of death or lung transplant after a diagnosis of idiopathic pulmonary fibrosis: insights from the IPF-PRO Registry. Respir Res 2019;20(1):105.

37. Ratwani AP, Ahmad KI, Barnett SD, et al. Connective tissue disease-associated interstitial lung disease and outcomes after hospitalization: a cohort study. Respir Med 2019;154:1–5.

38. Khadawardi H, Mura M. A simple dyspnoea scale as part of the assessment to predict outcome across chronic interstitial lung disease. Respirology 2017;22(3):501–7.

39. Amano M, Izumi C, Baba M, et al. Progression of right ventricular dysfunction and predictors of mortality in patients with idiopathic interstitial pneumonias. J Cardiol 2020;75(3):242–9.

40. Hayes D Jr, Black SM, Tobias JD, et al. Influence of pulmonary hypertension on patients with idiopathic pulmonary fibrosis awaiting lung transplantation. Ann Thorac Surg 2016;101(1):246–52.

41. du Bois RM, Weycker D, Albera C, et al. Six-minute-walk test in idiopathic pulmonary fibrosis: test validation and minimal clinically important difference. Am J Respir Crit Care Med 2011;183(9): 1231–7.

42. Celli BR, Cote CG, Marin JM, et al. The body-mass index, airflow obstruction, dyspnea, and exercise capacity index in chronic obstructive pulmonary disease. N Engl J Med 2004;350(10):1005–12.

43. Bellou V, Belbasis L, Konstantinidis AK, et al. Prognostic models for outcome prediction in patients with chronic obstructive pulmonary disease: systematic review and critical appraisal. BMJ 2019; 367:l5358.

44. Reed RM, Cabral HJ, Dransfield MT, et al. Survival of lung transplant candidates with COPD: BODE score reconsidered. Chest 2018;153(3):697–701.

45. Pirard L, Marchand E. Reassessing the BODE score as a criterion for listing COPD patients for lung transplantation. Int J Chron Obstruct Pulmon Dis 2018;13:3963–70.

46. Thabut G, Ravaud P, Christie JD, et al. Determinants of the survival benefit of lung transplantation in patients with chronic obstructive pulmonary disease. Am J Respir Crit Care Med 2008;177(10): 1156–63.

47. Oswald-Mammosser M, Weitzenblum E, Quoix E, et al. Prognostic factors in COPD patients receiving long-term oxygen therapy. Importance of pulmonary artery pressure. Chest 1995;107(5):1193–8.

48. LaFon DC, Bhatt SP, Labaki WW, et al. Pulmonary artery enlargement and mortality risk in moderate to severe COPD: results from COPDGene. Eur Respir J 2020;55(2):1901812.

49. Martinez FJ, Foster G, Curtis JL, et al. Predictors of mortality in patients with emphysema and severe airflow obstruction. Am J Respir Crit Care Med 2006;173(12):1326–34.

50. Martinez FJ, Han MK, Andrei AC, et al. Longitudinal change in the BODE index predicts mortality in severe emphysema. Am J Respir Crit Care Med 2008;178(5):491–9.

51. Seneff MG, Wagner DP, Wagner RP, et al. Hospital and 1-year survival of patients admitted to intensive care units with acute exacerbation of chronic obstructive pulmonary disease. JAMA 1995; 274(23):1852–7.

52. Warwick M, Fernando SM, Aaron SD, et al. Outcomes and resource utilization among patients admitted to the intensive care unit following acute exacerbation of chronic obstructive pulmonary disease. J Intensive Care Med 2021;36(9):1091–7.

53. Heijerman HGM, McKone EF, Downey DG, et al. Efficacy and safety of the elexacaftor plus tezacaftor plus ivacaftor combination regimen in people with cystic fibrosis homozygous for the F508del mutation: a double-blind, randomised, phase 3 trial. Lancet 2019;394(10212):1940–8.

54. Barry PJ, Mall MA, Álvarez A, et al. Triple therapy for cystic fibrosis phe508del-gating and -residual function genotypes. N Engl J Med 2021;385(9): 815–25.

55. Burgel PR, Durieu I, Chiron R, et al. Rapid improvement after starting elexacaftor-tezacaftor-ivacaftor in patients with cystic fibrosis and advanced pulmonary disease. Am J Respir Crit Care Med 2021;204(1):64–73.

56. Middleton PG, Mall MA, Dřevínek P, et al. Elexacaftor-tezacaftor-ivacaftor for cystic fibrosis with a single phe508del allele. N Engl J Med 2019;381(19): 1809–19.

57. Flume PA, Biner RF, Downey DG, et al. Long-term safety and efficacy of tezacaftor-ivacaftor in individuals with cystic fibrosis aged 12 years or older who are homozygous or heterozygous for Phe508-del CFTR (EXTEND): an open-label extension study. Lancet Respir Med 2021;9(7):733–46.

58. McColley SA, Konstan MW, Ramsey BW, et al. Lumacaftor/Ivacaftor reduces pulmonary exacerbations in patients irrespective of initial changes in FEV(1). J Cyst Fibros 2019;18(1):94–101.

59. Kapnadak SG, Dimango E, Hadjiliadis D, et al. Cystic fibrosis foundation consensus guidelines for the care of individuals with advanced cystic fibrosis lung disease. J Cyst Fibros 2020;19(3): 344–54.

60. Kapnadak SG, Ramos KJ, Dellon EP. Enhancing care for individuals with advanced cystic fibrosis lung disease. Pediatr Pulmonol 2021;56(Suppl 1): S69–78.

61. Kerem E, Reisman J, Corey M, et al. Prediction of mortality in patients with cystic fibrosis. New Engl J Med 1992;326(18):1187–91.

62. Milla CE, Warwick WJ. Risk of death in cystic fibrosis patients with severely compromised lung function. Chest 1998;113(5):1230–4.

63. Ramos KJ, Quon BS, Heltshe SL, et al. Heterogeneity in survival in adult patients with cystic fibrosis with FEV(1) < 30% of predicted in the United States. Chest 2017;151(6):1320–8.

64. Hayes D Jr, Kirkby S, Whitson BA, et al. Mortality risk and pulmonary function in adults with cystic fibrosis at time of wait listing for lung transplantation. Ann Thorac Surg 2015;100(2):474–9.

65. Lehr CJ, Skeans M, Dasenbrook E, et al. Effect of including important clinical variables on accuracy of the lung allocation score for cystic fibrosis and chronic obstructive pulmonary disease. Am J Respir Crit Care Med 2019;200(8):1013–21.

66. Belkin RA, Henig NR, Singer LG, et al. Risk factors for death of patients with cystic fibrosis awaiting lung transplantation. Am J Respir Crit Care Med 2006;173(6):659–66.

67. de Boer K, Vandemheen KL, Tullis E, et al. Exacerbation frequency and clinical outcomes in adult patients with cystic fibrosis. Thorax 2011;66(8): 680–5.

68. Hayes D Jr, Tobias JD, Mansour HM, et al. Pulmonary hypertension in cystic fibrosis with advanced lung disease. Am J Respir Crit Care Med 2014; 190(8):898–905.

69. Hayes D Jr, Tumin D, Daniels CJ, et al. Pulmonary artery pressure and benefit of lung transplantation in adult cystic fibrosis patients. Ann Thorac Surg 2016;101(3):1104–9.

70. Martin C, Chapron J, Hubert D, et al. Prognostic value of six minute walk test in cystic fibrosis adults. Respir Med 2013;107(12):1881–7.

71. Flight WG, Barry PJ, Bright-Thomas RJ, et al. Outcomes following bronchial artery embolisation for haemoptysis in cystic fibrosis. Cardiovasc Intervent Radiol 2017;40(8):1164–8.

72. Ramos KJ, Hee Wai T, Stephenson AL, et al. Development and internal validation of a prognostic model of 2-year death or lung transplant for cystic fibrosis. Chest 2022;S0012-3692(22):01049–52.

73. Chalmers JD, Goeminne P, Aliberti S, et al. The bronchiectasis severity index. An international derivation and validation study. Am J Respir Crit Care Med 2014;189(5):576–85.

74. Galiè N, Humbert M, Vachiery JL, et al. 2015 ESC/ERS guidelines for the diagnosis and treatment of pulmonary hypertension: the joint task force for the diagnosis and treatment of pulmonary hypertension of the european society of cardiology (ESC) and the European respiratory society (ERS): endorsed by: association for European paediatric and congenital Cardiology (AEPC), international society for heart and lung transplantation (ISHLT). Eur Heart J 2016;37(1):67–119.

75. Hoeper MM, Kramer T, Pan Z, et al. Mortality in pulmonary arterial hypertension: prediction by the 2015 European pulmonary hypertension guidelines risk stratification model. Eur Respir J 2017;50(2): 1700740.

76. Benza RL, Gomberg-Maitland M, Elliott CG, et al. Predicting survival in patients with pulmonary arterial hypertension: the reveal risk score calculator 2.0 and comparison with ESC/ERS-Based Risk ASSESSMENT STrategies. Chest 2019;156(2): 323–37.

77. Chakinala MM, Coyne DW, Benza RL, et al. Impact of declining renal function on outcomes in pulmonary arterial hypertension: a REVEAL registry analysis. J Heart Lung Transpl 2018;37(6):696–705.

78. van de Veerdonk MC, Kind T, Marcus JT, et al. Progressive right ventricular dysfunction in patients with pulmonary arterial hypertension responding to therapy. J Am Coll Cardiol 2011; 58(24):2511–9.

79. Badagliacca R, Papa S, Poscia R, et al. The added value of cardiopulmonary exercise testing in the follow-up of pulmonary arterial hypertension. J Heart Lung Transpl 2019;38(3):306–14.

80. Galiè N, Channick RN, Frantz RP, et al. Risk stratification and medical therapy of pulmonary arterial hypertension. Eur Respir J 2019;53(1):1801889.

81. Montani D, O'Callaghan DS, Savale L, et al. Pulmonary veno-occlusive disease: recent progress and current challenges. Respir Med 2010;104(Suppl 1):S23–32.

82. Young A, Vummidi D, Visovatti S, et al. Prevalence, treatment, and outcomes of coexistent pulmonary hypertension and interstitial lung disease in systemic sclerosis. Arthritis Rheumatol 2019;71(8): 1339–49.

83. Chen H, Shiboski SC, Golden JA, et al. Impact of the lung allocation score on lung transplantation for pulmonary arterial hypertension. Am J Respir Crit Care Med 2009;180(5):468–74.

84. Gomberg-Maitland M, Glassner-Kolmin C, Watson S, et al. Survival in pulmonary arterial hypertension patients awaiting lung transplantation. J Heart Lung Transpl 2013;32(12):1179–86.

85. Savale L, Le Pavec J, Mercier O, et al. Impact of high-priority allocation on lung and heart-lung transplantation for pulmonary hypertension. Ann Thorac Surg 2017;104(2):404–11.

86. Lyu DM, Goff RR, Chan KM. The lung allocation score and its relevance. Semin Respir Crit Care Med 2021;42(3):346–56.

87. Demerouti E, Karyofyllis P, Manginas A, et al. Improving survival in patients with pulmonary arterial hypertension: focus on intravenous epoprostenol. Am J Cardiovasc Drugs 2019;19(2):99–105.

88. Garcia MVF, Souza R, Costa ELV, et al. Outcomes and prognostic factors of decompensated pulmonary hypertension in the intensive care unit. Respir Med 2021;190:106685.

89. Savale L, Vuillard C, Pichon J, et al. Five-year survival after an acute episode of decompensated pulmonary arterial hypertension in the modern management era of right heart failure. Eur Respir J 2021;58(3):2100466.

90. Hoeper MM, Benza RL, Corris P, et al. Intensive care, right ventricular support and lung transplantation in patients with pulmonary hypertension. Eur Respir J 2019;53(1):1801906.

91. McCarthy C, Gupta N, Johnson SR, et al. Lymphangioleiomyomatosis: pathogenesis, clinical features, diagnosis, and management. Lancet Respir Med 2021;9(11):1313–27.

92. McCormack FX, Inoue Y, Moss J, et al. Efficacy and safety of sirolimus in lymphangioleiomyomatosis. N Engl J Med 2011;364(17):1595–606.

93. Yao J, Taveira-DaSilva AM, Jones AM, et al. Sustained effects of sirolimus on lung function and

cystic lung lesions in lymphangioleiomyomatosis. Am J Respir Crit Care Med 2014;190(11):1273–82.

94. Gupta N, Lee HS, Ryu JH, et al. The NHLBI LAM registry: prognostic physiologic and radiologic biomarkers emerge from a 15-year prospective longitudinal analysis. Chest 2019;155(2):288–96.

95. Oprescu N, McCormack FX, Byrnes S, et al. Clinical predictors of mortality and cause of death in lymphangioleiomyomatosis: a population-based registry. Lung 2013;191(1):35–42.

96. Kirkil G, Lower EE, Baughman RP. Predictors of mortality in pulmonary sarcoidosis. Chest 2018; 153(1):105–13.

97. Meyer KC. Lung transplantation for pulmonary sarcoidosis. Sarcoidosis Vasc Diffuse Lung Dis 2019;36(2):92–107.

98. Le Pavec J, Valeyre D, Gazengel P, et al. Lung transplantation for sarcoidosis: outcome and prognostic factors. Eur Respir J 2021;58(2):2003358.

99. Akagi T, Matsumoto T, Harada T, et al. Coexistent emphysema delays the decrease of vital capacity in idiopathic pulmonary fibrosis. Respir Med 2009;103(8):1209–15.

100. Yoon HY, Kim TH, Seo JB, et al. Effects of emphysema on physiological and prognostic characteristics of lung function in idiopathic pulmonary fibrosis. Respirology 2019;24(1):55–62.

101. Ranieri VM, Rubenfeld GD, Thompson BT, et al. Acute respiratory distress syndrome: the Berlin Definition. JAMA 2012;307(23):2526–33.

102. Chang Y, Lee SO, Shim TS, et al. Lung transplantation as a therapeutic option in acute respiratory distress syndrome. Transplantation 2018;102(5): 829–37.

103. Kon ZN, Dahi S, Evans CF, et al. Long-term venovenous extracorporeal membrane oxygenation support for acute respiratory distress syndrome. Ann Thorac Surg 2015;100(6):2059–63.

104. Combes A, Hajage D, Capellier G, et al. Extracorporeal membrane oxygenation for severe acute respiratory distress syndrome. N Engl J Med 2018;378(21):1965–75.

105. Novick RJ, Stitt LW, Al-Kattan K, et al. Pulmonary retransplantation: predictors of graft function and survival in 230 patients. Pulmonary Retransplant Registry. Ann Thorac Surg 1998;65(1):227–34.

106. Kawut SM, Lederer DJ, Keshavjee S, et al. Outcomes after lung retransplantation in the modern era. Am J Respir Crit Care Med 2008;177(1): 114–20.

107. Verleden SE, Todd JL, Sato M, et al. Impact of CLAD phenotype on survival after lung retransplantation: a multicenter study. Am J Transpl 2015; 15(8):2223–30.

108. Hall DJ, Belli EV, Gregg JA, et al. Two decades of lung retransplantation: a single-center experience. Ann Thorac Surg 2017;103(4):1076–83.

109. Wallinder A, Danielsson C, Magnusson J, et al. Outcomes and long-term survival after pulmonary retransplantation: a single-center experience. Ann Thorac Surg 2019;108(4):1037–44.

110. Young JS, Coppolino A. Esophageal disease in lung transplant patients. Ann Transl Med 2021; 9(10):900.

111. Davis RD Jr, Lau CL, Eubanks S, et al. Improved lung allograft function after fundoplication in patients with gastroesophageal reflux disease undergoing lung transplantation. J Thorac Cardiovasc Surg 2003;125(3):533–42.

112. Hartwig MG, Anderson DJ, Onaitis MW, et al. Fundoplication after lung transplantation prevents the allograft dysfunction associated with reflux. Ann Thorac Surg 2011;92(2):462–8. discussion; 468-469.

113. Hoppo T, Jarido V, Pennathur A, et al. Antireflux surgery preserves lung function in patients with gastroesophageal reflux disease and end-stage lung disease before and after lung transplantation. Arch Surg 2011;146(9):1041–7.

114. ASTS/AST/ISHLT. Joint statement about COVID-19 vaccination in organ transplant candidates and recipients. Available at: https://ishltorg/ishlt/media/documents/ISHLT-AST-ASTS_Joint-Statement_COVID19-Vaccination_13Marchpdf.

115. Rosenberger EM, Dew MA, DiMartini AF, et al. Psychosocial issues facing lung transplant candidates, recipients and family caregivers. Thorac Surg Clin 2012;22(4):517–29.

116. Smith PJ, Blumenthal JA, Snyder LD, et al. Depressive symptoms and early mortality following lung transplantation: a pilot study. Clin Transpl 2017; 31(2):e12874.

117. Smith PJ, Blumenthal JA, Trulock EP, et al. Psychosocial predictors of mortality following lung transplantation. Am J Transpl 2016;16(1):271–7.

118. Smith PJ, Snyder LD, Palmer SM, et al. Depression, social support, and clinical outcomes following lung transplantation: a single-center cohort study. Transpl Int 2018;31(5):495–502.

119. Dobbels F, Verleden G, Dupont L, et al. To transplant or not? The importance of psychosocial and behavioural factors before lung transplantation. Chron Respir Dis 2006;3(1):39–47.

120. Pradère P, Tudorache I, Magnusson J, et al. Lung transplantation for scleroderma lung disease: an international, multicenter, observational cohort study. J Heart Lung Transpl 2018;37(7):903–11.

121. Chan EY, Goodarzi A, Sinha N, et al. Long-term survival in bilateral lung transplantation for scleroderma-related lung disease. Ann Thorac Surg 2018;105(3):893–900.

122. Jennerich AL, Pryor JB, Wai TYH, et al. Low body mass index as a barrier to lung transplant in cystic fibrosis. J Cyst Fibros 2022;21(3):475–81.

123. Ramos KJ, Kapnadak SG, Bradford MC, et al. Underweight patients with cystic fibrosis have acceptable survival following lung transplantation: a united Network for organ sharing registry study. Chest 2020;157(4):898–906.

124. Hayanga AJ, Aboagye JK, Hayanga HE, et al. Contemporary analysis of early outcomes after lung transplantation in the elderly using a national registry. J Heart Lung Transpl 2015;34(2):182–8.

125. Perez AA, Singer JP, Schwartz BS, et al. Management and clinical outcomes after lung transplantation in patients with pre-transplant Mycobacterium abscessus infection: a single center experience. Transpl Infect Dis 2019;21(3):e13084.

126. Raats D, Lorent N, Saegeman V, et al. Successful lung transplantation for chronic Mycobacterium abscessus infection in advanced cystic fibrosis, a case series. Transpl Infect Dis 2019;21(2):e13046.

127. Al-Adra DP, Hammel L, Roberts J, et al. Pretransplant solid organ malignancy and organ transplant candidacy: a consensus expert opinion statement. Am J Transpl 2021;21(2):460–74.

128. Al-Adra DP, Hammel L, Roberts J, et al. Preexisting melanoma and hematological malignancies, prognosis, and timing to solid organ transplantation: a consensus expert opinion statement. Am J Transpl 2021;21(2):475–83.

129. Lanken PN, Terry PB, Delisser HM, et al. An official American Thoracic Society clinical policy statement: palliative care for patients with respiratory diseases and critical illnesses. Am J Respir Crit Care Med 2008;177(8):912–27.

130. Ruggiero R, Reinke LF. Palliative care in advanced lung diseases: a void that needs filling. Ann Am Thorac Soc 2018;15(11):1265–8.

131. Halpin DMG. Palliative care for people with COPD: effective but underused. Eur Respir J 2018;51(2): 1702645.

132. Hayanga AJ, Aboagye J, Esper S, et al. Extracorporeal membrane oxygenation as a bridge to lung transplantation in the United States: an evolving strategy in the management of rapidly advancing pulmonary disease. J Thorac Cardiovasc Surg 2015;149(1):291–6.

133. Benazzo A, Schwarz S, Frommlet F, et al. Twenty-year experience with extracorporeal life support as bridge to lung transplantation. J Thorac Cardiovasc Surg 2019;157(6):2515–25. e2510.

134. Hoetzenecker K, Donahoe L, Yeung JC, et al. Extracorporeal life support as a bridge to lung transplantation-experience of a high-volume transplant center. J Thorac Cardiovasc Surg 2018; 155(3):1316–28.e1311.

135. Fuehner T, Kuehn C, Hadem J, et al. Extracorporeal membrane oxygenation in awake patients as bridge to lung transplantation. Am J Respir Crit Care Med 2012;185(7):763–8.

136. Lafarge M, Mordant P, Thabut G, et al. Experience of extracorporeal membrane oxygenation as a bridge to lung transplantation in France. J Heart Lung Transpl 2013;32(9):905–13.

137. Biscotti M, Gannon WD, Agerstrand C, et al. Awake extracorporeal membrane oxygenation as bridge to lung transplantation: a 9-year experience. Ann Thorac Surg 2017;104(2):412–9.

138. Hayanga JW, Lira A, Aboagye JK, et al. Extracorporeal membrane oxygenation as a bridge to lung transplantation: what lessons might we learn from volume and expertise? Interact Cardiovasc Thorac Surg 2016;22(4):406–10.

139. Mattar A, Chatterjee S, Loor G. Bridging to lung transplantation. Crit Care Clin 2019;35(1):11–25.

140. Aversa M. Approaches to the management of sensitized lung transplant candidates: findings from an international survey. J Heart Lung Transpl 2020;39(4):S315.

141. Abrams D, Javidfar J, Farrand E, et al. Early mobilization of patients receiving extracorporeal membrane oxygenation: a retrospective cohort study. Crit Care 2014;18(1):R38.

142. Georges G, Kalavrouziotis D, Mohammadi S. Commentary: walking wounded: role of ambulatory femoral venovenous extracorporeal membrane oxygenation. JTCVS Tech 2021;9:204–5.

143. Pasrija C, Mackowick KM, Raithel M, et al. Ambulation with femoral arterial cannulation can Be safely performed on venoarterial extracorporeal membrane oxygenation. Ann Thorac Surg 2019;107(5): 1389–94.

144. Tang A, Thuita L, Siddiqui HU, et al. Urgently listed lung transplant patients have outcomes similar to those of electively listed patients. J Thorac Cardiovasc Surg 2020;S0022-5223(20):30997–1001.

145. Gan CT, Hoek RAS, van der Bij W, et al. Long-term outcome and bridging success of patients evaluated and bridged to lung transplantation on the ICU. J Heart Lung Transpl 2022;41(5):589–98.

146. Bharat A, Querrey M, Markov NS, et al. Lung transplantation for patients with severe COVID-19. Sci Transl Med 2020;12(574):eabe4282.

147. Bush EL, Krishnan A, Chidi AP, et al. The effect of the cystic fibrosis care center on outcomes after lung transplantation for cystic fibrosis. J Heart Lung Transpl 2022;41(3):300–7.

Listing Dilemmas
Age, Frailty, Weight, Preexisting Cancers, and Systemic Diseases

Darya Rudym, MD[a],*, Jake G. Natalini, MD, MSCE[a], Anil J. Trindade, MD[b]

KEYWORDS

- Lung transplantation • Advanced age • Frailty • Body mass index • Preexisting cancers
- Systemic autoimmune rheumatic disease

KEY POINTS

- Older patients may be safely considered for lung transplantation.
- Frailty in lung transplant candidates is a complex entity that requires better assessment tools and may be predictive of outcomes posttransplant.
- Low and high body mass index is associated with worse outcomes in lung transplant recipients.
- Patients with a history of preexisting malignancies may be carefully considered for lung transplantation on individual bases.
- Evaluation of patients with the systemic autoimmune rheumatic disease requires a multi-specialty approach pre- and post-lung transplantation.

INTRODUCTION

Selection of lung transplant candidates is an evolving field that pushes the boundaries of what is considered the norm. Candidate characteristics once thought to be prohibitive are continually questioned, making listing decisions more challenging as programs consider more marginal candidates. Little evidence exists to support decisions in more complex scenarios, leaving many to debate these dilemmas in the listing. Given the continually changing demographics of the typical lung transplant recipient as well as the growing list of risk factors that predispose patients to poor posttransplant outcomes, we explore the dilemmas in lung transplant candidate selections pertaining to older age, frailty, low and high body mass index, preexisting cancers, and systemic diseases.

Older Age

Elderly patients continue to represent a significant percentage of lung transplant candidates. In fact, in the past 20 years, the proportion of candidates greater or equal to 60 years who underwent lung transplantation doubled from 20% to 40%.[1]

Several factors have led to an increased age of wait-listed candidates. First, the general population is aging. In 2019, the United States population greater or equal to 65 years was 54 million (16%). Yet by 2040, the estimated population greater or equal to 65 years is expected to be 85 million (21.6%). Next, life expectancy is increasing. Although in 2000, the expected survival for a 62-year-old in the United States was 19 years for men and 22 years for women, by 2040, it is projected to be 22 and 24 years, respectively.[2] Further, the leading indications for lung transplantation are interstitial lung disease (ILD) and chronic obstructive lung disease (COPD), which naturally select for an older demographic. As the population continues to age, and with the advent of newer medical therapies for cystic fibrosis (CF) and pulmonary vascular disease, a further separation in the age gap among lung transplant candidates will likely occur.[3]

a Division of Pulmonary and Critical Care Medicine, New York University, Langone Health, 530 First Avenue, HCC-4A, New York, NY 10016, USA; b Division of Allergy, Pulmonary, and Critical Care Medicine, Vanderbilt University Medical Center, Oxford House, Room 539, 1313 21st Avenue South, Nashville, TN 37232, USA
* Corresponding author.
E-mail address: Darya.Rudym@nyulangone.org

Clin Chest Med 44 (2023) 35–46
https://doi.org/10.1016/j.ccm.2022.10.002
0272-5231/23/© 2022 Elsevier Inc. All rights reserved.

chestmed.theclinics.com

Concerns regarding poor recipient outcomes have historically curtailed candidate age.[4,5] Moreover, other non-pulmonary age-associated comorbidities have limited survival, including cardiovascular disease, chronic kidney disease (CKD), and malignancy. For example, increased recipient age is one of the major risk factors for developing CKD within the first-year post-lung transplantation.[6] CKD, in turn, increases the risk of mortality fourfold.[7] Advanced recipient age is also associated with increased cardiovascular complications including arrhythmias, which significantly reduce posttransplant survival.[8] In addition, older age is associated with increased likelihood of developing certain types of malignancies, including skin and lung cancers.[9]

Nevertheless, recent studies suggest that lung transplantation in candidates of advanced age is associated with acceptable outcomes. In an analysis of the United Network for Organ Sharing (UNOS) Registry between 2005 and 2012 examining 11,776 patients, 1-year survival was similar across all age strata for recipients of single lung transplants, though for bilateral transplants, 1-year survival was markedly lower for patients ≥75 years (84% vs 51%). Similarly, 3- to 5-year survival was significantly decreased for patients ≥75 years (26%). Not surprisingly, the etiology of mortality shifted by age group with increased frequencies of cardiovascular and oncologic disease in older patients.[10] More recently, a retrospective analysis of 14,253 patients in the UNOS Registry between 2006 and 2015, found age to be the most significant risk factor for mortality posttransplant, with the impact becoming more prominent as time from transplant increased.[11] Finally, a very recent study evaluating risk factors among 5815 recipients age ≥65 years in the UNOS Registry between 2005 and 2018 found a median survival for this older cohort of 4.41 years, which worsened with increasing age strata (**Fig. 1**). The most significant risk factors for mortality on multivariate regression analysis were older age strata, single lung transplant, cytomegalovirus mismatch, pretransplant hospitalization, and pretransplant steroid use.[12]

Most studies regarding age and transplantation are retrospective in nature and, therefore, are subject to implicit biases present at the time of transplant. For example, it remains debatable whether older patients are better suited for single versus bilateral transplant.[13] Retrospective studies regarding age are ostensibly biased as healthier patients with a longer expected posttransplant survival are more likely to be listed for bilateral transplant.[14] There is a need for well-designed retrospective studies, or better-yet, multicenter prospective studies, that account for these biases. Notably, many of the larger transplant centers prefer bilateral lung transplantation for most of their recipients and do not consider age, by itself, as a criteria for the type of transplant procedure. Ultimately, chronologic age is a surrogate for physiologic function and reserve.[15] Ideally, the transplant community would have better markers for identifying how well a person can withstand major surgery, resultant deconditioning, side effects of immunosuppression, and other insults to the body. Age alone insufficiently conveys that vital information. Whether frailty, markers of immune function, cellular age (telomere length), or senescence, are adequate indicators of vitality, either alone or in conjunction, remains worthy of discussion.[16] Similarly, studies comparing the impact of age on functional outcomes and quality of life measures posttransplant may be just as important as survival statistics.[17,18]

Undoubtedly, the push to extend current age limitations and make lung transplantation available to as many as possible will provoke debate regarding the ethical implications of the use of scarce resources. In particular, there may be debate regarding the crossroads of the ethical principle of utility (is there an aggregate good or overall benefit to society by transplanting recipients of advanced age?) versus justice (is there equitable access of a limited resource to candidates of all ages?).19,20

In summary, extending the age criterion for recipient acceptability to at least age 74 years, if not beyond, is supported by the literature. There should be a movement toward using more objective markers of vitality and physical reserve, as opposed to chronologic age that may not provide an accurate representation of physiologic function. Finally, the ability to transplant older patients with advanced lung disease should not be at the detriment of access to lung transplantation for younger patients.

Frailty

The topic of frailty and its role in listing dilemmas has gained momentum in recent years. Defined as a state of low physiologic reserve and generalized vulnerability to stressors, frailty remains a challenging construct, historically leaving clinicians to apply "an eyeball test" in lieu of an objective assessment.

Frailty is very common in lung transplant patients, estimated to affect anywhere between a fifth to nearly a half of candidates, depending on which means are used to define frailty.[21–23] No single defining measure has been agreed upon due to

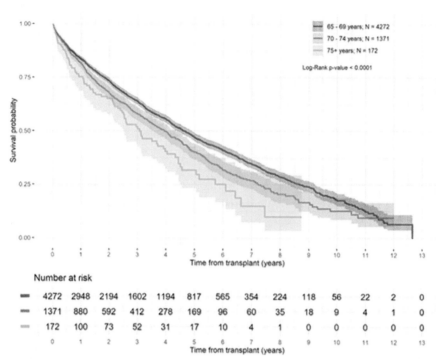

Fig. 1. Kaplan–Meier plot displaying time to allograft failure by age strata in patients ≥65 years. Shaded areas represent the 95%CI bands. (*From* Mosher CL, Weber JM, Frankel CW, Neely ML, Palmer SM. Risk factors for mortality in lung transplant recipients aged ≥65 years: A retrospective cohort study of 5815 patients in the scientific registry of transplant recipients. *J Heart Lung Transplant.* 2021;40(1):42 to 55.)

multiple mechanisms innate to frailty pathogenesis. These mechanisms include genetic and environmental triggers that in conjunction with nutritional deficiencies and physical deconditioning, may lead to poor outcomes in the setting of an additional stressor.[24,25] Given such multifaceted nature and inherent overlap in pathogenesis, frailty associated with chronic respiratory failure and age-related frailty share similarities (**Fig. 2**).[24,26,27] Thus, most frailty assessment tools, including the Short Physical Performance Battery (SPPB), the Fried Frailty Phenotype (FFP), and the Frailty Index, originate from geriatric literature studying community-dwelling older adults.[28,29] Assessment tools specific to advanced lung diseases, such as Duke Activity Status Index (DASI) and Lung Transplant Valued Life Activities (LT-VLA), are far and few.[30,31] SPPB and FFP are most widely used and studied in lung transplantation yet their validity in this population is not well established.[32]

Other quantifiable markers have been studied to characterize and define frailty, yet distinguishing between age-associated and lung disease-related physiologic changes remains difficult. These measurable surrogates include markers of chronic inflammation such as interleukin-6 (IL-6),

C-reactive protein (CRP), and tumor necrosis factor receptor 1 (TNFR1), cachexia (low leptin levels), sarcopenia (low muscle mass and function, often measured as loss of appendicular skeletal muscle mass), hypoalbuminemia, and reduced 6-min walk distance (6MWD).[33–38] Mechanisms by which these markers are implicated in pathogenesis of frailty are still speculative and further research is needed to adjudicate their predictive value, jointly or individually.

Frailty carries several prognostic implications. Preoperatively, frailty is associated with decreased exercise capacity, and postoperatively, has been suggested to lead to longer length of stay, higher risk of re-hospitalization, and a greater risk of being discharged to a skilled nursing facility.[33,39,40] More importantly, frailty is associated with an increased risk of delisting and has been shown to increase mortality in lung transplant patients on the waitlist as well as those who have been transplanted.[21,22,29,41,42] Specifically, a single center study of 102 lung transplant recipients found frail patients (identified using the frailty index) to be at an increased risk of death with an adjusted hazard ratio (HR) of 2.24 (95% confidence interval [CI], 1.22–4.19; $P = .0089$).[22] More recently, a multicenter analysis of 386 patients

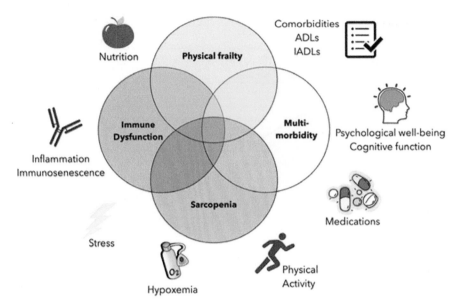

Fig. 2. Conceptual framework of frailty and aging-associated dysfunction in lung transplant candidates. Venn diagram demonstrating the age-related constructs that may overlap with frailty, including multi-morbidity, sarcopenia, and immune system dysfunction, along with health-related issues that may contribute to these manifestations of aging. (*From* Schaenman JM, Diamond JM, Greenland JR, et al. Frailty and aging-associated syndromes in lung transplant candidates and recipients. Am J Transplant. 2021;21(6):2018 to 2024.)

examining frailty, as measured by SPPB, in association with mortality after transplant, found frail patients to have an absolute increased risk of death within the first year of 12.2% (95% CI, 3.1%–21%), compared with non-frail patients. Furthermore, per 1 unit increase in SPPB, there was a 20% increased risk of longer-term death after lung transplantation.[21]

Recent studies suggest pretransplant frailty could improve after transplantation, albeit quantification of such improvement is dependent on the assessment modality chosen for the study.[32,43] Notably, intensive rehabilitation, both pretransplant (so-called prehabilitation) and posttransplant, has been shown to improve patient outcomes and is widely recommended.[44–46] Approaches to prehabilitation may be multifaceted, targeting exercise, nutritional, as well as psychological factors, and may include novel methodologies such as home-based interventions.[47]

Importantly, many recognize the need for standardized frailty evaluation and assessment. In a recent report on frailty, surveying 257 physicians, surgeons, and allied health professionals, an overwhelming majority (93%) agreed that frailty is a critical part of pretransplant evaluation and should be incorporated into the decision-making with regard to candidate selection.[48] Yet no unified approach to the measurement of frailty has been recommended by the International Society of Heart and Lung Transplantation (ISHLT)

guidelines. Further, although many constructs are being actively studied, none are yet validated and thus cannot be generally applied. Future research should focus on improving validity and predictive value of frailty assessments, and further characterizing the interplay between frailty, cognitive function, nutrition, exercise, and chronic inflammation while identifying modifiable risk factors. Until then, frail patients should be approached very cautiously given the association of frailty with decreased survival as well as short- and long-term complications.

Body Mass Index

The effects of body mass index (BMI) on outcomes in lung transplantation have repeatedly shown that patients with BMI in the normal range do best, whereas underweight and obese patients have varying outcomes.

Lung transplant candidates who are underweight pretransplant, defined as BMI $\leq$ 18 kg/m^2, have a higher risk of posttransplant mortality.[49,50] In a meta-analysis of seven observational cohort studies, underweight status was associated with mortality compared with normal BMI with a relative risk (RR) of 1.36 (95% CI 1.11–1.66, I^2 = 0%).[51] Interestingly, one large study examining evolution of BMI reported no difference in posttransplant outcomes in listed underweight candidates who gained weight pretransplant compared with those who stayed underweight.[52] Patients with CF with BMI < 17 kg/m^2 notably have similar posttransplant mortality compared with patients with COPD, idiopathic pulmonary fibrosis (IPF) as well as normal-weight CF recipients.[53] As such, current ISHLT guidelines recognize BMI < 16 kg/m^2 as "high or substantially increased risk" recipient characteristic but do not consider underweight status a contraindication to lung transplant.[54]

Although trajectories of underweight patients have been more consistent in recent years, the decisions regarding listing obese patients have become more complex, partly owing to changing recipient population. With the prevalence of obesity nearly tripling worldwide in the past half century, lung transplant candidate characteristics reflect these trends in the obesity epidemic.[55,56] In fact, the most recent ISHLT registry report describes a gradual increase in recipient BMI over the last three decades with median BMI steadily rising from 25 kg/m^2 in the 1990s to 26.5 kg/m^2 in the most recent years ($P < .0001$).[57]

The approach to examining obesity in the literature has also evolved. One of the earlier studies on the subject, showed obesity, defined as BMI $\geq$ 30 kg/m^2, to be an independent risk factor for death in the first year posttransplant.[50] Specifically, the adjusted odds of death in obese patients were 40% greater (95% CI, 11%–75%, $P = .0004$) in the first year posttransplant and 29% greater after 5 years among survivors, relative to normal weight recipients. Studies that followed further stratified obesity groups, examining Class I obesity (BMI 30–34.9 kg/m^2) separately from Class II (BMI 35–39.9 kg/m^2) and Class III (BMI $\geq$ 40 kg/m^2) obesity. Whereas recipients with Class I obesity did not have an increase in 1-year mortality, Class II and III obesity was associated with a nearly twofold increase in mortality with an HR of 1.9 (95% CI, 1.3–2.8) (Fig. 3). Further, examining BMI per unit increase showed predicted probability of death to be lowest at BMI of 26 kg/m^2 with a quantifiable increase in mortality per unit change of BMI, in either direction.[58] Studies suggest that some of the mortality risk can be ameliorated with pretransplant efforts focusing on weight loss and intensive pulmonary rehabilitation.[59,60] Thus, recommendations for consideration of obese patients have continued to evolve, with the ISHTL updating the consensus document for the selection of lung transplant candidates from considering BMI $\geq$ 35 kg/m^2 an absolute contraindication to now being considered a relative contraindication.[54,61]

Differences in outcomes between classes of obesity question the underlying mechanisms to explain the discrepancy and further underscore that BMI is not a well-suited surrogate for body mass composition. The shortcomings of BMI as a measure of adipose tissue have long been recognized.[49,62–64] Other markers of obesity and novel methods to characterize adipose tissue are continually studied to optimize risk stratification in lung transplant candidates. For example, a study examining the levels of leptin (a satiety hormone generated by adipose tissue and postulated to be a better correlate of total body adipose tissue mass than BMI) in lung transplant recipients and found higher levels to be associated with increased mortality.[49,65] Another study showed greater abdominal subcutaneous adipose tissue area, as measured on abdominal computed tomography (CT) scans and indexed to height, to be associated with an increased risk of primary graft dysfunction after lung transplantation.[66] Such studies and others ongoing are encouraging that 1 day, there may be better ways to understand, characterize, and risk stratify patients according to their body composition.

In summary, both ends of the spectrum, high as well as low BMIs, have been associated with increased mortality but an increasing amount of caveats exist suggesting that BMI cut-offs might evolve to be less rigid and may be considered in conjunction with other measures such as molecular analysis and radiographic evidence when selecting the appropriate candidates for lung transplantation.

Preexisting Cancers

One of the most evolved fields in candidate selection and listing has been in the consideration of patients with a history of malignancy. Both preexisting and treated, as well active and low-grade, malignancies are being considered on more frequent basis.[67–70] The most recent ISHLT report describes a historical increase in incidence of malignancy in potential candidates, quoting a history of malignancy in about 2.7% of candidates in the 1990s, compared with 7.9% of candidates in the 2010s ($P < .0001$).[57] Further, a more recent analysis of the UNOS registry of 18,032 patients noted an increase in recipients who carry a diagnosis of pretransplant malignancy from 5.7% in mid-2000s to 8.1% in mid-2010s.[71]

Most of the evidence supporting the guidelines for transplanting patients with preexisting cancers stems from experience in other solid organ transplants.[72,73] Original lung transplant-specific recommendations universally advised waiting a minimum of 5 years before transplantation in any patient with a history of malignancy.[74] Since

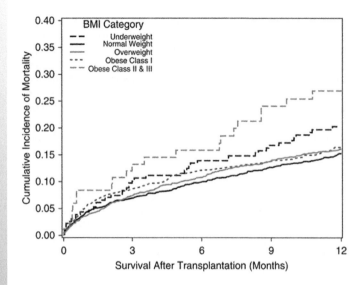

Fig. 3. Kaplan–Meier curve demonstrating survival separated by body mass index (BMI, in kg/m²). Underweight is BMI < 18.5 kg/m², normal weight is BMI 18.5 to 24.9 kg/m², overweight is BMI 25 to 29.9 kg/m² and obese is BMI > 30 kg/m². (*From* Singer JP, Peterson ER, Snyder ME, et al. Body composition and mortality after adult lung transplantation in the United States. Am J Respir Crit Care Med. 2014;190(9):1012-1021. Reprinted with permission of the American Thoracic Society. Copyright © 2022 American Thoracic Society. All rights reserved.)

then, guidelines for candidate selection have evolved from first suggesting a 2 to 5-year disease-free interval to now advising to consider distinct risks associated with pretransplant malignancies and to view malignancy with high risk of recurrent or death related to cancer as an absolute contraindication.[57,61]

Not all malignancies carry the same risk. The makeup of the preexisting cancers in lung transplant candidates is vastly heterogeneous, with prostate, breast, and non-melanoma skin cancers being most common (**Table 1**).[71,75,76] Each malignancy calls for a distinct approach in surveillance and management as each carries its own signature regarding recurrence and associated mortality. Recently, two consensus statements detail approaches to pretransplant solid organ malignancy and hematological malignancies, considering staging at the time of transplant and advances in cancer therapeutics.[77,78]

The altered immune system in chronically immunosuppressed patients has long been implicated in carcinogenesis.[79–81] Underlying mechanisms have included impaired immunosurveillance of neoplastic cells, direct carcinogenic effects of immunosuppressive medications, and subpar defense against oncogenic viruses.[82,83] The latter category namely includes Epstein-Barr virus (EBV) causing posttransplant lymphoproliferative disorder (PTLD), human herpesvirus 8 (HHV-6) causing Kaposi sarcoma, and human papillomavirus (HPV) causing nonmelanoma skin cancer and anogenital cancers.[80,81,84] It is well recognized that chronic immunosuppression is associated with an increased likelihood of de novo malignancies.[9,85,86] Yet immunosuppression has

also been implicated in the recurrence of preexisting cancers and the development of cancers transmitted via donor, albeit pathogenic mechanisms are less understood.[83,87,88]

Nevertheless, recurrence of preexisting cancers is common.[89–91] By extension, it has been postulated that patients with previous malignancy would have worse survival after lung transplantation. Interestingly, in the most recent report of ISHLT registry evaluating candidate characteristics in 35,214 patients, survival to 5-year posttransplant conditional on survival to 1 year in recipients with a history of malignancy did not differ from those without such history (P = .1106), albeit this analysis did not solely represent pretransplant cancers and included de novo malignancies and those transmitted from donor.[57] However, a large study of the UNOS Registry focusing specifically on pretransplant malignancy found that patients with preexisting cancers are more likely to die within 5 years than patients without (HR 1.16, P = .003).[71] In addition, patients with preexisting malignancy were more likely to die from posttransplant malignancy, an effect that was particularly pronounced in those with active malignancy at the time of transplant.[71] Further, a recent single-center study reported pretransplant malignancy to be significantly associated with an increased risk of developing posttransplant malignancy (HR 3.24, P < .001), notably with the majority of posttransplant cancers being unrelated to pretransplant cancers.[75]

In the recent years, it has become apparent that although some cancers have a reasonably low risk of recurrence or progression, others pose a more substantial risk once exposed to

Table 1
Malignancy type in patients with pretransplant malignancy

Pretransplant Malignancy	Recipients (*N* = 18,032)
None	16,711 (92.7%)
Any pretransplant malignancy	1,321 (7.3%)
Type	
Skin	468 (35.4%)
Genitourinary	142 (10.7%)
Breast	152 (11.5%)
Thyroid	22 (1.7%)
Tongue/throat/ laryngeal	19 (1.4%)
Lung	42 (3.2%)
Leukemia	120 (%)
Other	282 (21.3%)
Multiple	74 (5.6%)
Active malignancy at transplant	58 (0.3%)

From Rudasill SE, Iyengar A, Sanaiha Y, et al. Pretransplant malignancy among lung transplant recipients in the modern era. Surgery. 2019;165(6):1228-1233.

immunosuppression. Deciphering whether the risk of recurrence is "low enough" and would not subject the recipient to less than the median life expectancy posttransplant remains a challenge. Each listing of preexisting cancer warrants a thorough evaluation with respective consultants, either in oncology or hematology. In select patients in whom risk of recurrence is deemed to be sufficiently low and who go on to receive a transplant, aggressive surveillance and frequent specialty follow-up is imperative in minimizing cancer-related risk postoperatively.

Systemic Diseases

Careful candidate selection is critical when considering patients with systemic autoimmune rheumatic diseases such as rheumatoid arthritis (RA), systemic sclerosis (SSc), systemic lupus erythematosus, and dermato- and polymyositis. ILD and pulmonary arterial hypertension (PAH) in such patients strongly contribute to increased morbidity and mortality.[92] For patients with rapidly progressive or end-stage connective tissue disease (CTD)-associated ILD and PAH (hereafter, CTD-ILD and CTD-PAH, respectively), lung transplantation provides a potentially life-saving therapeutic intervention. However, many transplant centers may be reluctant to offer lung transplantation to patients with CTD due to underlying concerns that extrapulmonary manifestations of their disease may limit long-term survival.[93] In fact, CTD-associated lung disease only accounted for less than 1% of lung transplants performed in the United States between the years 2015 to 2018, with RA and undifferentiated CTD being the most common indications.[94] However, several studies to date have shown comparable outcomes relative to IPF and idiopathic PAH, two widely accepted indications for transplant.[95–100] Thus, carefully selected patients with CTD-ILD and CTD-PAH can safely undergo lung transplantation, although referral to a transplant center should occur early as candidacy evaluation often requires multidisciplinary expertise (eg, rheumatology and gastroenterology) and additional testing beyond a standard assessment.[54]

The ISHLT recently published guidelines on how to comprehensively evaluate patients with CTD being considered for lung transplantation.[101] As an example, RA typically manifests as a symmetric, inflammatory polyarthritis of the peripheral joints that leads to cartilaginous and bony destruction, although other synovial joints of the upper and lower extremities such as the elbows and knees are also commonly affected.[102] Thus, it is important to evaluate for symptomatic arthropathy despite optimal treatment with disease-modifying antirheumatic drugs (DMARDs) as poorly controlled articular symptoms could impede patients' ability to ambulate and participate in posttransplant rehabilitation. In addition, RA patients are at risk for cricoarytenoid joint arthritis which, in severe cases, can result in upper airway obstruction. Finally, patients should be screened for atlantoaxial joint instability, as it poses risk for subluxation and spinal cord compression.[101]

SSc is another excellent example of a CTD that requires input from multiple specialists when a transplant is being considered. Diffuse cutaneous SSc, more commonly associated with ILD than PAH, is a multisystem autoimmune disease characterized by fibrosis and vasculopathy of the skin and visceral organs.[103] Limited cutaneous SSc (also known as "CREST syndrome") is more commonly associated with PAH than ILD and manifests as cutaneous calcinosis, Raynaud's phenomenon, esophageal dysmotility, digital sclerodactyly, and telangiectasias.[103] Among patients with SSc, ILD and PAH are the most common causes of death.[104] Disease manifestations that may affect transplant candidacy include oropharyngeal dysphagia with recurrent aspiration, underlying esophageal dysfunction, gastroparesis, small bowel hypomotility with intestinal pseudo-obstruction, and active myocarditis.[101] Given the myriad of possible gastrointestinal manifestations, conversations regarding a patient's willingness to comply with a strict "nothing by mouth" protocol in which nutrition is exclusively provided via a feeding tube for several months after transplant may be warranted. In addition, poorly controlled skin manifestations may lead to refractory digital ulcers that pose risk for infection posttransplant, as well as chest wall tightness that can cause persistent physiologic restriction despite having undergone lung transplantation.[101] Lastly, microstomia may result in difficulties intubating with a double-lumen endotracheal tube, needed for selective single-lung ventilation during the transplant itself.

Both RA and SSc are mentioned to highlight the complexities of evaluating patients with CTD for lung transplantation. The recent ISHLT guidelines referenced above provide comprehensive disease-specific transplant considerations when assessing a patient's candidacy.[101] Above all else, it is important to consider early referral in this patient population, anticipating that the involvement of multiple specialists and assessment of CTD-specific disease manifestations will be warranted.

SUMMARY

The dilemmas in listing lung transplant candidates are so-called because often the answers are not clear and evidence to support decision-making is lacking. These decisions are highly individualized, challenging to make, and carry significant implications. More research and experience are needed to further our understanding of these complex scenarios and to improve patient outcomes.

CLINICS CARE POINTS

- Little evidence exists to support decision-making in lung transplant candidate selection.With regard to age, frailty, body mass index, pre-existing cancers, and systemic diseases affecting candidacy, guidelines and select studies may provide support yet decisions to list patients for lung transplantation should remain highly individualized.

DISCLOSURE

The authors have no conflicts of interest to report.

REFERENCES

1. Benden C, Edwards LB, Kucheryavaya AY, et al. The registry of the international society for heart and lung transplantation: sixteenth official pediatric lung and heart-lung transplantation report–2013; focus theme: age. J Heart Lung Transpl 2013; 32(10):989–97.
2. Medina LD, Sabo S, Vespa J. Living longer: historical and projected life expectancy in the United States, 1960 to 2060. In: Current population reports. U.S. Census Bureau; 2020. p. 1125–45.
3. Avdimiretz N, Benden C. The changing landscape of pediatric lung transplantation. Clin Transpl 2022; 36(4):e14634.
4. Chambers DC, Yusen RD, Cherikh WS, et al. The registry of the international society for heart and lung transplantation: thirty-fourth adult lung and heart-lung transplantation report-2017; focus theme: allograft ischemic time. J Heart Lung Transpl 2017;36(10):1047–59.
5. Colvin MM, Smith CA, Tullius SG, et al. Aging and the immune response to organ transplantation. J Clin Invest 2017;127(7):2523–9.
6. Canales M, Youssef P, Spong R, et al. Predictors of chronic kidney disease in long-term survivors of lung and heart-lung transplantation. Am J Transpl 2006;6(9):2157–63.
7. Ojo AO, Held PJ, Port FK, et al. Chronic renal failure after transplantation of a nonrenal organ. N Engl J Med 2003;349(10):931–40.
8. D'Angelo AM, Chan EG, Hayanga JW, et al. Atrial arrhythmias after lung transplantation: incidence and risk factors in 652 lung transplant recipients. J Thorac Cardiovasc Surg 2016;152(3):901–9.
9. Shtraichman O, Ahya VN. Malignancy after lung transplantation. Ann Transl Med 2020;8(6):416.
10. Biswas Roy S, Alarcon D, Walia R, et al. Is there an age limit to lung transplantation? Ann Thorac Surg 2015;100(2):443–51.
11. Lehr CJ, Blackstone EH, McCurry KR, et al. Extremes of age decrease survival in adults after lung transplant. Chest 2020;157(4):907–15.
12. Mosher CL, Weber JM, Frankel CW, et al. Risk factors for mortality in lung transplant recipients aged ≥65 years: a retrospective cohort study of 5,815 patients in the scientific registry of transplant recipients. J Heart Lung Transpl 2021; 40(1):42–55.
13. Meyer DM, Edwards LB, Torres F, et al. Impact of recipient age and procedure type on survival after lung transplantation for pulmonary fibrosis. Ann Thorac Surg 2005;79(3):950–7. ; discussion 957-958.
14. Puri V, Patterson GA, Meyers BF. Single versus bilateral lung transplantation: do guidelines exist? Thorac Surg Clin 2015;25(1):47–54.

15. Artz AS. Biologic vs physiologic age in the transplant candidate. Hematol Am Soc Hematol Educ Program 2016;2016(1):99–105.
16. Wigfield CH, Buie V, Onsager D. Age" in lung transplantation: factors related to outcomes and other considerations. Curr Pulmonol Rep 2016;5:152–8.
17. Genao L, Whitson HE, Zaas D, et al. Functional status after lung transplantation in older adults in the post-allocation score era. Am J Transpl 2013;13(1):157–66.
18. Singer JP, Katz PP, Soong A, et al. Effect of lung transplantation on health-related quality of life in the era of the lung allocation score: a U.S. Prospective cohort study. Am J Transpl 2017;17(5):1334–45.
19. Lawrence EC. Ethical issues in lung transplantation. Am J Med Sci 1998;315(3):142–5.
20. Network OPaT. Ethical principles in the allocation of human organs. In:2015.
21. Singer JP, Diamond JM, Anderson MR, et al. Frailty phenotypes and mortality after lung transplantation: a prospective cohort study. Am J Transpl 2018;18(8):1995–2004.
22. Wilson ME, Vakil AP, Kandel P, et al. Pretransplant frailty is associated with decreased survival after lung transplantation. J Heart Lung Transpl 2016;35(2):173–8.
23. Rozenberg D, Mathur S, Wickerson L, et al. Frailty and clinical benefits with lung transplantation. J Heart Lung Transpl 2018;37(10):1245–53.
24. Schaenman JM, Diamond JM, Greenland JR, et al. Frailty and aging-associated syndromes in lung transplant candidates and recipients. Am J Transpl 2021;21(6):2018–24.
25. Chen X, Mao G, Leng SX. Frailty syndrome: an overview. Clin Interv Aging 2014;9:433–41.
26. Koons B, Anderson MR, Smith PJ, et al. The Intersection of aging and lung transplantation: its impact on transplant evaluation, outcomes, and clinical care. Curr Transplant Rep 2022;9(3):149–59.
27. Fried LP, Tangen CM, Walston J, et al. Frailty in older adults: evidence for a phenotype. J Gerontol A Biol Sci Med Sci 2001;56(3):M146–56.
28. Dent E, Kowal P, Hoogendijk EO. Frailty measurement in research and clinical practice: a review. Eur J Intern Med 2016;31:3–10.
29. Singer JP, Diamond JM, Gries CJ, et al. Frailty phenotypes, disability, and outcomes in adult candidates for lung transplantation. Am J Respir Crit Care Med 2015;192(11):1325–34.
30. Baldwin MR, Singer JP, Huang D, et al. Refining low physical activity measurement improves frailty assessment in advanced lung disease and survivors of critical illness. Ann Am Thorac Soc 2017;14(8):1270–9.
31. Singer JP, Blanc PD, Dean YM, et al. Development and validation of a lung transplant-specific disability questionnaire. Thorax 2014;69(5):445.
32. Venado A, McCulloch C, Greenland JR, et al. Frailty trajectories in adult lung transplantation: a cohort study. J Heart Lung Transpl 2019;38(7):699–707.
33. Courtwright AM, Zaleski D, Gardo L, et al. Causes, preventability, and cost of unplanned rehospitalizations within 30 Days of discharge after lung transplantation. Transplantation 2018;102(5):838–44.
34. Halpern AL, Boshier PR, White AM, et al. A Comparison of frailty measures at listing to predict outcomes after lung transplantation. Ann Thorac Surg 2020;109(1):233–40.
35. Hsu J, Krishnan A, Lin CT, et al. Sarcopenia of the psoas muscles is associated with poor outcomes following lung transplantation. Ann Thorac Surg 2019;107(4):1082–8.
36. Maheshwari JA, Kolaitis NA, Anderson MR, et al. Construct and predictive validity of sarcopenia in lung transplant candidates. Ann Am Thorac Soc 2021;18(9):1464–74.
37. Cruz-Jentoft AJ, Baeyens JP, Bauer JM, et al. Sarcopenia: european consensus on definition and diagnosis: report of the european working group on sarcopenia in older people. Age and Ageing 2010;39(4):412–23.
38. Wilson D, Jackson T, Sapey E, et al. Frailty and sarcopenia: the potential role of an aged immune system. Ageing Res Rev 2017;36:1–10.
39. Layton AM, Armstrong HF, Baldwin MR, et al. Frailty and maximal exercise capacity in adult lung transplant candidates. Respir Med 2017;131:70–6.
40. Makary MA, Segev DL, Pronovost PJ, et al. Frailty as a predictor of surgical outcomes in older patients. J Am Coll Surg 2010;210(6):901–8.
41. Varughese RA, Theou O, Li Y, et al. Cumulative deficits frailty index predicts outcomes for solid organ transplant candidates. Transplant Direct 2021;7(3).
42. Rozenberg D, Singer LG, Herridge M, et al. Evaluation of skeletal muscle function in lung transplant candidates. Transplantation 2017;101(9):2183–91. Paper presented at.
43. Montgomery E, Macdonald PS, Newton PJ, et al. Reversibility of frailty after lung transplantation. J Transpl 2020;2020:3239495.
44. Wickerson L, Rozenberg D, Janaudis-Ferreira T, et al. Physical rehabilitation for lung transplant candidates and recipients: an evidence-informed clinical approach. World J Transpl 2016;6(3):517–31.
45. Li M, Mathur S, Chowdhury NA, et al. Pulmonary rehabilitation in lung transplant candidates. J Heart Lung Transpl 2013;32(6):626–32.

46. Langer D. Rehabilitation in patients before and after lung transplantation. Respiration 2015;89(5):353–62.

47. Singer JP, Soong A, Bruun A, et al. A mobile health technology enabled home-based intervention to treat frailty in adult lung transplant candidates: a pilot study. Clin Transplant 2018;32(6):e13274.

48. Kobashigawa J, Dadhania D, Bhorade S, et al. Report from the American Society of Transplantation on frailty in solid organ transplantation. Am J Transpl 2019;19(4):984–94.

49. Singer JP, Peterson ER, Snyder ME, et al. Body composition and mortality after adult lung transplantation in the United States. Am J Respir Crit Care Med 2014;190(9):1012–21.

50. Lederer DJ, Wilt JS, D'Ovidio F, et al. Obesity and underweight are associated with an increased risk of death after lung transplantation. Am J Respir Crit Care Med 2009;180(9):887–95.

51. Upala S, Panichsillapakit T, Wijarnpreecha K, et al. Underweight and obesity increase the risk of mortality after lung transplantation: a systematic review and meta-analysis. Transpl Int 2016;29(3):285–96.

52. Jomphe V, Mailhot G, Damphousse V, et al. The impact of waiting list BMI changes on the short-term outcomes of lung transplantation. Transplantation 2018;102(2):318–25.

53. Ramos KJ, Kapnadak SG, Bradford MC, et al. Underweight patients with cystic fibrosis have acceptable survival following lung transplantation: a united Network for organ sharing registry study. Chest 2020;157(4):898–906.

54. Leard LE, Holm AM, Valapour M, et al. Consensus document for the selection of lung transplant candidates: an update from the International Society for Heart and Lung Transplantation. J Heart Lung Transpl 2021;40(11):1349–79.

55. Centers for Disease Control and Prevention. Adult obesity facts. 2022. Available at: https://www.cdc.gov/obesity/data/adult.html. Accessed August 17, 2022.

56. World Health Organization. Obesity and overweight. 2021. Available at: https://www.who.int/en/news-room/fact-sheets/detail/obesity-and-overweight. Accessed August 17, 2022.

57. Chambers DC, Perch M, Zuckermann A, et al. The international thoracic organ transplant registry of the international society for heart and lung transplantation: thirty-eighth adult lung transplantation report - 2021; focus on recipient characteristics. J Heart Lung Transpl 2021;40(10):1060–72.

58. Fernandez R, Safaeinili N, Kurihara C, et al. Association of body mass index with lung transplantation survival in the United States following implementation of the lung allocation score. J Thorac Cardiovasc Surg 2018;155(4):1871–1879 e1873.

59. Clausen ES, Frankel C, Palmer SM, et al. Pretransplant weight loss and clinical outcomes after lung transplantation. J Heart Lung Transpl 2018;37(12):1443–7.

60. Chandrashekaran S, Keller CA, Kremers WK, et al. Weight loss prior to lung transplantation is associated with improved survival. J Heart Lung Transpl 2015;34(5):651–7.

61. Weill D, Benden C, Corris PA, et al. A consensus document for the selection of lung transplant candidates: 2014–an update from the pulmonary transplantation council of the international society for heart and lung transplantation. J Heart Lung Transpl 2015;34(1):1–15.

62. Shah NR, Braverman ER. Measuring adiposity in patients: the utility of body mass index (BMI), percent body fat, and leptin. PloS one 2012;7(4):e33308.

63. Romero-Corral A, Somers VK, Sierra-Johnson J, et al. Accuracy of body mass index in diagnosing obesity in the adult general population. Int J Obes (Lond) 2008;32(6):959–66.

64. Kuk JL, Janiszewski PM, Ross R. Body mass index and hip and thigh circumferences are negatively associated with visceral adipose tissue after control for waist circumference. Am J Clin Nutr 2007;85(6):1540–4.

65. Considine RV, Sinha MK, Heiman ML, et al. Serum immunoreactive-leptin concentrations in normal-weight and obese humans. N Engl J Med 1996;334(5):292–5.

66. Anderson MR, Udupa JK, Edwin E, et al. Adipose tissue quantification and primary graft dysfunction after lung transplantation: the Lung Transplant Body Composition study. J Heart Lung Transpl 2019;38(12):1246–56.

67. Whitson BA, Shelstad RC, Hertz MI, et al. Lung transplantation after hematopoietic stem cell transplantation. Clin Transpl 2012;26(2):254–8.

68. Van Raemdonck D, Vos R, Yserbyt J, et al. Lung cancer: a rare indication for, but frequent complication after lung transplantation. J Thorac Dis 2016;8(Suppl 11):S915–24.

69. Copur MS, Wurdeman JM, Nelson D, et al. Normalization of elevated tumor marker CA27-29 after bilateral lung transplantation in a patient with breast cancer and idiopathic pulmonary fibrosis. Oncol Res 2018;26(3):515–8.

70. Beaty CA, George TJ, Kilic A, et al. Pretransplant malignancy: an analysis of outcomes after thoracic organ transplantation. J Heart Lung Transpl 2013;32(2):202–11.

71. Rudasill SE, Iyengar A, Sanaiha Y, et al. Pretransplant malignancy among lung transplant recipients in the modern era. Surgery 2019;165(6):1228–33.

72. Kasiske BL, Cangro CB, Hariharan S, et al. The evaluation of renal transplantation candidates:

clinical practice guidelines. Am J Transpl 2001; 1(Suppl 2):3–95.

73. Penn I. Evaluation of the candidate with a previous malignancy. Liver Transpl Surg 1996;2(5 Suppl 1): 109–13.

74. Orens JB, Estenne M, Arcasoy S, et al. International guidelines for the selection of lung transplant candidates: 2006 update–a consensus report from the pulmonary scientific council of the international society for heart and lung transplantation. J Heart Lung Transpl 2006;25(7):745–55.

75. Sekowski V, Jackson K, Halloran K, et al. Pretransplant malignancy is associated with increased risk of de novo malignancy post-lung transplantation. Respir Med 2022;197:106855.

76. Parada MT, Sepulveda C, Alba A, et al. Malignancy development in lung transplant patients. Transpl Proc 2011;43(6):2316–7.

77. Al-Adra DP, Hammel L, Roberts J, et al. Pretransplant solid organ malignancy and organ transplant candidacy: a consensus expert opinion statement. Am J Transpl 2021;21(2):460–74.

78. Al-Adra DP, Hammel L, Roberts J, et al. Preexisting melanoma and hematological malignancies, prognosis, and timing to solid organ transplantation: a consensus expert opinion statement. Am J Transpl 2021;21(2):475–83.

79. Nair N, Gongora E, Mehra MR. Long-term immunosuppression and malignancy in thoracic transplantation: where is the balance? J Heart Lung Transpl 2014;33(5):461–7.

80. Campistol JM, Cuervas-Mons V, Manito N, et al. New concepts and best practices for management of pre- and posttransplantation cancer. Transpl Rev (Orlando) 2012;26(4):261–79.

81. Engels EA, Pfeiffer RM, Fraumeni JF Jr, et al. Spectrum of cancer risk among US solid organ transplant recipients. JAMA 2011;306(17):1891–901.

82. Krisl JC, Doan VP. Chemotherapy and transplantation: the role of immunosuppression in malignancy and a review of antineoplastic agents in solid organ transplant recipients. Am J Transpl 2017;17(8):1974–91.

83. Katabathina VS, Menias CO, Tammisetti VS, et al. Malignancy after solid organ transplantation: comprehensive imaging review. Radiographics 2016;36(5):1390–407.

84. Dantal J, Soulillou JP. Immunosuppressive drugs and the risk of cancer after organ transplantation. N Engl J Med 2005;352(13):1371–3.

85. Noone AM, Pfeiffer RM, Dorgan JF, et al. Cancer-attributable mortality among solid organ transplant recipients in the United States: 1987 through 2014. Cancer 2019;125(15):2647–55.

86. Billups K, Neal J, Salyer J. Immunosuppressant-driven de novo malignant neoplasms after solid-organ transplant. Prog Transpl 2015;25(2):182–8.

87. Rudasill SE, Iyengar A, Sanaiha Y, et al. Donor history of malignancy: a limited risk for heart transplant recipients. Clin Transpl 2020;34(2):e13762.

88. Bennett D, Fossi A, Refini RM, et al. Posttransplant solid organ malignancies in lung transplant recipients: a single-center experience and review of the literature. Tumori 2016;102(6):574–81.

89. Acuna SA, Huang JW, Dossa F, et al. Cancer recurrence after solid organ transplantation: a systematic review and meta-analysis. Transpl Rev (Orlando) 2017;31(4):240–8.

90. Acuna SA, Sutradhar R, Kim SJ, et al. Solid organ transplantation in patients with preexisting malignancies in remission: a propensity score matched cohort study. Transplantation 2018;102(7):1156–64.

91. Brattstrom C, Granath F, Edgren G, et al. Overall and cause-specific mortality in transplant recipients with a pretransplantation cancer history. Transplantation 2013;96(3):297–305.

92. Antin-Ozerkis D, Highland KB. Thoracic manifestations of rheumatic disease. Clin Chest Med 2019; 40(3). xiii.

93. Lee JC, Ahya VN. Lung transplantation in autoimmune diseases. Clin Chest Med 2010;31(3): 589–603.

94. Chambers DC, Cherikh WS, Harhay MO, et al. The international thoracic organ transplant registry of the international society for heart and lung transplantation: thirty-sixth adult lung and heart-lung transplantation report-2019; focus theme: donor and recipient size match. J Heart Lung Transpl 2019;38(10):1042–55.

95. Courtwright AM, El-Chemaly S, Dellaripa PF, et al. Survival and outcomes after lung transplantation for non-scleroderma connective tissue-related interstitial lung disease. J Heart Lung Transpl 2017;36(7):763–9.

96. Crespo MM, Bermudez CA, Dew MA, et al. Lung transplant in patients with scleroderma compared with pulmonary fibrosis: short- and long-term outcomes. Ann Am Thorac Soc 2016;13(6):784–92.

97. Khan IY, Singer LG, de Perrot M, et al. Survival after lung transplantation in systemic sclerosis. A systematic review. Respir Med 2013;107(12):2081–7.

98. Bernstein EJ, Bathon JM, Lederer DJ. Survival of adults with systemic autoimmune rheumatic diseases and pulmonary arterial hypertension after lung transplantation. Rheumatology (Oxford) 2018;57(5):831–4.

99. Bernstein EJ, Peterson ER, Sell JL, et al. Survival of adults with systemic sclerosis following lung transplantation: a nationwide cohort study. Arthritis Rheumatol 2015;67(5):1314–22.

100. Natalini JG, Diamond JM, Porteous MK, et al. Risk of primary graft dysfunction following lung transplantation in selected adults with connective tissue disease-associated interstitial lung disease. J Heart Lung Transpl 2021;40(5):351–8.

101. Crespo MM, Lease ED, Sole A, et al. ISHLT consensus document on lung transplantation in patients with connective tissue disease: Part I: epidemiology, assessment of extrapulmonary conditions, candidate evaluation, selection criteria, and pathology statements. J Heart Lung Transpl 2021;40(11):1251–66.

102. McInnes IB, Schett G. The pathogenesis of rheumatoid arthritis. N Engl J Med 2011;365(23): 2205–19.

103. van den Hoogen F, Khanna D, Fransen J, et al. 2013 Classification criteria for systemic sclerosis: an American college of rheumatology/European league against rheumatism collaborative initiative. Ann Rheum Dis 2013;72(11):1747–55.

104. Solomon JJ, Olson AL, Fischer A, et al. Scleroderma lung disease. Eur Respir Rev 2013; 22(127):6–19.

Lung Transplant Procedure of Choice

Bilateral Transplantation Versus Single Transplantation Complications, Quality of Life, and Survival

Melanie Subramanian, MD, Bryan F. Meyers, MD, MPH*

KEYWORDS

- Bilateral lung transplantation • Single lung transplantation • Health-related quality of life
- Survival analysis • Comparative outcomes studies

INTRODUCTION

Since the first successful isolated lung transplant performed by Cooper and colleagues[1] in Toronto in 1983, lung transplantation has been considered a suitable therapy for multiple causes of end-stage pulmonary disease.

The initial isolated transplant operations were single lung transplants performed on patients with severe idiopathic pulmonary fibrosis (IPF). At the time, the rationale was that the increased pulmonary vascular resistance in the remaining native lung, along with the poor pulmonary parenchymal compliance of that native lung, would set up an ideal situation of preferential ventilation and perfusion of the new graft lung. Since then, lung transplantation has been used to treat patients with multiple conditions including interstitial lung disease (ILD), chronic obstructive pulmonary disease (COPD), cystic fibrosis (CF), pulmonary hypertension, and more.[2] During the past several decades, changes in donor selection, intraoperative and postoperative care, and immunosuppression therapy have broadened the use of lung transplant and improved outcomes for transplant recipients.[3] Although constantly evolving guidelines exist to guide transplant candidate selection and management, there has been continuous debate surrounding the utilization of single (SLT) versus bilateral lung transplantation (BLT) for patients eligible for either strategy.[2,4,5] To date, much of the decision-making regarding the use of single versus bilateral lung transplant is based on individual institutional case series experience or retrospective review of large lung transplant registries. There is a lack of randomized, prospective data to provide clear criteria favoring SLT or BLT for patients for whom either strategy is possible. Furthermore, there is a lack of consensus on the philosophical dilemma: should a bilateral operation with better palliation be offered to fewer patients, or should a less effective but simpler unilateral operation be offered to more recipients? The purpose of this article is to review the existing literature regarding SLT and BLT to help form an answer to those questions. Specifically, this review will highlight the following subjects: disease-specific indications for SLT versus BLT; the impact of procedure type on posttransplantation functional status; the impact of procedure type on posttransplantation quality of life (QOL); common complications and chronic rejection after lung transplantation; ethical challenges facing the choice between single and bilateral transplants; and novel strategies in this arena.

The authors have nothing to disclose.
Washington University, School of Medicine, Barnes-Jewish Hospital, Saint Louis, MO, USA
* Corresponding author.
E-mail address: meyersb@wustl.edu

chestmed.theclinics.com

DISEASE-SPECIFIC INDICATIONS FOR LUNG TRANSPLANTATION

The many indications for lung transplantation include end-stage COPD, ILD, pulmonary hypertension, CF and bronchiectasis, and others.[2] Because patients with septic lung disease (including CF and bronchiectasis) and primary pulmonary hypertension almost always undergo BLT, these indications will not be discussed further in this review.[6]

The International Society for Heart and Lung Transplantation (ISHLT) provides the most comprehensive data on long-term survival associated with BLT and SLT for all recipients.[7] In the 2019 ISHLT report, summarizing survival trends from 1992 to 2017, recipients of a lung transplantation operation had a median survival of 6.7 years. In an unadjusted analysis, the overall and conditional to 1-year survival posttransplant in BLT recipients was better (7.8 and 10.2 years, respectively) compared with SLT recipients (4.8 and 6.5 years, respectively). This difference can be first seen at 1-year postop but increases during a 14-year follow-up period. Survival for BLT and SLT groups were 90% and 88% at 3 months, 83% and 79% at 1 year, 70% and 62% at 3 years, 61% and 48% at 5 years, and 42% and 23% at 10 years, respectively. The simple, unadjusted comparison between strategies represents the opening salvo of the discussion because there are multiple issues of selection bias and confounding that cloud the comparison of single versus bilateral transplantation outcomes. Additional literature has focused on short and long-term outcomes associated with transplantation type within subgroups of patients with specific diagnoses. The bulk of the existing literature examines the use of SLT and BLT in patients with either advanced COPD or ILD. It seems widely agreed on that those 2 diagnoses represent the "battleground" for the single versus bilateral dispute.

Chronic Obstructive Pulmonary Disease

Emphysema was the most common indication for lung transplantation until the introduction of the lung allocation score (LAS).[2] The first successful experience with transplantation in the COPD population involved isolated SLT, initially described by Cooper and his team.[1] However, with the development of BLT and improvements in surgical techniques, anesthesia management, ECMO support, and postoperative management, BLT has received increased clinical adoption for patients with COPD.[6,8] The prevailing physiologic reasoning supporting the use of BLT is that the technique reduces the risk of early ventilation/perfusion mismatch and eliminates the risk of late hyperinflation in the unresected emphysematous native lung that occurs after SLT.[8]

During the accumulation of the early experience, there was a tendency to offer BLT to younger patients for several reasons. It was thought that the younger patients might have greater physiologic reserve and fewer comorbidities, attributes that would make them better able to withstand the increased stress of a more prolonged BLT surgery.[1,4,6] That selection bias may have been appropriate but it might have also burdened the SLT cohort with an older and frailer group of recipient patients who would be at greater risk for premature death regardless of the differential contribution of the SLT versus BLT. Early retrospective analysis of the ISHLT/United Network for Organ Sharing (UNOS) registry of patients with COPD compared BLT and SLT in the COPD population and assessed the correlation between transplantation technique (SLT vs BLT) and survival while stratifying by age groups (41–50, 51–60, 61–70 years).[4] Among all transplant recipients, recipient age and procedure type (SLT vs BLT) were associated with increased risk for mortality with advanced age, SLT, and their interaction demonstrating significant associations. The authors demonstrated that BLT was associated with higher survival in both the 41–50 and 51–60 years age categories across all time points, with a more pronounced survival benefit occurring further out from surgery. Survival rates among younger patients (<50 years) who underwent SLT were 93.6%, 80.2% and 43.6% at 30 days, 1 year, and 5 years, respectively, compared with 94.9%, 84.7%, and 68.2% in the young BLT group. Among those aged 51–60 years, the differences in long-term survival were less pronounced. When using risk ratios to calculate risk of mortality across all ages, the authors noted an increased probability of mortality for recipients of SLT between ages 40 and 57 years. At approximately age 57, however, the trend reversed. No significant differences were observed between BLT and SLT in the rates of rejection, onset of bronchiolitis obliterans (BOS), bronchial artery complications, and hospitalizations for infections. However, the study did not measure variables associated with short-term morbidity, which may be more relevant in older patients. The study concluded that BLT was associated with greater short-term and long-term survivals in patients aged less than 60 years. At the time of that study, most recipients were indeed aged less than 60 years.

In a later survival analysis of the ISHLT registry between 1987 and 2006, which included 9883 patients with COPD, the proportion of patients who underwent BLT more than doubled from the 1990s to the close of the studied time interval (21.6% in 1993 to 56.2% in 2006). The median survival was significantly longer for those who received BLT (6.41 years) compared with the median survival for those who received SLT (4.59 years). However, the survival advantage associated with BLT did not hold true for patients aged older than 60 years. The practical conclusion was common wisdom of the time: offer BLT to younger patients with COPD but accept the lack of a difference in older recipients and perhaps use other criteria to choose the transplantation strategy in that population.[9]

In a 13-year review of 306 patients undergoing lung transplantation for COPD at the authors' institution, 220 (72%) patients received BLT, reflecting a strong institutional preference for the method.[10] The report emphasized that the preference for BLT was due to increased survival and the ease of postoperative ventilator management and weaning. When examining long-term survival, patients with COPD who received BLT had 5-year survival of 66.7% compared with 44.9% for patients who received single lung replacement.

Conversely, a retrospective study at the University of Colorado examined 5-year survival rates between patients receiving SLT (206 patients) and BLT (30 patients) from 1992 to 2012. During this period, this institution observed transplant guidelines to perform SLT on emphysema patients aged older than 55 years.[11] As expected, the SLT cohort tended to skew older and had lower pretransplant pulmonary function and poorer physical conditioning compared with the BLT cohort. Within this institution, 30-day, 1-year, and 5-year survival estimates between treatment cohorts were similar, with long-term survival trending slightly higher for patients with BLT. Due to their small pool of patients with BLT, they also compared their institutional data to the outcomes of patients with SLT and BLT in the UNOS registry. When comparing institutional data to SLT and BLT patients in the UNOS registry, patients with SLT had similar preoperative risk in terms of age, comorbid conditions, and pulmonary function. The institution's SLT short-term and long-term survival rates were similar to those of the UNOS registry's BLT subset. They concluded that although BLT may provide an individual survival benefit, SLT had substantial utility and should be promoted, given the overall influence it can have by increasing the number of potential patients receiving transplantation.

In a more recent series, 186 patients with end-stage COPD undergoing lung transplantation from 2012 to 2020 at Temple University Hospital, the decision to perform SLT versus BLT was left to the operating surgeon, although there was a general tendency to offer SLT for patients with advanced age or significant comorbidity in an institution in which SLT is by far the most offered procedure.[12] Approximately 38% of the cohort underwent BLT while the remainder (62%) underwent SLT. Interestingly, patients who underwent BLT tended to have a significantly higher LAS. Unadjusted survival was similar between patients with SLT and patients with BLT at 1 year, 3 years, and 5 years posttransplantation. This observation persisted when stratifying patients by age (older than 65 years). On Cox proportional hazard analysis, adjusting for multiple factors including age, gender, LAS (among others), there was no differences in survival risk by transplant type.

Several studies of BLT versus SLT have been performed on institutional or national databases that captured data before the 2005 implementation of the LAS. Before LAS, it was quite common to see COPD as the most common indication for transplant because these recipients were often listed early in their physiologic decline and their survival on the wait list was comparably good. A retrospective analysis of the UNOS registry from 2005 to 2012, compared graft survival between transplantation strategies after the implementation of the LAS in the United States.[13] Graft survival represented a composite of posttransplantation mortality and graft failure rates. These patients were propensity-matched to reduce the impact of treatment selection bias on the results of the study. Among 3174 patients with COPD, 1299 underwent SLT and 1875 underwent BLT. The median follow-up was during 2 years posttransplant, and there was no significant association found between the type of transplant and median graft survival (67.7 months for BLT vs 64.0 months for SLT). The distinction from previous study results may be explained by the novel way that patients were selected for transplantation using the LAS. Compared with the pre-LAS era, during which time on the waiting list gave priority for transplantation, patients with COPD in the LAS era have been more impaired to achieve a higher and more competitive and transplantable allocation score.[14] The use of the LAS to prioritize recipients for transplantation, and the use of propensity matching to account for bias, may have trimmed the apparent, measurable benefit of BLT for patients with COPD.

INTERSTITIAL LUNG DISEASES

The use of BLT in patients with IPF has increased over time. In 2017, approximately 82% of lung transplant operations among patients with IPF were BLT.[15] Despite the increasing number of BLTs in patients with IPF, there is no definitive survival advantage consistently shown to be associated with either BLT or SLT.

A retrospective institutional case series performed at Cleveland Clinic, compared overall 30-day, 1-year, and 5-year survival among 82 patients who underwent lung transplantation.[16] Overall survival among patients with IPF was significantly worse at all time points compared with their non-IPF matched counterparts. Importantly, they calculated that BLT conferred a survival advantage among patients with IPF (81% vs 67% at one year and 55% vs 34% at 5 years). However, they could only compare BLT versus SLT in 10 matched pairs due to the strong selection bias attributed to an institutional preference to perform BLT in younger patients. Interestingly, they were unable to point to advanced age as an independent risk factor for mortality in BLT.

Additional studies have also supported the use of BLT in patients with IPF because of an apparent survival advantage. A study with 1256 patients listed in the UNOS registry between 2005 and 2007 examined all-cause mortality 1-year after transplant in patients with IPF after the institution of the LAS score.[17] Additionally, it examined the effect of pretransplant disease severity on mortality outcomes by stratifying patients into LAS quartiles. Quartiles 1–3 indicated lower risk patients with IPF, whereas quartile 4 contained the highest risk patients with IPF. They determined that patients with IPF with higher LAS were more likely to receive BLT. They observed a trend toward greater usage of BLT in sicker patients, with 21% more patients receiving BLT in the highest LAS quartile compared with the lowest (59.5% vs 38.4%). Within the highest quartile, SLT was associated with a 14.4% increased risk in cumulative mortality compared with BLT. However, in the lowest quartile, SLT was found to be an independent protective factor in terms of mortality. There was no demonstrated short-term survival benefit associated with either transplantation type. Their findings are counterintuitive to the notion that BLT should be reserved for younger patients with more physiologic reserve, and instead suggest a role for BLT specifically for those with potentially higher preoperative risk.

Similarly, a large retrospective review of lung transplantation in 3860 (2431 SLT and 1429 BLT) patients from the UNOS registry from 1987 to 2008 using propensity score matching demonstrated a survival advantage when a 1-year conditional survival analysis was performed. BLT had significantly better long-term survival (12.08 vs 6.8 years).[18] When analyzing for risk factors for death within the BLT group, they reported recipient age, donor age, and year of transplantation to be significant predictors of mortality. Specifically, they observed that patients aged older than 57 years had higher first year posttransplant mortality risk. Based on the conditional survival analysis and the significant correlation between advanced age and mortality risk, the authors concluded that younger patients with IPF would most likely benefit from BLT to enhance long-term survival.

Not all available studies found a survival advantage associated with BLT in the IPF cohort. In a unique approach, studying 1001 lung transplant recipients with IPF concurrently listed for BLT and SLT of the UNOS registry from 2001 to 2009, 434 (43%) of these patients underwent SLT while the remaining 57% underwent BLT. There were significant differences in baseline comorbidities, functional status, pulmonary function tests, and recipient disease severity. Despite these baseline differences, there were no observed differences in short-term or long-term graft survivals. Based on these comparable outcomes, the authors advocated for more liberal use of SLT among patients with IPF.[19] However, they did note that a major limitation of their study was the assumption that single or bilateral organ assignment was random and based solely on the availability of 1 or 2 donor lungs. At the institutional level, or even the surgeon level, there may be great variability in willingness to accept any individual donor lung based on several donor and recipient characteristics. For example, a hospital may list a patient for either SLT or BLT, suggesting equipoise but that same group may have an easier threshold to decline a single lung donor for graft quality. This idea effectively challenges the authors' original assumption about the equivalence of the transplanted lungs.

Another retrospective review of the early UNOS registry experience in 2001 included a cohort of 821 lung transplant patients (636 SLT, 185 BLT) with pulmonary fibrosis. In the univariate analysis, younger patients with IPF (30–49 years) with SLT had better short-term and long-term survivals posttransplant than similar patients after BLT (90.9% vs 77.1% at 1 month; 63.8% vs 46.2% at 3 years; $P = .02$). The same trend favoring single lung replacement was observed in older patients. However, when a 1-month posttransplant conditional survival analysis was performed, there were no significant subsequent differences seen between procedure types at any age group. This pattern suggests that there may be greater periprocedural mortality associated with BLT. Propensity score matching and multivariate regression analysis failed to show survival differences between procedure types.[5]

A more updated analysis of the UNOS registry of patients with IPF undergoing SLT and BLT examined 9191 patients with IPF who underwent lung transplantation between 1987 and 2015.[20] The analysis found an overall growth in the utilization of BLT over time for patients with IPF. A steady increase was observed in the use of BLT since 2004, with BLT overtaking SLT by 2008. In unadjusted analysis, survival was similar between cohorts within the first-year posttransplant. However, after the first year, survival rates diverged with a 10-year survival significantly better for BLT compared with SLT (55% vs 32%, $P < .001$). These trends persisted after propensity-matched subgroup analysis and held true for both the pre-LAS and post-LAS eras. When examining the interaction effect of age, the authors noted a survival advantage for patients who underwent BLT up until the age of 70 years, after which survival rates for the 2 groups were similar. Interestingly, BLT demonstrated superior survival compared with SLT regardless of LAS score or mean PA pressures. In fact, for patients undergoing SLT, 10-year survival for those with mean PA pressures greater than 30 mm Hg and those with PA pressures greater than 40 mm Hg were only 25% and 17%, respectively. The authors concluded that for patients with IPF undergoing lung transplantation, BLT should be considered as the procedure of choice for those aged younger than 70 years. Meanwhile, they suggested that SLT not be considered for patients with mean PA pressures greater than 30 mm Hg or an allocation score greater than 45, which is contrary to previous assumptions that SLT be reserved for sicker patients.[20]

A systematic review of SLT vs BLT for fibrotic lung disease analyzed the survival outcomes in 5601 patients from 7 studies (including some of the studies reported above) that stratified survival data by transplant type.[21] Several studies presented conflicting results with respect to short-term transplantation outcomes; however, the BLT conferred an improved long-term survival (5 years or more) over that of SLT. They found that 5-year, 10-year, and 15-year survival estimates were 50%, 27.8%, and 13.9%, respectively, for patients with SLT. These values were lower than the survival rates for BLT, which were 57%, 35.3%, and 24% for 5, 10, and 15 years, respectively. Although the authors were able to accumulate a large pool of patients, their analysis did not allow for risk adjustment. Additionally, they included studies dating back to 1989, thus the results may not reflect subsequent advances in surgical technique or perioperative care.

In summary, when examining diagnosis-specific survival outcomes for BLT versus SLT, the existing literature demonstrates mixed findings. Comparing bilateral and single lung transplant effects by indication is crucial because the underlying pathophysiology of each disease is quite different and could greatly alter outcomes. Despite the mixed findings of these single center and registry studies, the use of bilateral transplant for both COPD and IPF is increasing over time. Both techniques have been used in younger and older populations despite previous notions that older individuals may "lack the reserve" to tolerate the procedure. Some data have demonstrated a greater advantage for using bilateral transplant in younger COPD populations but the evidence in COPD is still conflicting. The picture is even more mixed in analyses of patients with IPF. A randomized control trial is neither practical nor feasible in this setting. High-quality data prospectively collected from a variety of institutions that comprehensively consider the effects of age and multiple comorbidities will be useful in further unmasking the effect of transplantation type for patients with advanced COPD and IPF. Until that time, the data are diverse and conflicting enough to simply state that there is equipoise between the 2 strategies. Factors other than patient survival or graft survival must be considered as well.

BEYOND SURVIVAL: POSTTRANSPLANT FUNCTIONAL STATUS AND PROCEDURE TYPE

In addition to collecting data on short-term and long-term survivals, it is equally important to assess the functional status after transplantation. This key aspect of postlung transplant outcome is commonly quantified by spirometry, which has been correlated often with functional status, as well as other measures such as the 6-minute walk test (6MWT) and comprehensive surveys on a patient's ability to perform daily activities.

A single-institution study of 509 adult transplant recipients with 9471 postoperative forced 1-second expiratory volume (FEV_1) and forced vital capacity (FVC) values evaluated the impact of lung transplantation on recipient pulmonary function, with a particular focus on measuring percent-predicted FEV_1%.[22] For both patients with BLT and SLT, FEV_1% typically peaked at 1 year after transplant. FEV_1% increased from 50% in the immediate postoperative period to 55% at 1 year postoperatively in SLT recipients, and then gradually declined to 47% by 3 years. BLT recipients exhibited a similar trend but had higher overall FEV_1% values than the SLT cohort at every time point (60% immediately posttransplant, 75% 1 year posttransplant, and 65% 3 years posttransplant). Although patients undergoing either SLT or BLT exhibited increased risk of death with declining FEV1, this association in BLT recipients was notably tempered. The authors suggested that BLT may confer a protective effect on FEV_1—and thus survival—by providing recipients with enhanced pulmonary reserve.

In a single center and retrospective study of 130 patients with emphysema with similar baseline FEV1, FVC, and 6-minute walk scores, 84 patients underwent SLT, and 46 patients underwent BLT. The authors favored the use of SLT in older recipients, so the BLT recipients were measurably younger (51.1 vs 56.2 years). BLT was rarely used for recipients aged older than 60 years. The authors measured secondary outcomes of spirometry and 6-minute walk distances preoperatively, and at 3-month to 6-month intervals postoperatively. At all posttransplantation timepoints during a 4-year observation period, BLT recipients exhibited higher FEV_1 and FVC values compared with SLT recipients, despite having similar baseline pulmonary function. Additionally, patients with BLT had a higher mean 6-minute walk distance at all follow-up time points compared with patients with SLT, with the difference ranging from 100 to 400 ft. The SLT cohort was preferentially burdened by a group of patients with more advanced age, and presumably more comorbidities and frailty. Further assessment of comorbidity or pretransplant disease severity was not performed. The authors concluded with their preference for BLT in younger recipients was due to the superior functional results and quality-of-life payoff the bilateral approach affords. The degree to which their a priori programmatic adoption of a BLT strategy for younger recipients created this appearance of an improved postop function is impossible to measure.[23]

A prospective analysis of posttransplantation functional status and QOL targeted spirometry and 6-minute walk distance and prospectively enrolled 44 patients before lung transplantation.[24] Fourteen (32%) eventually received SLT, whereas the remainder (68%) received BLT. Spirometry and exercise assessment were performed before the transplant, as well as 6 and 12 months posttransplantation. Patients included in the report were required to be followed for at least 2 years posttransplantation, raising some concerns about "survivor bias" and challenging the degree to which the result apply to patients on the waiting list. Although lung transplantation provided higher FEV_1% predicted compared with baseline in all patients, this positive effect was dramatically lower among SLT recipients. At each time point

during 4 years posttransplantation, patients with SLT consistently had spirometry values at least 20% lower than spirometry scores of BLT recipients. However, 6MWT distances were not significantly different between cohorts.

POSTTRANSPLANTATION QUALITY OF LIFE OUTCOMES

For most patients with end-stage lung disease, lung transplantation cannot only provide a survival advantage but can also influence dramatic changes in health-related QOL (HRQL). The most significant gains in HRQL are expected to be seen in physical health and functioning, and the greatest improvements are expected to occur early (within the first 6 months) after transplant.[24] After 1 year, the risk of onset of BOS and the effect of other patient comorbidities can blunt the effect of transplantation on HRQL.[25] Research into patient-centered outcomes in lung transplantation has received increasing attention during recent years. However, the available literature on this topic is lacking, and there are even fewer studies that attempt to examine the influence of transplantation type on QOL.

Certain cross-sectional studies have asserted a positive effect of BLT on HRQL measures. A European multicenter cross-sectional study of 255 lung transplant recipients administered the EuroQOL5D (EQ5D) and visual analog scale (VAS) health-utility instruments to patients who received bilateral (n = 79), single (n = 106), and heart–lung (n = 70) transplants.[26] The EQ5D defines health quality in 5 dimensions: mobility, selfcare, usual activities, pain and discomfort, and anxiety or depression. Utility scores can then be assigned to each of these health states using regression analysis. The VAS allows participants to subjectively assess their own health on a scale of 0 to 100 (worst possible health to best possible health). In addition to stratifying results by transplant type, the authors repeated surveys at 4 different posttransplant time periods: 0–6, 7–18, 19–36, and greater than 36 months. Problems in all 5 EQ5D domains in all time periods were more common among patients with SLT than patients with BLT. Those who received bilateral or combined heart–lung transplants had significantly higher EQ5Dand VAS scores than their SLT counterparts in all time groups after 6 months (P = .001). However, this study was limited by the lack of controlling for age and pretransplant diagnosis.[26]

The positive impact of BLT on HRQL was not demonstrated by all studies. A study of 34 patients who had undergone SLT (n = 14), or BLT (n = 20) assesses HRQL with the use of the VAS in combination with St. George's Respiratory Questionnaire (SGRQ).[24] The SGRQ primarily addresses respiratory symptoms, accomplishment of routine activities and disease impact on daily life. These patients were followed for at least 2 years (when the authors believed average onset of BOS occurs) and all data were collected prospectively. The SGRQ and VAS scores were significantly improved after transplant compared with pretransplant in both SLT and BLT groups. However, posttransplant, there was no significant differences in QOL scores between SLT and BLT groups. Scores were also independent of the underlying disease that led to transplantation. As described in the previous section, the authors also collected spirometry and 6MWTdata and found that the posttransplantation improvement in FEV$_1$% predicted and QOL scores were significantly less in SLT versus BLT recipients. 6MWTs were comparable between cohorts. The authors suggested that pulmonary function had limited influence on objective and subjective parameters of patient HRQOL (24). A similar study used the Medical Outcomes Study 36-Item Short-Form Health Survey (SF-36) to measure QOL. As a part of the SF-36, scores are assigned to develop the Physical Component Survey and Mental Component Survey. When stratified by transplant type, bilateral operations did not confer a significant advantage in gains in physical component scores over single lung transplant.[27] Given that the functional outcome benefit conferred by bilateral procedures has been shown to be greater in the long term (>1 year), it would be interesting to see if there would be a clinically important difference in QOL scores if they were longitudinally followed over a longer period of time.

ASSOCIATIONS BETWEEN PROCEDURE TYPE, CHRONIC REJECTION AND OTHER COMMON COMPLICATIONS

Although the exact physiological mechanism behind the development of BOS is unknown, multiple studies have reported SLT as a risk factor for the development of BOS.[24,28,29] After controlling for other patient comorbidities and characteristics, SLT was found to be significantly associated with BOS onset in multivariable regression analysis. Other variables including transplant center, recipient age, and underlying end-stage lung disease diagnosis were not associated with the risk of BOS development.[29] As diagnosis of BOS depends on the decline in FEV$_1$%, it makes sense that patients with SLT are at an increased risk of BOS development. Unlike patients with BLT, patients with SLT still have a diseased native lung,

and its deterioration over time contributes to their overall FEV$_1$%. Moreover, as described above, the FEV$_1$% achieved after SLT is lower than with BLT giving patients with a SLT a higher baseline risk for meeting the threshold of a BOS diagnosis compared with a BLT patient simply due to a lower best FEV$_1$ posttransplant and/or progressive native lung dysfunction. Not all studies have demonstrated the same association between transplantation type and onset of BOS. In a much larger UNOS database analysis of 2260 lung transplant recipients with primary diagnosis of COPD, the authors did not observe a difference in BOS incidence between SLT and BLT cohorts during the 3-year follow-up period.[4] Given the enormous morbidity and mortality burden that BOS imposes on lung transplant recipients, further research is warranted to investigate the physiologic mechanism of BOS and any possible link there may be to the transplantation type.

Most of the studies described previously in this review are evaluating the impact of procedures in different indications and measuring the postprocedure mortality and functional status. There are limited available data looking at other meaningful clinical outcomes such as time to weaning from mechanical ventilation, need for tracheostomy, length of stay, and overall clinical outcomes. Most early posttransplant complications not directly associated to the actual SLT or BLT procedure, such as pneumonia, bronchial anastomotic stenosis or dehiscence, pleural effusions, chylothorax, and postsurgical paralysis or paresis of the diaphragm are often associated with devastating clinical implications and poorer QOL and outcomes after SLT when compared with BLT recipients. The obvious explanation is that these rare complications almost never occur bilaterally, so when they do take place at all, the buffering effect of a second transplanted lung mitigates the negative impact.

ETHICAL AND POPULATION-BASED CONSIDERATIONS

Much of the debate surrounding the use of BLT or SLT stems from the ethical challenge of how best to make use of a limited resource: donor lungs. The persistent ethical dilemma surrounding lung transplantation is whether the possible broader societal benefits of splitting a pair of donor lungs and thus reducing the overall wait list time and wait list mortality outweighs the cost to the individual recipient who is forced to forego a BLT. In reality, this theoretical concern has not proven to be true. Data from the ISHLT have shown an increase in the numbers of transplants performed from 1709 in 2000 to 4673 performed in 2016.

This almost exponential growth in the number of transplants has been exclusively because of increasing in the number of BLTs. During this entire time frame, although the number of SLTs has remained stable with an average of 958 transplants, the BLT numbers have increased from 884 in the year 2000 to 3759 in 2016. In the United States, several institutions, including our own, routinely use BLT for most lung transplant recipients.[10] Today, BLT is the most practiced lung operation and pulmonary fibrosis is the most common indication for transplantation. A review from the UNOS lung transplant recipient data including 5171 lung transplants performed between 2019 and 2020 shows that 3926 (76%) were BLT, a practice that is even more common in the largest lung transplant programs by volume (>40 lung transplants per year) where 80% of their operations are BLTs with only 2 of these 21 centers showing a predilection for SLT.

One study used the UNOS registry to study lung block utilization in all SLTs performed between 1987 and 2011. There were 7232 unique SLT donors identified. Of these donors, only 3129 (43%) had both lungs used for SLT. The authors reported that more than 200 potential donor lungs went unused annually since 2005. This study challenged one of the long-standing utilitarian arguments in favor of SLT.[30] At our own institution, there is a greater preference to perform BLT in part due to the prevailing notion that 2 lungs provide patients with greater physiologic reserve.[10] Given this assumption, surgeons often use what might be considered "extended" donor lungs for BLT for patients—mildly flawed donor organs that would otherwise might be wasted if considered individually in single lung blocks and thus declined. Similarly, the ability to use 2 lungs might allow a physically small donor to provide lung transplantation for a much larger recipient. Therefore, it is possible that there are common situations, based on quality and size, in which the use of specific donor lungs is either "both or none." In this sense, BLT may expand donor lung utilization. It is also true that some pairs of donor lungs become available in which one lung seems pristine and clearly useful for transplantation, yet the second lung may have parenchymal flaws that would raise concerns about using it for a SLT. There is little concern about using this second lung as a "plus one," when it is accompanied by its healthier donor twin. In such circumstances, the choice may not be between one bilateral operation versus 2 single lung transplants for difference recipients. Instead, the choice is whether to do one bilateral operation versus one single lung operation—a much easier dilemma to solve.

A study looking at the cost-effectiveness of transplantation included additional comparisons of SLT and BLT.[31] They determined that during a theoretical 15-year period, transplantation (compared with remaining on the waitlist with medical therapy) provided 2.1 and 3.3 quality-adjusted life-years (QALY) for SLT and BLT, respectively. The costs per each QALY gained were US$48,241 for SLT and US$32,803 for BLT. Based on the cost per QALY gained, the authors concluded that SLT was the least cost-effective form of therapy for patients with an end-stage lung disease. Moreover, it may be possible that the cost to society would be more accurately measured in total cost and not cost per QALY. The broad use of single rather than bilateral operations could increase the total cost of lung transplantation programs to a society or a payer. Other views considered not only the ethical challenges in offering 1 versus 2 lungs but also the effect of many patients remaining on the transplant waiting list longer with the hopes to undergo bilateral transplantation.[32]

THE NATIVE LUNG: POTENTIAL COMPLICATIONS AND RISK OF CANCER

One special consideration for the use of SLT is the risk of potential complications in the untransplanted native lung. Native lungs already have diminished lung function secondary to underlying disease process, and the use of SLT can potentially impose the additional complications. These complications included overinflation, pneumothorax, hemothorax, pneumonia, invasive aspergillosis, and malignancy in the native lung. In some of these patients, a pneumonectomy is required for the management of these complications. This experience was reported in a study in 180 single lung transplants performed from 1998 to 2008, 25 patients (14%) experienced significant native lung complications.[33] Of these, 11 patients went on to receive a pneumonectomy for nonsmall cell lung cancer, aspergilloma, bronchopleural fistula, and recurrent infection. Complication rates after receiving pneumonectomy were high (36.4%) but there was no hospital mortality. Additionally, when comparing patients who received a pneumonectomy for a complication to those who did not experience a complication, there was no statistically significant difference in median survival (4.3 vs 5.1 years).[33] Although early recognition and management of native lung complications is important, the possibility of developing a native lung complication does not necessarily weigh in as evidence opposing the use of SLT.

One additional concern regarding SLT is the risk of cancer development in the native lung. Citing increased risk associated with long-term chronic lung disease, recipient smoking history, increased age, and potential adverse effects of immunotherapy, one review documented a 9% prevalence of primary lung cancer found in native lungs after SLT.[34] Presumably, leaving a second lung untransplanted would expose a recipient to a risk of cancer in the second native lung, although this risk has yet to be clearly demonstrated in broad clinical practice. Finally, in some selected patients, mostly with underlying diagnosis of pulmonary fibrosis, cough is a major factor in the decision for transplantation, and this should be considered at the time of listing because chronic cough may not significantly improve after SLT.

Bilateral Sequential Lung Transplantation: Two single-lung transplantations as Good as a bilateral lung transplantation?

To mitigate perioperative morbidity and mortality risk and to preserve the observed long-term benefit of BLT, an alternative strategy is the utilization of SLT in selected recipients and then quickly relist them for a subsequent contralateral SLT at a future date.[35] Typically, an institution using this strategy will list individuals deemed to have higher perioperative risk (by age or comorbidity) to undergo the safer SLT. After transplantation, these patients are reviewed for relisting and all individuals who were noted to have acceptably low perioperative complications and reasonable functional status were thus considered. Relisting for contralateral transplant was performed as soon as was clinically appropriate (as determined by adequate functional recovery and the absence of infection or rejection). The authors performed a matched cohort analysis with a primary outcome of survival. Twelve patients underwent bilateral sequential lung transplantation (BSLT), and matches were selected in a 1:2:2 ratio from SLT and BLT recipients with ILD and similar LAS score. When comparing characteristics between the first and second stages of the BSLT procedure, there were no significant differences between donor characteristics. LASs were significantly higher in the first stage operation compared with the second stage (48.6 vs 24.5, $P < .01$). When comparing matched cases, the authors found no significant differences in survival. The authors thus proposed SBLT as an alternative to SLT and BLT. The concept of SBLT is intriguing but the strategy itself is fraught with potential complications and ethical challenges. It is unclear with the current risk stratification of cardiac diseases, the modern intraoperative and surgical techniques, and the ready availability of both VA and VV ECMO support for lung transplant recipients, which patients are at sufficient risk during a BLT to benefit from 2 SLT operations instead. Additionally, the existing knowledge on the immunologic consequences of receiving a second lung from a separate donor is limited. It is unclear whether these patients will be at greater or reduced risk for developing lung allograft dysfunction long-term. From an ethical perspective, it is unclear whether SBLT truly results in a better redistribution of a limited resource. Although more lungs would be available for use if individuals underwent a unilateral first stage operation instead of a BLT, many would ultimately reappear on the waitlist. The previously discussed issues about the fact that one bilateral lung transplant donor does not always translate into 2 single lung transplants still pertain here.

SUMMARY

Although isolated lung transplantation began as a single lung replacement for pulmonary fibrosis, BLT has grown in utilization among most lung transplant centers and presents the best option for patients with a variety of end-stage lung disease diagnoses. The increased adoption of BLT is reflective of increased comfort in practice among transplant surgeons and recognition of benefits measured by long-term survival and improvements in functional and QOL outcomes. However, much of the literature that examines the use of BLT versus SLT is conflicting, and the clinical picture is further nuanced by disease indication, age of recipient, donor lung quality, and patient disease severity. Although BLT has become the preferred practice in the authors' institution and many other largest transplant centers, with probably better survival and clinical outcomes, we cannot recommend to others one procedure type over another given the lack of high-quality evidence. Transplantation strategy will continue to be determined on an individual basis and by surgeons centers experience, with some of these centers having comparable outcomes and recommending strongly SLT for most of their patients. The current clinical picture of transplantation in the post-LAS era is certainly different than before but much of the existing data available are not yet reflective of this change. The ethical concerns about the best utilization of organs and the increased surgical risk of BLT over SLT are questionable and probably not supported by current practices. There will likely never be a randomized trial to clarify the respective roles of BLT and SLT. However, further large database analyses and prospective observational studies will be instrumental to bring better clarity to this debate.

REFERENCES

1. Toronto Lung Transplant Group. Unilateral lung transplantation for pulmonary fibrosis. N Engl J Med 1986;314:1140–5.

2. Yusen RD, Edwards LB, Dipchand AI, et al. The registry of the international society for heart and lung transplantation: thirty-third adult lung and heart-lung transplant report-2016; focus theme: primary diagnostic indications for transplant. J Heart Lung Transplant 2016;35:1170–84.

3. Puri V, Patterson GA. Adult lung transplantation: technical considerations. Semin Thorac Cardiovasc Surg 2008;20:152–64.

4. Meyer DM, Bennett LE, Novick RJ, et al. Single vs bilateral, sequential lung transplantation for end-stage emphysema: influence of recipient age on survival and secondary end-points. J Heart Lung Transplant 2001;20:935–41.

5. Meyer DM, Edwards LB, Torres F, et al. Impact of recipient age and procedure type on survival after lung transplantation for pulmonary fibrosis. Ann Thorac Surg 2005;79:950–7.

6. Puri V, Patterson GA, Meyers BF. Single versus bilateral lung transplantation: do guidelines exist? Thorac Surg Clin 2015;25:47–54.

7. Chambers DC, Cherikh WS, Harhay MO, et al. The registry of the international society for heart and lung transplantation: thirty-sixth adult lung and heart-lung transplantation report-2019; focus theme:donor and recipient size match. J Heart Lung Transplant 2019;38:1042–55.

8. Aigner C, Klepetko W. Bilateral lung transportation. Oper Tech Thorac Cardiovasc Surg 2012;17: 181–93.

9. Thabut G, Christie JD, Ravaud P, et al. Survival after bilateral versus single lung transplantation for patients with chronic obstructive pulmonary disease: a retrospective analysis of registry data. Lancet 2008;371:744–51.

10. Cassivi SD, Meyers BF, Battafarano RJ, et al. Thirteen-year experience in lung transplantation for emphysema. Ann Thorac Surg 2002;74:1663–9 [discussion: 9-70].

11. Bennett DT, Zamora M, Reece TB, et al. Continued utility of single-lung transplantation in select populations: chronic obstructive pulmonary disease. Ann Thorac Surg 2015;100:437–42.

12. Mutyala S, Kashem MA, Kanaparthi J, et al. Comparing outcomes in patients with end-stage chronic obstructive pulmonary disease: single versus bilateral lung transplants. Interact Cardiovasc Thorac Surg 2021;33:807–13.

13. Schaffer JM, Singh SK, Reitz BA, et al. Single- vs double-lung transplantation in patients with chronic obstructive pulmonary disease and idiopathic pulmonary fibrosis since the implementation of lung allocation based on medical need. JAMA 2015;313:936–48.

14. Lane CR, Tonelli AR. Lung transplantation in chronic obstructive pulmonary disease: patient selection and special considerations. Int J Chron Obstruct Pulmon Dis 2015;10:2137–46.

15. Weill D, Benden C, Corris PA, et al. A consensus document for the selection of lung transplant candidates: 2014–an update from the pulmonary transplantation council of the international society for heart and lung transplantation. J Heart Lung Transplant 2015;34:1–15.

16. Mason DP, Brizzio ME, Alster JM, et al. Lung transplantation for idiopathic pulmonary fibrosis. Ann Thorac Surg 2007;84:1121–8.

17. Weiss ES, Allen JG, Merlo CA, et al. Survival after single versus bilateral lung transplantation for high-risk patients with pulmonary fibrosis. Ann Thorac Surg 2009;88:1616–25 [discussion: 25-6].

18. Force SD, Kilgo P, Neujahr DC, et al. Bilateral lung transplantation offers better long-term survival, compared with single-lung transplantation, for younger patients with idiopathic pulmonary fibrosis. Ann Thorac Surg 2011;91:244–9.

19. Chauhan D, Karanam AB, Merlo A, et al. Post-transplant survival in idiopathic pulmonary fibrosis patients concurrently listed for single and double lung transplantation. J Heart Lung Transplant 2016; 35:657–60.

20. Villavicencio MA, Axtell AL, Osho A, et al. Single-versus double-lung transplantation in pulmonary fibrosis: impact of age and pulmonary hypertension. Ann Thorac Surg 2018;106:856–63.

21. Wilson-Smith AR, Kim YS, Evans GE, et al. Single versus double lung transplantation for fibrotic disease-systematic review. Ann Cardiothorac Surg 2020;9(1):10–9.

22. Mason DP, Rajeswaran J, Li L, et al. Effect of changes in postoperative spirometry on survival after lung transplantation. J Thorac Cardiovasc Surg 2012;144:197–203.

23. Pochettino A, Kotloff RM, Rosengard BR, et al. Bilateral versus single lung transplantation for chronic obstructive pulmonary disease: intermediate-term results. Ann Thorac Surg 2000;70:1813–8 [discussion: 8-9].

24. Gerbase MW, Spiliopoulos A, Rochat T, et al. Health-related quality of life following single or bilateral lung transplantation: a 7-year comparison to functional outcome. Chest 2005;128:1371–8.

25. Vermeulen KM, Ouwens JP, van der Bij W, et al. Long-term quality of life in patients surviving at least 55 months after lung transplantation. Gen Hosp Psychiatry 2003;25:95–102.

26. Anyanwu AC, McGuire A, Rogers CA, et al. Assessment of quality of life in lung transplantation using a simple generic tool. Thorax 2001;56:218–22.

27. Finlen Copeland CA, Vock DM, Pieper K, et al. Impact of lung transplantation on recipient quality of life: a serial, prospective, multicenter analysis through the first posttransplant year. Chest 2013; 143:744–50.

28. Neurohr C, Huppmann P, Thum D, et al. Potential functional and survival benefit of double over single lung transplantation for selected patients with idiopathic pulmonary fibrosis. Transpl Int 2010;23:887–96.

29. Hadjiliadis D, Angel LF. Controversies in lung transplantation: are two lungs better than one? Semin Respir Crit Care Med 2006;27:561–6.

30. Speicher PJ, Ganapathi AM, Englum BR, et al. Single-lung transplantation in the United States: what happens to the other lung? J Heart Lung Transplant 2015;34:36–42.

31. Anyanwu AC, McGuire A, Rogers CA, et al. An economic evaluation of lung transplantation. J Thorac Cardiovasc Surg 2002;123:411–8 [discussion: 8-20].

32. Wang Q, Rogers CA, Bonser RS, et al. Assessing the benefit of accepting a single lung offer now compared with waiting for a subsequent double lung offer. Transplantation 2011;91:921–6.

33. King CS, Khandhar S, Burton N, et al. Native lung complications in single-lung transplant recipients and the role of pneumonectomy. J Heart Lung Transplant 2009;28:851–6.

34. Olland AB, Falcoz PE, Santelmo N, et al. Primary lung cancer in lung transplant recipients. Ann Thorac Surg 2014;98:362–71.

35. Hartwig MG, Ganapathi AM, Osho AA, et al. Staging of bilateral lung transplantation for high-risk patients with interstitial lung disease: one lung at a time. Am J Transplant 2016;16:3270–7.

The Past, Present, and Near Future of Lung Allocation in the United States

Wayne M. Tsuang, MD MHS[a], Erika D. Lease, MD[b],
Marie M. Budev, DO, MPH[a],*

KEYWORDS

- Lung transplantation • Lung allocation • Lung allocation score • Continuous distribution

KEY POINTS

- The implementation of the lung allocation score (LAS)-based allocation system led to a decrease in waitlist mortality and an increase in lung transplants performed in the United States.
- International adoption of the LAS-based allocation system can be seen worldwide.
- The continuous distribution (CD) organ allocation system based on composite allocation score (CAS) composed of attributes including medical urgency, outcomes, efficiency, and patient access is a points-based system unlike the LAS classification-based system.
- CD allows the elimination of hard "boundaries" in donor lung allocation and promotes better transparency as to the role of the various factors within the candidate score.
- The CAS for the allocation of donor lungs is divided into five goals: medical urgency, posttransplant outcomes, biological disadvantages limiting patient access (blood type, height, and allosensitization), other patient access factors (promoting access for pediatric candidates and prior living organ donors), and efficiency (promoting efficient management of the organ allocation and placement system).
- The CD-based allocation system is aligned with the ideals expressed in the Final Rule.

INTRODUCTION

Over the last several decades, lung transplantation has emerged as a viable therapeutic option for patients suffering from end-stage lung disease. In 1998, the US Department of Health and Human Services (DHHS) issued the Final Rule to address organ allocation in transplantation. The Final Rule went into effect in 2000 and required that existing organ allocation policies needed to address several factors including broader geographical sharing of organs, the reduction of waitlist (WL) time as a factor in allocation, and the use of objective medical criteria and medical urgency to allocate donor organs.[1,2] Before the implantation of the lung allocation score (LAS) in 2005, the initial lung allocation policy guidelines were relatively simple with donor organs being offered to candidates based on individual cumulative waiting time and ABO. This resulted in increased WL mortality and a limited number of lung transplants performed annually. With the implementation of the LAS, WL mortality was reduced, and the number of transplants performed increased.[3] The implementation of LAS has a great success compared with previous polices and has been adopted as

No conflicts of interest to report.
Of note: All authors WT, EL, MB serve as volunteers on committees within the United Network of Organ Sharing (UNOS).
[a] Lerner College of Medicine, Respiratory Institute, Cleveland Clinic, 9500 Euclid Avenue, Cleveland, OH 44195, USA; [b] Division of Pulmonary, Critical Care, and Sleep Medicine, University of Washington, 1959 NE Pacific Street, Box 356175, Seattle, Washington 98195, USA
* Corresponding author.
E-mail address: budevm@ccf.org

Clin Chest Med 44 (2023) 59–68
https://doi.org/10.1016/j.ccm.2022.10.004

the foundation for allocation systems worldwide. A review of the current allocation system by Organ Procurement and Transplantation Network (OPTN) led to the approval for the development of a continuous organ distribution framework for lung organ allocation. Lung was the first organ to participate in the creation of the new continuous distribution (CD) organ allocation system implemented early in the year of 2023. In this review, the authors describe the history of lung allocation, history of the development and composition of CD lung allocation system, and then finally the various lung allocation systems that exist throughout the world.

The History of Lung Allocation in the United States

In 1984, the National Organ Transplant Act established the OPTN. The OPTN role is to provide oversight for organ allocation policies that are developed in the United States.[1] In 1998, The DHHS issued the Final Rule on organ transplantation, creating the regulatory framework for the structure and operations of the OPTN, including guidance around policy development.[2] Importantly, the Final Rule requires that the OPTN develops policies for the equitable allocation of deceased donor organs that among other conditions:

- "Shall be based on sound medical judgment"
- "Shall seek to achieve the best use of donated organs"
- "Shall be designed to avoid wasting organs, avoid futile transplants, promote patient access to transplantation, and promote the efficient management of organ placement"
- "Shall not be based on the candidate's place of residence or place of listing, except to the extent required" to achieve the other conditions as above.

The first official donor lung allocation system in the United States was initiated by the United Network of Organ Sharing (UNOS) in 1990. The initial policy for lung allocation adopted by UNOS was simple with donor lungs allocated based on ABO match and the amount of time the candidates accrued on the waiting list. Donor offers were first given to candidates within the geographic bounders of the local organ procurement organization (OPO) donor service area (DSA) of the local hospital where the donor was located. DSAs were established in 1984, with the goal of minimizing organ cold ischemic times by reducing the distance to the transplant hospital within the same geographic area. In the early allocation system, if the lungs were not placed with the DSA, the organs would then allocated to concentric 500 nautical mile (NM) circles from the donor hospital designated as Zones A-D until the organ was placed.[3] Priority in the early allocation system was primary based on geography and waiting time. As a result, patients with rapidly progressive disease died while waiting on the list for an appropriate organ offer. In addition, transplant centers would list patients early in their disease course to help accrue time on the waiting list and to ensure if a decline in clinical status should occur, the patient would not miss the opportunity to receive an organ.[4] As the waiting transplant list had more patients, it become more evident that patients with pulmonary fibrosis who were listed for lung transplant had a much higher chance of dying on the waiting list than patients listed with emphysema.[5] This lead to the first amendment to the allocation system in 1995, which provided an additional 90-day credit to the waiting time at the time of listing for patients with the diagnosis of pulmonary fibrosis in the hopes to address the increased WL mortality in this population. The result of this amendment was never evaluated in terms of its impact.[6]

The Final Rule went into effect in March 2000, and in the same year, a report was commissioned from the Institute of Medicine (IOM) to comment on the Final Rule. The IOM agreed that organ allocation should be based on measures of medical urgency, however, avoiding futile transplants while waiting time should not be used as a criteria and encourage broader geographic sharing as part of an allocation system.[7] Despite the 90-day credit for idiopathic pulmonary fibrosis (IPF) patients on the waiting list, WL mortality and WL size continued to steadily rise.[8] Based on the ideals outlined by Final Rule, the OPTN Thoracic Transplant Committee formed the Lung Allocation Sub- Committee (Thoracic Organ Allocation Modeling Sub- Committee) to study and model an allocation system which would prioritize the allocation of lung donors based on recipient urgency rather than cumulative WL time.[9] The OPTN Thoracic Organ Transplant Committee was also in agreement that waiting time should only be considered as part of the framework of an organ allocation system which should include other factors including medical urgency and cold ischemic time. Over a half decade later in March 2005, the first major change to the lung allocation system occurred with the implementation of the LAS.[8] The LAS is based on an algorithm to estimate transplant benefit by calculating a WL urgency measure (WLAUC) or the WL mortality and posttransplant survival measure (PTAUC). WLAUC is weighted twice as much compared with post-transplant survival (PT) which is only weighted once in the calculation of transplant measure and raw allocation score. The raw score is normalized and subsequently the LAS is generated that ranges from 0 to 100 (**Table 1**).[10] The Committee realized that distinct types of lung diseases had unique natural histories and rates of progression. An analysis of WL survival probability, PT probability, and other factors impacting survival were applied to four disease-specific categories that compromised almost 80% of waitlisted patients. These four disease-specific categories included *Group A:* obstructive lung disease (chronic obstructive pulmonary disease [COPD] and emphysema due to α-1-antitrypsin deficiency; *Group B:* pulmonary hypertension (primary or secondary); *Group C:* cystic fibrosis; and *Group D:* restrictive lung disease/interstitial lung disease. The reference cohort used for the analysis included patients added to the lung transplant waiting list between January 1, 1997 and June 30, 1999. A variety of different 3-year cohorts of listed and post-lung transplant patients were analyzed initially by logistic regression and then by Cox's proportional hazard models.[6] Results of the analysis yielded different rates of WL mortality and PT for each diagnosis group. In addition, variables including forced vital capacity, oxygen use, and 6-minute walk distance (6 MW) were weighted differently within each diagnosis group, with different coefficients assigned to each variable depending on the diagnosis group. Final models combined hazard ratios for identified predictive factors in separate diagnosis groups. These predictive factors, which have been adjusted over the past few years, were ultimately selected to calculate WL mortality and PT. The current list of factors used to calculate WL mortality and PT is shown in **Table 2**.[3]

As dynamic changes in a candidate's clinical status may occur over time, a requirement for updating the LAS every 6 months exists.[3,11] Analysis of the updated data every 6 months would have allowed for confirmation of relevant hazards for WL and PT and to identify new factors that may be relevant. However, there existed a lag of 5 years after implementation where no analysis of WL or posttransplant data was undertaken. Since the implementation of the LAS allocation system, one major revision of the LAS calculation has taken place and several minor updates. In 2006, the incorporation of partial pressure of carbon dioxide ($PaCO_2$ mm Hg) as a factor in the WL mortality model that was first minor update based on evidence that noted an increase in the $PaCO_2$ could impact higher WL mortality leading

to a more urgent need for a transplant.[12] Also in 2006, amid concerns that the LAS did not appropriately represent medical urgency in the pulmonary hypertension population (Group B), an exception request of an LAS at the 90th percentile of the current WL could be requested from the national OPTN Lung Review Board if the following criteria were present: clinical deterioration despite maximal medical therapy with hemodynamic measurements of right atrial pressure greater than 15 mm Hg or cardiac index less than 1.8 L/min/m². In February 2015, a major revision to the LAS calculation was implemented with the addition of serum creatinine, change in $PaCO_2$, total bilirubin, and cardiac index.[6] In the 3-year post-2015 LAS revision OPTN monitoring report (2/19/2015–1/18/2018), there was an increase in median LAS at listing for diagnosis Group B that was seen, and a slight decrease in the median LAS in diagnosis Group D.[13]

An OPTN Lung Review Board also was created with the primary mission to review requests for LAS exceptions if a center believed that the calculated LAS did not represent their candidate's acuity of illness.[14] In 2011, OPTN required that candidates with LAS greater than 50 have updated clinical variables including assisted ventilation, supplemental 02 requirements, $PaCO_2$ every 2 weeks. It was believed that candidates with LAS greater than 50 are generally hospitalized with higher degree of illness. Therefore, an updated LAS may reflect the urgency for the need for transplant in this population.[11]

Regarding the pediatric population, when the LAS was implemented in 2005, pediatric candidates from age 0 to 11 were allocated organs based on time on the waiting list rather than the LAS. Later in 2010, for patients between the ages of 0 and 11, priority was based on disease severity either as a priority 1 or priority 2 followed by time on the WL within the priority 1 patients or total wait time on the list for priority 2 pediatric patients. In 2010, greater access to pediatric donors for pediatric recipients through broader sharing was implemented by the elimination of DSA and first 500 nm first zone. For a child donor 0 to 11 years old, the offer would first be given to a priority 1 pediatric recipient within 1,000 NM then to priority 2 pediatric recipients within 1,000 NM and then to adolescent recipients, ages 12 to 17 years old within 500 NM.[15]

Overall, the implementation of the LAS has been successful; however, it did not address broader sharing and geographic variability in organ availability. The second major change in the lung allocation system occurred in 2017 because of a successful lawsuit filed by the parents of a 10-

Table 1
Definitions of terms used and calculation of the lung allocation score

Waitlist Urgency Measure (WLAUC)	Defined expected days lived during additional 1 y on the waiting list • Weighted 2x
Posttransplant Survival Measure (PTAUC)	Defined expected days lived during 1 y after transplant • Weighted 1x
Raw Allocation Score	Posttransplant Survival Measure—2x Waitlist Urgency Measure • Ranges from −730 to 365
Normalization Raw Score = LAS	LAS 0–100 • Raw Score −730 = LAS 0 • Raw Score 365 = LAS 100

Data from A guide to calculating the lung allocation score. UNOS. Available at: https://unos.org/wp-content/uploads/unos/lung-allocation-score.pdf. Accessed June 14 2022.

year-old cystic fibrosis patient; the OPTN Executive Committee approved a temporary policy, the Adolescent Classification Exception for Pediatric Candidates, for candidates less than 12 years old. This policy made it permissible for pediatric candidates ages 0 to 12 who are medical priority 1 or 2 to apply to the national OPTN Lung Review Board for an LAS exception score. This exception value would create a second registration based on the LAS exception and not on the pediatric priority allowing the pediatric population access to adolescent and adult donor lungs. In addition, in the same year, a new policy allowed candidates less than 12 years old to receive a deceased donor organ of any compatible blood type. This policy change grouped all donors as either under the age 18 or over the age of 18. A pediatric donor under the age of 18 would first be offered to a priority 1 child recipient within 1,000 NM in addition to wait time on the list and then be offered to a priority to child candidate in addition to wait time within 1,000 NM and followed by offering the organ to a 12 to 17-year-old adolescent candidates within 1,000 NM and finally offered to adults within the DSA. The implementation of this policy improved the likelihood that a pediatric donor offer would be given to pediatric candidate.[11] Another recent minor change in the LAS 2020 occurred because of changes in lung candidates in comparison to previous era candidates with more recent candidates being older and sicker. The transplant community voiced that there needed to be an effort to update the coefficients to accurately estimate 1-year waiting list and PT. As a result of this modeling exercise, several covariates were recommended to be dropped due to small sample size and subsequent limited results.[16]

Several positive effects were noted as a result of the LAS-based allocation system implementation. Initially, the number of lung transplants performed increased from an average 1,063 lung transplants performed per year during the 5 years before implementation of the LAS (2000–2004) to 1,920 during the 5 years after implementation (2006–2011), an 80% increase in the number of lung transplants.[8] More impactful was the drop in WL mortality by 40% (from 500/year to 300/year). In addition, a shift was noted in the most common indication for transplantation changing from COPD to restrictive forms of lung disease. Although sicker patients were being transplanted no change in 1-year survival posttransplant was seen. The number of lungs offers before center acceptance also decreased from a median of 10 calls to 3 calls after the implementation of the LAS.[17] Despite the successes of the LAS implementation, concerns have been raised by the transplant community about the overall transplant benefit in older, sicker individuals with higher LAS and the impact on longer term survival. The LAS does not account for survival beyond 1 year. Concerns have been raised going back to the change in the allocation system in 2005, including the greater use of resources for patients with higher LAS, such as the use of bridging techniques such as extracorporeal membrane oxygenation (ECMO) and increased utilization of ECMO posttransplant, and notable increases in hospital charges and health care costs.[18,19]

Continuous Distribution

In response to the 2017 successful lawsuit filed against the lung allocation systems, the OPTN Board of Directors convened the Ad Hoc Geography Committee to establish principles and a framework to guide how OPTN policies may consider the use of geographic constraints in organ allocation. Ultimately, the committee recommended organ distribution without geographic

Table 2
Covariant factors used in the calculation of lung allocation score since 2022[3]

Waitlist List Mortality Factors	Posttransplant Survival Factors
Age (years) at time of offer	Age (years) at time of offer
Bilirubin mg/dL	Cardiac index (L/min/m^2) at rest
Increase in bilirubin of at least 50% if diagnosis Group B	Creatinine mg/dL
Body mass index kg/m^2	Increase in creatinine $\geq$ 150%
Cardiac index (L/min/m^2) at rest	If hospitalized—need for continuous mechanical ventilation
Central venous pressure mm Hg	*Diagnosis Group*
If hospitalized—need for continuous mechanical ventilation	Group A: Obstructive lung disease
Creatinine mg/dL	Group B: Pulmonary hypertension
Diagnosis Group	Group C: Cystic fibrosis
Group A: Obstructive lung disease	Group D: Restrictive lung disease
Group B: Pulmonary hypertension	A 6-min walk distance (feet)
Group C: Cystic fibrosis	Supplemental oxygen need at rest (L/min) to maintain oxygen saturation $\geq$88% or higher
Group D: Restrictive lung disease	
• Sarcoidosis with pulmonary artery pressure > 30 mm Hg (Group D)	
• Sarcoidosis with pulmonary artery pressure < 30 mm Hg (Group A)	
Forced vital capacity % predicted	
Supplemental oxygen need at rest (L/min) to maintain oxygen saturation $\geq$88% or higher	
PCO$_2$ mm Hg	
PCO$_2$ mm Hg increase of at least 15% (▲ change)	
Pulmonary artery (PA) systolic pressure at rest mm Hg	
A 6-min walk distance (feet)	

Modified from Egan TM. How should lungs be allocated for transplant? Semin Respir Crit Care Med 2018;39:126-137.

boundaries, organ allocation as geographically broad as possible, and the geographic constraints must be rationally determined and consistently applied.[20]

Arbitrary geographic boundaries were not the only arbitrary "boundaries" in the historical LAS classification-based allocation system that precluded a patient from being prioritized ahead of another patient on the other side of the "boundary." Another example of a classification-based allocation process included the allocation of donor lungs first to all identical blood type candidates only after which then compatible blood type candidates could be considered, irrespective of medical urgency and without medical necessity to do so. In addition, the historical LAS-based lung allocation system did not consider many clinical issues relating to patient access to organ transplantation.

The CD organ allocation system results in a composite allocation score (CAS) based on medical urgency, outcomes, efficiency, and patient access (**Fig. 1**).[21] This points-based system, as opposed to the previous classification-based system, allows the elimination of hard "boundaries" in donor lung allocation and promotes better transparency as to the role of a range of factors within the candidate score. The CAS for the allocation of donor lungs is divided into five goals: medical urgency (prioritizing medically urgent candidates to achieve the best use of donated organs), posttransplant outcomes (improving posttransplant outcomes and avoiding futile transplants), biological disadvantages limiting patient access (promoting patient access by addressing biological disadvantages such as blood type, height, and allo-sensitization), other patient access factors (promoting patient access for pediatric candidates and prior living organ donors), and efficiency (promoting efficient management of the organ allocation and placement system) (**Fig. 2**).[22]

The attributes within each goal of the CAS are assigned points when combined comprise the score by which candidates on the lung transplant waiting list are ranked. Although geographic constraints are considered regarding the practical

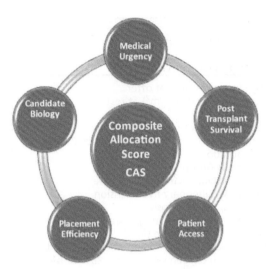

Fig. 1. Goals of the composite allocation score (CAS).

and logistical efficiency of the organ allocation and placement system, there are no geographic hard boundaries limiting candidates' access to donor lungs purely based on their geographic location. Points are distributed based on medical urgency and PT using the individual components of the LAS-based WL and PT cox proportional hazard models calculating areas under the curve (AUC), WLAUC, and PTAUC, respectively. In addition, points are allotted for blood type, height, and allo-sensitization in a way that reflects the proportional limitations of access to donor lungs by candidates based on these attributes. The binary

attributes of pediatric or prior living donor status are allotted points fully or not at all. Finally, points are assigned for placement efficiency and proximity understanding the logistics of donor organ procurement becomes more difficult the further the distance the candidate is from the donor hospital while still allowing the sickest or those with disadvantaged access wider geographic access.

Although data are incorporated whenever possible to support the proportional allocation of points in the CAS, inherently the weighting of the attributes against each other is a value-based decision. As a larger community, for example, is it more important to allocate donor lungs to those who are the most medically urgent irrespective of pediatric status? Or is it more important to prioritize PT over accounting for biological disadvantages limiting access of candidates to donor lungs? These questions cannot be based on data nor is there a "right" answer to how the attributes compared with each other for priority. The decision of how to weight the attributes against each other must be driven by community values.

There are several methods for multi-criteria decision-making within operations research that allow for participants to express the relative importance of categories, or in this case attributes, to achieve a given goal. For the development of CD, the Analytical Hierarchy Process was chosen given its history of use in other health care scenarios involving multiple parties in clinical decision-making.[21] By involving transplant

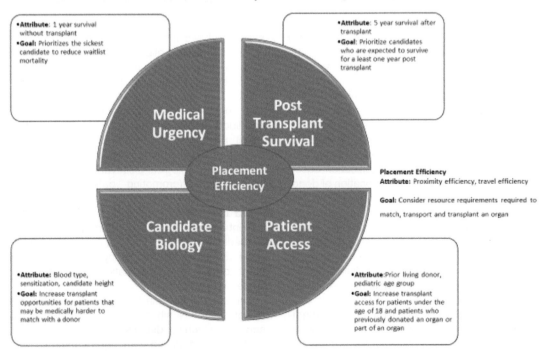

Fig. 2. Lung attributes and supporting goals.

Table 3
Lung composite allocation score

Attribute	Lung CAS Points
Waitlist survival (WLAUC)	25
Posttransplant survival (PTAUC)	25
Biological disadvantages	15 (total)
Blood type	5
Height	5
Allo-sensitization	5
Patient access (binary)	25 (total)
Pediatric status	20
Prior living donor status	5
Efficiency	10 (total)
Travel efficiency	5
Proximity efficiency	5
Total points	100

professionals, patients, donor families, and OPO professionals, and among others, community values were revealed regarding the preferred weighting of the various attributes against each other.

The current iteration of the Lung CAS, based on a total of 100 points, allots a maximum of 25 points for medical urgency, 25 points for PT, 15 points for biological disadvantages (5 for each attribute of blood type, height, and allo-sensitization), 20 binary points for pediatric status, 5 binary points for a candidate who was a prior living donor, and 10 points for efficiency of the organ placement system based on a travel efficiency and proximity efficiency score (5 of the 10 points for each) (**Table 3**). One of the benefits to the Lung CAS, however, is that it is a modular system allowing for adjustments as needed much more easily than the historical LAS system, such as changing of the weighting and adding attributes

Another distinction from the historical LAS system is the change of the posttransplant component of the LAS (PTAUC) to be based on a 5-year survival instead of the previous 1-year survival metric. Despite overall medical advances, survival after lung transplantation has plateaued with a 5-year survival of about 60%.[23] The historical LAS-based allocation system used a 1-year survival metric which, when combined with twice the weighting of WL survival over PT, may have inadvertently allowed for increased transplant rates for those candidates who were critically ill but at the expense of longer term outcomes. Although prediction of PT is notoriously difficult and imprecise, simulation modeling showed that predictive capabilities of 1-year PT was equivalent to the predictive capabilities of a 5-year PT metric. In addition, simulation modeling showed a significant increase in transplant rates for candidates less than 65 years of age.[24]

As the Lung CAS was being developed, several simulation models were created to assess as best as possible the impact, and possible unintended consequences, of the newly designed system. Importantly, simulation modeling showed a significant reduction in WL deaths in general and across many clinical factors such as female sex, ethnicity, insurance status, and for pediatric candidates.[22] As anticipated, simulation modeling showed the median distance traveled by a lung transplant program to be farther than with the LAS-based allocation system particularly for those candidates of the highest medical urgency while the distance traveled remained similar for candidates of lower medical urgency.

Although time passes following the implementation of the Lung CAS, close monitoring at many time points will allow for confirmation of the improvements in donor lung allocation predicted by simulation modeling. In addition, further refinements may be considered early while also allowing for future modifications to be implemented much more easily and quickly.

Worldwide Donor Lung Allocation Systems

There is wide variation in how deceased donor lungs are allocated across the world. Allocation systems are often unique to a specific country or region, and international agreements on donor lung sharing are common. Nations which have recently published their experiences are reviewed here, but this list is not meant to be all-inclusive.

After the United States' implementation of the LAS in 2005, the next country to use the (LAS was Germany in 2011.[23] Gottlieb and colleagues reviewed 3 years before and after adoption of the LAS and found a significant increase in the number of patients transplanted for restrictive lung disease (41% vs 32%; $P < 0.001$) which was similar to the trend seen in the United States[23] The overall number of waitlisted patients decreased 29%, along with a 26% decrease in WL mortality, and a shortening of the median WL time from 199 days pre-LAS to 84 days post-LAS. In addition, the number of transplants increased 21% and 1-year PT improved from 76% pre-LAS to 81% post-LAS. For patients less than 12 years of age and listed for lung transplant, the allocation system automatically assigns the highest possible LAS of 100 regardless of clinical acuity. This is in recognition of the fact that it is more difficult for children to access donor lungs as well as the advocacy of the German lung transplant system on behalf of a vulnerable population, which cannot advocate for itself.[24]

In 2014, the third country to adopt an LAS was the Netherlands. Over a 10-year period from 2010 to 2019, there were 1,276 patients. A study comparing the period before and after the LAS and found that the annual number of transplants did not change, nor did WL mortality. However, much like in Germany and the United States, the proportion of patients with pulmonary fibrosis increased from 22% to 39% and the chance of transplant increased significantly for patients with pulmonary fibrosis. PT did not change.[25]

In a regional approach to donor lung allocation, several European nations participate in Eurotransplant, which is a unique partnership between Austria, Belgium, Croatia, Germany, Hungary, Luxembourg, the Netherlands, and Slovenia.[26] Eurotransplant manages the matching between donor hospitals and transplant centers for all solid organ types, and in 2021, there were 1,231 lung transplants facilitated through Eurotransplant. Of note, in 2011, the Eurotransplant LAS was implemented. Like the LAS used in other countries, there are over a dozen clinical variables which are imputed to calculate the LAS and the numeric result is used to prioritize patients for donor lungs. The LAS is used primarily to establish if the LAS is ≥ 50, which places a waitlisted patient into a high priority category. The data for these high LAS patients must be updated every 3 days. Once a patient is established as high priority, if there is a negative balance between the country of the waitlisted patient and the country of the donor, the waitlisted patient will be placed at the top of the donor's country match list. For waitlisted patients, where the LAS is less than 50 and her/his/their country has a negative balance with the donor country, the waitlisted patient will be allocated per the donor country's allocation system which may be LAS-based or waiting time-based.[26] Like the United States, health care providers may also advocate to Eurotransplant's Lung Review Board if it is thought the calculated LAS does not accurately represent the clinical acuity of a patient and that a higher score is needed to improve a patient's chances of transplant.[26]

There are other regions where allocation is driven not by the LAS but by a clinical assessment of urgency. Scandiatransplant encompasses Demark, Finland, Norway, and Sweden, and in 2009, the Scandiatransplant Urgent Lung Allocation System was implemented to prioritize high urgency patients. Each of the five transplant centers in Scandiatransplant on its own decides which patients have urgent status. When this occurs, the patient has priority for donors throughout the entire Scandiatransplant region. Each center is limited to three such urgent listings per year. Since implementation of this system, recipients were found to more likely be younger, have suppurative lung disease, and more likely to be on life support before transplant which may have contributed to a shorter survival.[27]

In Australia, potential donors are referred to one of the four individual transplant centers based on geographic location. Matching between donor and waitlisted patient is based on a combination of ABO blood group, size compatibility, antibody match, clinical urgency, logistics, potential recipient long-term outcome, and WL time. The median wait time in Australia is 116 days, and there is an average of more than 200 lung transplants per year.[28] Recently, an LAS algorithm has been developed at St Vincent's Hospital in Sydney, with a goal toward implementation of the algorithm at the center to help streamline donor lung allocation.[29]

In Canada, waitlisted patients are assigned either a status 1 (stable) or status 2 (deteriorating), which is determined by a multidisciplinary team at the transplant center. The assignment of status may have different thresholds at the differing Canadian transplant centers. Within each status rank, donor lungs are offered to the transplant center in the jurisdiction of the donor hospital. Declined donor offers go on to the next nearest transplant center until all centers have declined.[30] Interestingly, donor lungs in the United States, which have been declined by all US centers may then be allocated to Canada. In a recent report, Cypel and colleagues reviewed the experience at the University of Toronto and found that 124/1424 (8.7%) of lung transplants done at their center used donors from the United States with similar short- and long-term outcomes compared with donor lungs from Canada.[31]

Worldwide, there has been growth in the number of lung transplants. This highlights the need to have rigorous and transparent donor lung allocation systems. The allocation systems highlighted here are only a few among many. As the lung transplant field continues to grow, shared experiences and collaboration between countries will be key to advance the field of allocation so that all donor lungs are optimally used.

SUMMARY

The implementation of the LAS-based allocation system was a significant improvement over previous allocation systems based on WL time and ABO. The LAS implementation led to reduction in WL mortality and an increase in the number of transplants performed in the United States. The success of the LAS in the US allocation system has led to its adoption and adaption in various allocation systems throughout the world. Despite the many positive aspects of the LAS, issues including geographic constraints leading to hard boundaries of the allocation of lungs and the lack of consideration of the many clinical issues or biological disadvantages that limit patient access to transplant made the LAS an archaic system that needed to evolve. As a result, the CD lung allocation system implemented in 2023 eliminates the geographic constraints, includes points for placement efficiency, WLAU and PTAUC and biological disadvantages, patient access if applicable, and results in the CAS. The lung CAS is nimble enough to allow for adjustments easier than the LAS allocation system. As CD is implemented close monitoring for issues because of the new system will allow for timely modifications.

CLINICS CARE POINTS

- The lung allocation score (LAS)-based allocation system led to a decrease in waitlist mortality and an increase in lung transplants performed in the United States but was hindered by the arbitrary "boundaries" that precluded a patient from being prioritized ahead of another patient on the other side of the "boundary."

- International adoption of the LAS-based allocation system can be seen worldwide due to the early success showing waitlist mortality reduction.

- The continuous distribution (CD) organ allocation system based on composite allocation score (CAS) composed of attributes including medical urgency, outcomes, efficiency, and patient access is a points-based system unlike the LAS classification-based system.

- CD allows the elimination of hard "boundaries" in donor lung allocation and promotes better transparency as to the role of the several factors within the candidate score.

- The CAS for the allocation of donor lungs is divided into five goals: medical urgency, post-transplant outcomes, biological disadvantages limiting patient access (blood type, height, and allo-sensitization), other patient access factors (promoting access for pediatric candidates and prior living organ donors), and efficiency (promoting efficient management of the organ allocation and placement system).

- The CD-based allocation system is aligned with the ideals expressed in the Final Rule.

FUNDING SOURCE

WMT is supported by K23HL138191-04.

REFERENCES

1. National organ transplant Act. Available at: https://www.gpo.gov/fdsys/pkg/STATUTE-98/pdf/STATUTE-98-Pg2339.pdf. Accessed June 13th, 2022.
2. Organ procurement and transplantation Network. Final Rule. Available at: https://www.ecfr.gov/current/title-42/chapter-I/subchapter-K/part-121. Accessed June 14, 2022.
3. Egan TM, Murray S, Bustami RT, et al. Development of the new lung allocation system in the United States. Am J Transplant 2006;6(5 Pt 2):1212–27.
4. Eberlein M, Garrity ER, Orens JB, et al. Lung allocation in the United States. Clin Chest Med 2011;32:213–22.
5. Hosenpud JD, Bennett LE, Keck BM, et al. Effect of diagnosis on survival benefit of lung transplantation for end-stage lung disease. Lancet 1998;351:24–7.
6. Egan TM. How should lungs be allocated for transplant? Semin Respir Crit Care Med 2018;39:126–37.
7. Institute of Medicine, Committee on Non- Heart-Beating Transplantation II. Non-heart- beating organ transplantation: practice and protocols. Washington DC: National Academy Press; 2000.
8. Egan TM, Edwards LB. Effect of the lung allocation on lung transplantation in the United States. J Heart Lung Transplant 2016;35:433–9.
9. Organ Procurement and Transplantation Network Thoracic Organ Transplant Committee Chaired by Cliff H. Van Meter Jr. Report of the Thoracic Organ Transplant Committee to the UNOS Board of Directors. Baltimore, MD: November 18-19, 1999.
10. A guide to calculating the lung allocation score. UNOS. Available at: https://unos.org/wp-content/uploads/unos/lung-allocation-score.pdf Accessed June 14,2022.
11. Lyu DM, Goff RR, Chan KM. The lung allocation score and its relevance. Semin Respir Crit Care Med 2021;42:346–56.
12. OPTN Thoracic Organ Transplantation Committee. Proposed modification to OPTN/UNOS policy 3.7.6 (Lung Allocation) addition of PaC02 in lung allocation system (Thoracic Organ Transplantation Committee), 2006.
13. OPTN Thoracic Transplantation Committee. Analysis of LAS by diagnosis groups before and after LAS modification in February 2015.2019.
14. Wille KM, Edwards LB, Callahan LR, et al. Characteristics of lung allocation score exception requests submitted to the national Lung Review Board. J Heart Lung Transplant 2017;36:812–4.
15. Colvin-Adams M, Valapour M, Hertz M. Lung and heart allocation in the United States. AJT 2012;12:3213–34.

16. Update cohort for calculation of lung allocation score (LAS). 2020. https://optn.transplant.hrsa.gov/media/4206/bp_202012_update-cohort-for-calculation-of-the -lung- allocation- score.pdf. [Accessed 18 May 2022].

17. McCurry KR, Shearon TH, Edwards LB, et al. Lung transplantation in the United States, 1998-2007. AJT 2009;9:942–58.

18. Valapour M, Lehr CJ, Skeans MA, et al. OPTN/SRTR 2017 annual data report:lung. AJT 2019;19:404–84.

19. Snyder JJ, Salkowski N, Wey A, et al. Organ distribution without geographic boundaries: a possible framework for organ allocation. Am J Transplant 2018;18:2635–40.

20. Organ Procurement and Transplantation Network. Geographic organ distribution principles and models recommendation report. Available at: https://optn.transplant.hrsa.gov/media/2506/geography_recommendations_report_201806.pdf. Accessed May 18, 2022.

21. Organ Procurement and Transplantation Network. Continuous distribution of lungs. Available at: https://optn.transplant.hrsa.gov/media/3111/thoracic_publiccomment_201908.pdf. Accessed May 18, 2022.

22. Organ Procurement and Transplantation Network. Establish continuous distribution of lungs. Available at: https://optn.transplant.hrsa.gov/media/4772/continuous_distribution_of_lungs-public_comment.pdf. Accessed May 18, 2022.

23. Gottlieb J, Greer M, Sommerwerck U, et al. Introduction of the lung allocation score in Germany. Am J Transplant 2014;14(6):1318–27.

24. Gottlieb J, Smits J, Schramm R, et al. Lung transplantation in Germany since the introduction of the lung allocation score. Dtsch Arztebl Int 2017;114(11):179–85.

25. Hoffman TW, Hemke AC, Zanen P, et al. Waiting list dynamics and lung transplantation outcomes after introduction of the lung allocation score in The Netherlands. Transpl Direct 2021;7(10):e760.

26. Eurotransplant. Available at: http://www.eurotransplant.org/wp-content/uploads/2020/01/LAS_professionals.pdf. Accessed last May 5 2022.

27. Auråen H, Schultz HHL, Hämmäinen P, et al. Urgent lung allocation system in the Scandiatransplant countries. J Heart Lung Transplant 2018;37(12):1403–9.

28. Paraskeva MA, Levin KC, Westall GP, et al. Lung transplantation in Australia, 1986-2018: more than 30 years in the making. Med J Aust 2018;208(10):445–50.

29. Hwang B, E. Granger, P. Jansz, M et al. Development of a Donor-Recipient Matching Algorithm for Lung Transplantation in Australia. 2021;4: S-68.

30. Hirji A, Zhao H, Ospina MB, et al. Clinical judgment versus lung allocation score in predicting lung transplant waitlist mortality. Clin Transplant 2020;34(7):e13870.

31. Cypel M, Yeung J, Donahoe L, et al. Outcomes of lung transplantation at a Canadian center using donors declined in the United States. J Thorac Cardiovasc Surg 2022;164(6):1661–8.

Organ Donation, the Non-Perfect Lung Donor, and Variability in Conversion to Transplant

Melissa B. Lesko, DO[a],*, Luis F. Angel, MD[b]

KEYWORDS

• Organ donation • Lung transplant • Donor management

KEY POINTS

- The attitudes of health care workers and other ancillary hospital staff can have a significant impact on the decision of family members to pursue organ donation. Providing additional education about the donation to hospital employees may prove to be beneficial.
- Key features of donor management include protective ventilator strategies targeting volumes around 8 mL/kg, lung recruitment protocols, euvolemic volume status, and bronchoscopic evaluation for microbial data and airway clearance.
- Organ acceptance practices are influenced by a combination of programmatic factors relating to the staff's experience with higher risk donors but are also significantly affected by prior Transplant Centers refusals for donor quality (RDQ).
- Recipients of higher sequence organs, even those previously refused for donor quality, were not shown to have any difference in mortality or incidence of primary graft dysfunction.
- Standardizing both donor management protocols by organ procurement organizations and organ acceptance practices by transplant centers would increase lung transplant rates and decrease wait times for lung transplantation.

INTRODUCTION

Transplant activity decreased in 2020 due to geographic restrictions that were self-imposed by lung transplant programs and organ procurement organizations (OPOs) during the coronavirus disease (COVID) pandemic,[1] but returned to normal ranges in 2021 and 2022. In 2020, there were 3064 candidates awaiting transplants with 2524 transplants performed in the United States. Before the implementation of the lung allocation score (LAS) in 2005, one of the most significant factors affecting transplantation was the lack of available donor lungs with only 43% of the patients on the waiting list being transplanted annually. Since then, overall organ donation has increased from 7593 in 2005 to 13,863 in 2021 (83% increase) with a concomitant increase in lung allocation from these donors, from 1285 in 2005 to 2631 in 2021 (105% increase). Over the last 5 years, the need for donor's lungs and the availability of donors has been comparable with 86% of the patients listed being transplanted annually.[2]

The implementation of donor management protocols, the utilization of designated donor hospitals or centers by OPOs and the standardization for acceptance of extended donor criteria lungs among transplant centers will, in principle, yield enough donor lungs to significantly decrease both the wait time and mortality of transplant recipients. In the last 3 years (2020 to 2022), only

The authors have nothing to disclose.
[a] Division of Pulmonary & Critical Care Medicine, NYU Langone Medical Center, 550 First Avenue, New York, NY 10016, USA; [b] NYU Langone Medical Center, 550 First Avenue, New York, NY 10016, USA
* Corresponding author.
E-mail address: Melissa.Lesko@nyulangone.org

Clin Chest Med 44 (2023) 69–75
https://doi.org/10.1016/j.ccm.2022.10.005
0272-5231/23/© 2022 Elsevier Inc. All rights reserved.

10 of 44 large OPOs (>150 donors) had a lung allo-cation rate between 25% and 30%. An average rate of lung allocation of 25% for the other 34 large OPOs would increase the number of lung trans-plants enough to close the current disparity be-tween the number of available donor lungs and the number of patients waiting for transplantation.[2]

There are several factors that influence whether eligible donors are converted into actual trans-plants. This review explores the societal factors that contribute to organ availability, and the donor protocols that have improved procurement rates, and examines the variability in organ acceptance practices and how these issues influence conver-sion to transplant.

ORGAN DONATION

Definitions. It is difficult to measure the total number of actual donors available in the United States because of a lack of standardized definition of a "po-tential donor." Even the term "eligible donors," which should incorporate a pool of donors that transplant physicians agree to have the potential to be organ donors, is often disputed given the varying limits such as age that are acceptable in different in-stitutions. The scientific registry of transplant recipi-ents (SRTR) currently calculates the conversion rate using the number of eligible deaths.[3]

FACTORS AFFECTING ORGAN DONATION

A variety of factors affect the decision of patients and family members to donate their organs. A pro-spective cohort study at a large tertiary US Hospi-tal showed that families were more likely to donate organs of patients who had apnea testing for brain death confirmation. Race also played a role with African Americans 3.7 times less likely to consent for donation.[4] Consent rates were higher when an OPO Representative had the initial conversa-tion with the family and when discussion times were longer and in the same native language. However, the use of a translator was found to negatively affect a family's decision for an organ donation.[5] Overall, the family's perception about the quality of care that their loved one received significantly affected this decision.[6–8]

Owing to their interaction with patients and care-givers alike, the beliefs of health care workers also impacted the decision of family members to pursue donation. Positive attitudes of health care profes-sionals were associated with increased donation. This type of health care worker was more likely to have a higher educational level, a personal history of a chronic disease, experience with discussions about organ donation and a positive viewpoint about family in general.[9] Interestingly, there was a significant increase in negative attitudes among younger professionals, as well as nurses, who worked in Intensive Care.[10] Ancillary staff had a more negative viewpoint than nurses, which is important given his/her frequent interactions with the patient's family. This was attributed to a poten-tial lack of understanding about the concept of brain death as well as, a reluctance to accept it as actual death.[11] These studies suggest that addi-tional education for hospital employees about or-gan donation would be beneficial.

DONOR MANAGEMENT

Despite methods that have been used to expand the pool of potential organ donors, the shortage of donor lungs continues to be an issue. This problem could be addressed with more widespread donor management protocols, as well as improved coop-eration between critical care physicians and the OPO Coordinators. Protocols used for standard crit-ical care patients result in the best outcome for opti-mizing donation of these organs. The donation of other solid organs, in particular the liver and kidneys, is relatively close to the number of consented pa-tients for organ donation. Conversely, lungs are often the most difficult organ to maintain after brain death and are therefore only retrieved from the mi-nority of donors with a wide range of variation be-tween OPOs (10% to 30%). This is due in part to direct injury to the lungs from trauma, pulmonary edema, frequent aspiration, pneumonia, volume overload, and lower lobe atelectasis. These issues are often compounded by hemodynamic instability, as well as the physiologic derangements from brain death, especially cytokine release resulting in neuro-genic pulmonary edema.[12] The frequency of these findings results in approximately 10% of organ do-nors fulfilling ideal criteria for lung donation at the time of consent for organ donation.[2] Through the implementation of donor management protocols focusing on the optimization of extended criteria do-nors, lung procurement in OPOs with best practices is between 25% and 30%, but still significantly lower than other solid organs.[13] The recent addition of donor hospitals and recovery centers by the OPOs, where lung donor management protocols are consistently implemented, is associated with higher lung donation rates.

The term "ideal donor" was first used in the early days of transplantation to describe the criteria of the quintessential lung donor. As the "ideal" lung donor is rare (<10% of total lung donors), the increased demands for lung donors prompted mul-tiple programs to consider the use of "extended" donors. After undergoing donor management protocols, these donors meet most Major Lung Donor Criteria but may still fulfill some of the minor criteria.[14]

Major Lung Donor Criteria (modifiable with donor management protocols)

- PaO_2 greater than 300 mm Hg with 100% FiO_2 (PF ratio [PFR >300]) and with a positive end-expiratory pressure (PEEP) of 5 mm Hg
- Clear chest radiograph or at least significant improvement, in particular:
  - improvement of lower lobe atelectasis with lung recruitment
  - pulmonary edema with diuresis or better heart function
  - the presence of focal unilateral infiltrates consistent with single lobar pneumonia (on broad-spectrum antibiotics for > 24 h)
- Bronchoscopy assessment with no evidence of purulent secretions consistent with multi-lobar pneumonia or evidence of large aspiration

Minor donor criteria (not modifiable social or medical factors)

- age less than 55 years
- smoking history less than 20 pack years
- no significant chest trauma
- no evidence of multiorgan failure, septic shock, or bacteremia
- no prior cardiothoracic surgery
- no organisms in bronchoalveolar cultures, in particular invasive fungal or opportunistic infections
- no history of severe asthma, chronic obstructive pulmonary disease, or pulmonary fibrosis
- no evidence of pulmonary hypertension

In an effort to optimize potential organs for donation, management protocols have been created to provide guidance on ventilator management and recruitment, fluid management and bronchoscopy. In a study from Australia, implementing an aggressive donor protocol resulted in the goal PaO_2/FiO_2 of more than 300 mm Hg in 20 of 59 potential organ donors that were initially classified as marginal donors.[15] The San Antonio Lung Transplant (SALT) Protocol used Pressure Control Ventilation with an inspiratory pressure of 25 cm H_2O and a PEEP from 10 to 15 mm Hg for 2 h to aggressively recruit donor lungs. Of the 98 donor lungs studied, the Pao_2/Fio_2 in 1/3 was able to be augmented to more than 300 mm Hg. Of 98 actual lung donors during the protocol period, 53 (54%) had initially been considered poor donors; these donors provided 64 (53%) of the 121 lung transplants.[13] Similarly, a multicenter study demonstrated initiating a protocol to optimize lung donation resulted in an increase in the number of organs procured without any increase in the incidence of primary graft failure or change in early mortality posttransplant.[13,16]

Ventilator Management

For lung recruitment, lung protective ventilator strategies are recommended, but with volumes not as restrictive as those used in patients with acute respiratory distress syndrome (ARDS). A European multicenter randomized trial examined the use of a lung protective ventilator strategy using tidal volumes of 6-8 mL/kg, PEEP of 8 to 10 cm H_2O and a closed circuit for suctioning versus a protocol using 10 to 12 mL/kg, PEEP of 3-5 cm H_2O and an open circuit for suctioning and apnea testing. The lung-protective protocol doubled lung recovery rates (54% vs 27%, $P < .005$).[17] In terms of mode of ventilation, a single-center retrospective study compared lung transplantation rates after using a standard assist control versus airway pressure release mode to manage potential donors. Donors on the conventional mode of ventilation had lower organ recovery rates (18% vs 84%). The graft survival in both groups was comparable to the national average.[18]

A consensus statement on organ donor management validates standard donor management practices and recommends the following ventilator strategy for initial management, recruitment and maintenance of donor lungs:

- Protective Ventilation targeting tidal volumes of 8 mL/kg (ideal body weight)
- PEEP 8 to 10 cm H_2O for maintenance. PEEP up to 15 cm H_2O for lung recruitment based on oxygenation.
- Plateau pressure less than 30 cm H_2O
- Maximize the inspiratory time with an I:E ratio of 1:1 to 1:1.5
- Normal range respiratory rates between 10 and 18 according to the ventilatory requirement to keep a Pco_2 between 35 and 40 mm Hg[19]

Fluid Management

Owing to the mechanism of death, most organ donors have significant hemodynamic instability. Because of this, by the time they are declared brain dead, their fluid balance may be many liters positive, yet they are still on maintenance fluids. This clinical scenario is classically seen in trauma donors and those with severe renal failure. Later, because of peripheral vasodilation and central diabetes insipidus from brain death-related sympatholysis and hormone dysregulation, hypovolemia may be present.[20] We recommend assessing volume status by monitoring the pulse pressure variation (PPV) and, in particular, recommend diuresis and a decrease in maintenance fluids if the PPV is less than 13. This is a valuable test particularly in brain-dead donors who are all on positive pressure ventilation and have no spontaneous breathing, thereby meeting the optimal conditions for PPV to be valid. Fluid management protocols focus on the maintenance of euvolemia or a net negative fluid balance and avoiding hypervolemia, but still maintaining organ perfusion through the use of vasopressors.[21] As a part of the lung donor management protocol, the SALT protocol minimized the use of crystalloids and gave diuretics as necessary to maintain an even or negative fluid balance. This protocol resulted in an increase in lung procurement although it is unclear if it was due to a combination of factors rather than the fluid goal alone.[13] A study by Minambres and colleagues[22] proved that a strict fluid balance targeting a central venous pressure less than 6 mm Hg could increase the number of lungs suitable for transplant without compromising kidney graft survival.

Bronchoscopy

A bronchoscopy should be performed in all prospective lung donors. The timing for bronchoscopy is not standardized and unfortunately is often left as the final procedure before the allocation of organs. However, for maximal improvement, we recommend performing an early bronchoscopy particularly in "non-ideal" donors who may benefit from an early diagnosis of infection or clearance of secretions to optimize lung recruitment and ameliorate atelectasis. In addition, a large volume bronchoalveolar lavage is recommended to assess for purulent secretions and to aspirate distal mucus that will improve atelectasis. In cases in which the bronchoscopy is abnormal, this procedure should be repeated to evaluate for interval change before allocation, thereby providing a more thorough assessment.

This procedure allows for:

- An airway inspection.
- Evaluation for possible aspiration.
- Removal of secretions, purulence, and blood clots.
- Testing for infection and in particular for a severe acute respiratory syndrome coronavirus 2 polymerase chain reaction (PCR) test
- Guidance of antibiotic therapy for the care of the lung donor and potential recipient.[21]

Microbiology

Microbial data from the donor are essential in guiding the posttransplant management of the organ recipient. Despite the hesitancy of some programs to accept donors with infections, donor lung colonization rates do not correlate with the incidence of pneumonia. The group from the University of Birmingham looked at the correlation between a positive donor gram stain and the rates of pneumonia. In a group of 43 patients with a positive donor gram stain, 12% developed pneumonia compared with the 9% that developed pneumonia despite having a negative donor gram stain.[23] Similarly, a study from Barcelona found that the incidence of donor allograft infection was 52%. Donor-to-host transmission of infection occurred in 7.61% of the total number of transplants at this center. The most common organism identified in donors who died of a head injury was *Staphylococcal aureus*.[24] Infections with multidrug-resistant organisms and invasive fungal or mycobacterial organisms remain a relative contraindication to transplant.[25] Early in the management of prospective organ donors, it is imperative to use broad-spectrum antibiotics empirically and adjust treatment based on available culture results.

Coronavirus Disease Donor Screening Guidelines

Donor exposed to coronavirus disease-2019 (COVID-19) within the past 10 days.

- May consider donors with a known COVID-19 exposure for transplant if it has been greater than 7 days since the exposure and
- There is at least one negative PCR test from a lower respiratory sample within 24 h of the transplant
- Computed tomography (CT) chest negative for a pulmonary infection
- The recipient has a high risk of mortality without organ transplantation.

Donor with prior confirmed COVID-19:

- Clinical resolution of symptoms due to COVID-19 and greater than 21 days from the onset of symptoms in an immunocompetent donor
- No significant pulmonary disease secondary to COVID-19
- One negative COVID PCR
- CT chest which does not demonstrate any persistent disease secondary to COVID.
- Lower respiratory tract specimen.[26]

ORGAN UTILIZATION

A significant geographic disparity existed in the allocation system. In 2017, in response to a lawsuit from a Lung Transplant Candidate in New York

City, a Federal Court changed the geographic distribution of organs from a donor-specific area to a 250-mile radius of the donor hospital. This was found to significantly change a candidate's lung transplant rate and provided the bases for a new allocation system in the United States.[27]

Despite these changes, organ acceptance rates continue to vary significantly between lung transplant centers and impact survival to transplantation.[28] When reviewing data for organs that were previously declined, it was discovered that chest imaging was a poor predictor of pulmonary edema and histologic abnormalities, whereas, donor Pao_2 had a better correlation with recipient hypoxemia and complications posttransplant.[29] A retrospective US study concluded that a higher incidence of 1-year waitlist mortality was associated with lower transplant center acceptance rates. A 10% increase in the adjusted center accepted rate would result in a decreased waitlist mortality of 36.3% and increase the likelihood of transplant by 29.5%.[30] These results beget the question, should these practices be standardized? Using data from the United Network for Organ Sharing (UNOS), a study in the United States reviewed match-run outcomes for lung offers from May 2007 to June 2014. Acceptance of an organ later in the match run sequence was associated with abnormal imaging and bronchoscopies, high-risk donors, and donor smoking history.[31] Additional features of donors that were refused for quality included a male gender, a longer ischemic time, and older age.[32] Higher transplant center volume also influenced this decision. These centers are likely more willing to accept higher sequence organs due to programmatic experience, resources such as extracorporeal membrane oxygenation (ECMO) that are available, as well as, the comfort level of the physicians making these decisions.[31] Characteristics of donor recipients for these higher sequence organs included older age, a diagnosis of obstructive lung disease, and a lower LAS. The recipient characteristics were found to be more predictive of 1 year and overall mortality than those of the donor.[32] Also, there was no correlation pertaining to increased mortality or graft dysfunction with acceptance of higher sequence organs.[31–33]

The number of RDQ has also been examined. Recipients of high refusal donor lungs did not have a higher 1 year or overall mortality. In fact, even recipients with an organ that had an RDQ greater than 10 had a similar survival. Recipients who received organs from donors in the high RDQ group were more likely to be intubated at 72 h and require treatment for rejection within the first year. Other complications such as the need for hemodialysis as well as the overall length of stay were found to be equivalent.[32] The number or prior refusals should not factor into a program's decision to accept organs. The effect of programs declining organs that are eventually accepted by other institutions is that these organs are often going to lower-priority candidates. This practice results in an increase in waitlist mortality. When this process was reviewed on the institutional level and standardized, it resulted in an increase in donor utilization and transplant volume without a significant change in primary graft dysfunction (PGD) Grade 3 and 30-day mortality.[34] This is an area that should continue to be studied in an effort to maximize the utilization of organs with a goal of meeting the demand for organ transplantation.

CONCLUSION

The rates of lung donation have increased over the past several years as a result the optimization of lungs through the implementation of donor management protocols, the creation of donor hospitals or centers, and the now common utilization of donors with extended criteria. Although transplant programs vary significantly in their acceptance rates of these organs, there is not any apparent difference in the incidence of primary graft dysfunction or overall mortality for the recipient when higher match-run sequence organs are accepted. Yet, the level of comfort accepting these donors varies among transplant programs. Despite the lower rates of lung donation compared with other solid organs, a modest increase in lung procurement will allow the gap between the number of available donor lungs and the number of recipients on the transplant list to narrow.

CLINICS CARE POINTS

- Donor Management plays a critical role in increasing the number of available organs for lung donation.
- Key Features of Donor Mangement Include lung recruitment protocols, protective ventilator strategies targeting lung volumes of 8ml/kg, achieving a euvolemic fluid balance, and bronchoscopic evaluation for microbial data as well as airway clearance.
- Organ acceptance rates vary significantly between lung transplant centers and impact surival to transplantation.

- Recipients of higher sequence organs even those previously refused for donor quality, were shown to have no difference in mortality or incidence of primary graft dysfunction; therefore, the number of prior refusals should not factor into any program's decision to accept organs.

REFERENCES

1. Valapour M, Lehr CJ, Skeans MA, et al. OPTN/SRTR 2020 annual data report: lung. Am J Transpl 2022; 22(Suppl 2):438–518.
2. https://optn.transplant.hrsa.gov/data/view-data-reports/national-data/ (Accessed August 2022).
3. Scientific Registry of Transplant Recipients. Measuring donor conversion rates. Available at: Srtr. org/about-the-data/guide-to-key-opo-metrics/opoguidearticles/donor-conversion.
4. Kananeh MF, Brady PD, Mehta CB, et al. Factors that affect consent rate for organ donation after brain death: a 12-year registry. J Neurol Sci 2020; 416:117036.
5. Ebadat A, Brown CV, Ali S, et al. Improving organ donation rates by modifying the family approach process. J Trauma Acute Care Surg 2014;76(6): 1473–5.
6. Siminoff LA, Gordon N, Hewlett J, et al. Factors influencing families' consent for donation of solid organs for transplantation. JAMA 2001;286(1):71–7.
7. DeJong W, Franz HG, Wolfe SM, et al. Requesting organ donation: an interview study of donor and nondonor families. Am J Crit Care 1998;7(1):13–23. Available at: https://www.ncbi.nlm.nih.gov/pubmed/9429679.
8. Rodrigue JR, Cornell DL, Howard RJ. Organ donation decision: comparison of donor and nondonor families. Am J Transpl 2006;6(1):190–8.
9. Araujo C, Siqueira M. Brazilian health care professionals: a study of attitudes toward organ donation. Transpl Proc 2016;48(10):3241–4.
10. Damar HT, Ordin YS, Top FU. Factors affecting attitudes toward organ donation in health care professionals. Transpl Proc 2019;51(7):2167–70.
11. Zambudio AR, Conesa C, Ramirez P, et al. What is the attitude of hospital transplant-related personnel toward donation? J Heart Lung Transpl 2006;25(8): 972–6.
12. Munshi L, Keshavjee S, Cypel M. Donor management and lung preservation for lung transplantation. Lancet Respir Med 2013;1(4):318–28.
13. Angel LF, Levine DJ, Restrepo MI, et al. Impact of a lung transplantation donor-management protocol on lung donation and recipient outcomes. Am J Respir Crit Care Med 2006;174(6):710–6.
14. Van Raemdonck D, Neyrinck A, Verleden GM, et al. Lung donor selection and management. Proc Am Thorac Soc 2009;6(1):28–38.
15. Gabbay E, Williams TJ, Griffiths AP, et al. Maximizing the utilization of donor organs offered for lung transplantation. Am J Respir Crit Care Med 1999;160(1): 265–71.
16. Minambres E, Perez-Villares JM, Chico-Fernandez M, et al. Lung donor treatment protocol in brain dead-donors: a multicenter study. J Heart Lung Transpl 2015;34(6):773–80.
17. Mascia L, Pasero D, Slutsky AS, et al. Effect of a lung protective strategy for organ donors on eligibility and availability of lungs for transplantation: a randomized controlled trial. JAMA 2010;304(23): 2620–7.
18. Hanna K, Seder CW, Weinberger JB, et al. Airway pressure release ventilation and successful lung donation. Arch Surg 2011;146(3):325–8.
19. Copeland H, Hayanga JWA, Neyrinck A, et al. Donor heart and lung procurement: a consensus statement. J Heart Lung Transpl 2020;39(6):501–17.
20. Meyfroidt G, Gunst J, Martin-Loeches I, et al. Management of the brain-dead donor in the ICU: general and specific therapy to improve transplantable organ quality. Intensive Care Med 2019;45(3):343–53.
21. Kotloff RM, Blosser S, Fulda GJ, et al. Management of the potential organ donor in the ICU: Society of critical care medicine/American College of chest physicians/Association of organ procurement organizations consensus statement. Crit Care Med 2015;43(6):1291–325.
22. Minambres E, Rodrigo E, Ballesteros MA, et al. Impact of restrictive fluid balance focused to increase lung procurement on renal function after kidney transplantation. Nephrol Dial Transpl 2010; 25(7):2352–6.
23. Weill D, Dey GC, Hicks RA, et al. A positive donor gram stain does not predict outcome following lung transplantation. J Heart Lung Transpl 2002; 21(5):555–8.
24. Ruiz I, Gavalda J, Monforte V, et al. Donor-to-host transmission of bacterial and fungal infections in lung transplantation. Am J Transpl 2006;6(1): 178–82.
25. Arjuna A, Mazzeo AT, Tonetti T, et al. Management of the potential lung donor. Thorac Surg Clin 2022; 32(2):143–51.
26. Holm A MM, Vos R. . Deceased donor and recipient selection for cardiothoracic transplantation during the COVID-19 pandemic. 2021. International Society of Heart and Lung Transplantation (ishlt.org/governance/covid-19-information).
27. Kosztowski M, Zhou S, Bush E, et al. Geographic disparities in lung transplant rates. Am J Transpl 2019;19(5):1491–7.

28. Wey A, Valapour M, Skeans MA, et al. Heart and lung organ offer acceptance practices of transplant programs are associated with waitlist mortality and organ yield. Am J Transpl 2018;18(8):2061–7.

29. Ware YW L, Fang X, Warnock M, et al. Assessment of lungs rejected for transplantation and implications for donor selection. Lancet 2002;360:619–20.

30. Mulvihill MS, Lee HJ, Weber J, et al. Variability in donor organ offer acceptance and lung transplantation survival. J Heart Lung Transpl 2020;39(4): 353–62.

31. Harhay MO, Porcher R, Thabut G, et al. Donor lung sequence number and survival after lung transplantation in the United States. Ann Am Thorac Soc 2019;16(3):313–20.

32. Singh E, Schecter M, Towe C, et al. Sequence of refusals for donor quality, organ utilization, and survival after lung transplantation. J Heart Lung Transpl 2019;38(1):35–42.

33. Axtell AL, Moonsamy P, Melnitchouk S, et al. Increasing donor sequence number is not associated with inferior outcomes in lung transplantation. J Card Surg 2020;35(2):286–93.

34. G. Loor CL, J. Morrow, T. Grabowski, et al. Increasing lung utilization: Implementaion of a dedicated donor screening program jhtlonlineorg

Expanding the Lung Donor Pool

Donation After Circulatory Death, Ex-Vivo Lung Perfusion and Hepatitis C Donors

Sahar A. Saddoughi, MD, PhD[a], Marcelo Cypel, MD, MSc[b],*

KEYWORDS

- Donation after circulatory death • lung transplantation • Ex-Vivo Lung Perfusion
- Hepatitis C donors

KEY POINTS

- Innovative ways to increase the lung donor pool such as extended criteria and DCD donors help to decrease the waitlist morality and waitlist times for lung transplantation.
- Utilization of DCD lungs remain underutilized in the United States despite similar long-term outcomes.
- Implementation of EVLP has expanded the use of extended criteria and DCD lungs for transplantation.
- Use of Hepatitis C donors for lung transplantation are on the rise due to use of oral anti-viral treatments.

INTRODUCTION

Organ shortage remains a limiting factor in lung transplantation.[1] Traditionally, donation after brain death has been the main source of lungs used for transplantation; however, to meet the demand of patients requiring lung transplantation it is crucial to find innovative methods for organ donation. The implementation of extended donors,[2] lung donation after circulatory death (DCD),[3,4] the use of ex-vivo lung perfusion (EVLP) systems,[5–10] and more recently the acceptance of hepatitis C donors have started to close the gap between organ donors and recipients in need of lung transplantation.[11] This article focuses on the expansion of donor lungs for transplantation after DCD, the use of EVLP in evaluating extended criteria lungs, and the use of lung grafts from donors with hepatitis C.

Use of Lungs After Donation After Cardiac Death Procurement

The utilization of lungs after DCD remains low in the United States. A recent publication examining the UNOS database demonstrated that only 2.6% of lung transplants in the United States from 2005 to 2020 were from DCD donors.[12] DCD procurement is more labor and resource intensive and therefore requires significant investment from transplant programs in order to be successful. The Maastricht classification organizes DCD into 5 categories, ranging from controlled to uncontrolled donation (**Table 1**). Most of the organ

a Division of Thoracic Surgery and Department of Cardiovascular Surgery, Mayo Clinic, 200 First Street SW, Rochester, MN 55905, USA; b Toronto Lung Transplant Program, Toronto General Hospital, 200 Elizabeth Street, 9N983 Toronto, ON M5G 2C4, Canada
* Corresponding author.
E-mail address: Marcelo.Cypel@uhn.ca

Clin Chest Med 44 (2023) 77–83
https://doi.org/10.1016/j.ccm.2022.10.006
0272-5231/23/© 2022 Published by Elsevier Inc.

Table 1
Maastricht classification of DCD[19]

CLASS	Category	Definition
Uncontrolled	I	Death on arrival to hospital
	II	Death with Unsuccessful resuscitation
Controlled	III	Awaiting cardiac arrest
	IV	Unexpected cardiac arrest in a heart-beating donor
	V	Euthanasia

donation occurs with Maastricht classification III: controlled donation after cardiac arrest.[4] In this type of donation, the patient is not declared brain dead; however, it has been determined that there is no meaningful recovery possible and therefore consideration of withdrawal of life-sustained therapies (WLST) is considered as part of standard medical practice. When this is determined, the family or individual authorized to make health care decisions is approached for possible DCD organ donation followed by WLST, including extubation. The vital signs of the donor are closely monitored and recorded, once no pulse is felt, no electrical heart activity recorded, death is determined, and a period (usually 5 minutes) of hands off or no-touch period is started. The WLST is frequently done in the operating room (OR) or in the intensive care unit and followed by transport to the OR and reintubation. The unpredictability of the donor passing within a designated time frame also makes DCD procurement more challenging, as the yield of organ donation is lower than with brain-dead donors.[13] The time interval from withdrawal of life-sustaining support to declaration of death for a lung graft can vary from 60 minutes to 3 hours depending on the transplant program (**Fig. 1**). There is obvious concern regarding lung injury during this period, especially if blood pressure is very low, making some program less enthusiastic about using these organs. It is important to note that lungs are less prone to warm ischemic injury as long as they remain well ventilated. This is certainly an advantage of lung DCD procurement when compared with other organs that are more sensitive to warm ischemic injury such as the heart and liver. Importantly, 2 recent publications examined the relationship of agonal phase during DCD

procurement and recipient survival and found no significant differences in lung transplantation.[14,15] In addition, DCD procurement requires specialized training, as it can be more difficult to evaluate the lung function. Before withdrawal of life-sustaining support, the evaluation of the lung is the same for brain-dead and DCD donors. Importantly, heparin should be administered 5 minutes before withdrawal of life-sustaining support, although some European programs have not used heparin and have obtained good results. Once death has been confirmed by 2 independent physicians and after an important no-touch period, the chest can be opened and the patient reintubated. Ventilation is resumed and bronchoscopy performed. Pericardium is opened, the pulmonary artery cannulated, and prostaglandin E_1 administered with manual compression of the heart to circulate the drug. Pulmonary flush is administered, and from this point on, the procurement is similar to brain death donation. During the flush, the lungs are examined and recruited to eliminate atelectasis. Importantly, during DCD procurements, suitability of the lung for transplant can be more difficult to evaluate, as there is no arterial blood gas information, and it can be more difficult to fully appreciate the lung mechanics/function with no circulating blood. The evaluation of the lungs to properly deflate and manual palpation for edema/consolidation are critically important during lung DCD procurement.

Survival outcomes after transplantation with DCD lungs have been reported as single-institution experiences, meta-analysis, and database analysis.[16–19] The largest study reported uses the International Society for Heart and Lung Transplantation (ISHLT) Registry, examining controlled DCDs performed from 2003 to 2017. In this study 1090 cDCD (controlled DCD) lung transplants were performed, and there was no difference in 1- or 5-year survival rates when compared with brain-dead donors[18]; this is consistent with other published reports from single-institution experiences from around the world.[20–22]

Our knowledge of uncontrolled DCD, where donors come into the hospital already suffering from cardiac arrest is still in its infancy.[23–26] There have been several small case series demonstrating the proof of concept in procuring and transplanting these lungs. However, the logistics are quite complicated and obtaining consent for this type of procedure in a timely manner can be difficult. Despite these challenges, uDCD (uncontrolled DCD) has been successfully performed in several countries and presents a major opportunity for significant expansion of lung donation in the near future. It is important to note that utilization of EVLP is higher in this group, and the yield of suitable lungs is lower than cDCD.[23–26]

DCD type V occurs after euthanasia or medical assistance in dying[27,28] (see **Table 1**); this is a controversial topic and only accepted in a few countries such as Canada, Belgium, Netherlands, and Spain. The conventional assessment of lungs before procurement is usually not available in this group of donors. Very rarely would information such as arterial blood gases, computed tomography of the chest, or bronchoscopy be available. Despite this, it has been found that the quality of these lungs is often excellent and a valuable source of donor lungs with excellent recipient outcomes. The ethics surrounding this category of donation is particularly sensitive, and extra steps have been put in place to maintain the integrity of the donation process.[28] Importantly, the option of organ donation is only occurring after the process of medical assistance in dying is approved by a completely independent team.

Evaluating Lungs with Ex-Vivo Lung Perfusion

EVLP is an excellent tool to allow for further evaluation and physiologic assessment of lungs after procurement[29]; this additional testing is particularly useful for extended criteria lungs to help teams make a final decision on whether the lungs are appropriate for implantation.[30–32] The advantage of this technology is that it allows lung transplant programs to take calculated risk and as a result can help programs grow. Starting a DCD program or using extended lungs can create anxiety especially when transplant outcomes are highly scrutinized. However, having EVLP technology allows the transplant team to simulate lung implantation to ensure good lung function before recipient implantation; this includes bronchoscopic assessment, manual palpation of the lungs, arterial blood gas, ventilatory mechanics, pulmonary vascular mechanics, and chest radiograph (CXR) (**Fig. 2**). Through EVLP, lung transplant programs have reported a 15% to 20% increase in volume.[32–34] The most common indications used for EVLP include Pao_2 less than 300 mm Hg, declining P/F ratio, concerning bronchoscopy findings, concern for pneumonia or pulmonary edema, DCD procurement, and high-risk donor (**Table 2**). In general, contraindications for EVLP include severe pulmonary contusions resultant from mechanical trauma and established consolidative pneumonia. Importantly, the outcomes of lung transplant after EVLP assessment have been encouraging with no differences in primary graft dysfunction (PGD) grade 3 at 72 hours, 1-year survival, long-term survival, and chronic lung allograft dysfunction.[5,35] The NOVEL trial[36] and the EXPAND trial[37] were the first multicenter publications looking at 1-year outcomes following use of EVLP and reported no difference in survival at 1 year.

The Toronto Lung Transplant Program has a dedicated EVLP team on site that uses a well-developed and widely adopted protocol. Although

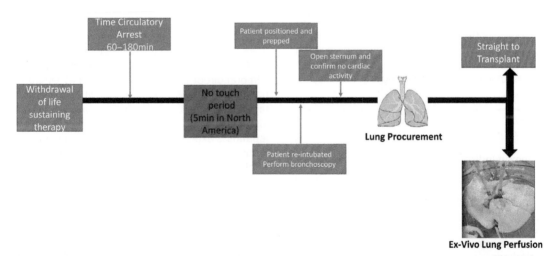

Fig. 1. Timeline for DCD lung procurement. Prior to withdrawal of life sustaining therapy, heparin is administered (100U/kg). Once the patient is extubated, vitals are closely monitored until circulatory arrest. Next, a 5 min no touch period begins and then two physicians will evaluate the donor and declare death. The donor will proceed to the OR to be re-intubated, and sternotomy is performed to allow for lung procurement. Once the lungs have been evaluated, they can proceed directly to transplant, or may need further evaluation with EVLP.

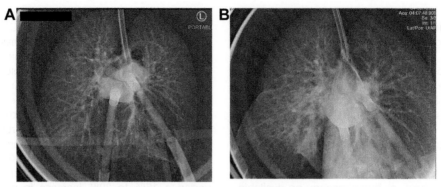

Fig. 2. Chest Xray assessment of donor lungs on EVLP. (*A*). The CXR demonstrates clear lung fields bilaterally after 3h of EVLP. All the parameters measured during EVLP were consistent with good performance of the lungs and they were accepted for transplantation. (*B*). This CXR demonstrates significant consolidation of the left lower lobe in lungs that were ultimately declined for transplantation.

it is certainly advantageous to have an onsite EVLP team, it does require specialized training and understanding of EVLP that may not be available at smaller transplant programs. To overcome this issue, centralized EVLP assessment sites (Baltimore, MD and Jacksonville, FL) were created in the United States.[38] At these locations, programs from all over the country can send their lungs after procurement for assessment. Surgeons who have expertise in EVLP are available to help assess the lungs and determine if they are appropriate for transplantation. One concern about these centralized centers is the fact that they can extend preservation time. However, numerous reports indicate that use of EVLP can safely extend overall preservation time without compromising short- and long-term survival outcomes.[39,40] Other reports suggest that there is an increased risk for PGD and 1-year mortality with increased cold preservation of the lungs after EVLP.[41] Understanding lung preservation time, temperature, and the role of EVLP is an important area of ongoing research.

Another unique aspect of EVLP is using it as a platform in the advancement of lung transplant science. EVLP can be used to study new drugs to recondition or treat lungs to make them suitable for transplantation. Examples include treatment of infection,[42,43] pulmonary embolism,[44] lung injury,[45] hepatitis C,[46] use of gene therapy,[47] or modifying organ blood type.[48] A unique aspect to EVLP treatment is the option of both inhaled treatments as well as intravenous treatments.[49,50] EVLP is an exciting option to evaluate high-risk donor lungs, leading to growth of lung transplant programs and also pushing the boundaries in the treatment of otherwise non-transplantable lungs.

Outcomes of Lung Transplantation with Use of Lung from Hepatitis C Donors

There is increasing utilization of lungs from hepatitis C donors, largely due to excellent outcomes with oral direct-acting antiviral agent (DAA) treatments for hepatitis C. A donor who has active hepatitis C infection will have a positive nucleic acid test (NAT+), whereas donors with recent hepatitis C exposure, treated infection, or spontaneous resolution may be NAT−, but antibody+[51] (**Table 3**). Knowing this information about the donor is important when explaining the risk of transmission to the lung transplant recipient. For example, there is very low risk of transmission for an NAT−/antibody+ donor, whereas donors that are NAT+ have a much higher transmission risk and require treatment. Thankfully, use of DAAs in the setting of NAT+ donors has led to similar short-term survival and graft function as hepatitis C−negative donor lung grafts.[52] A recent prospective, single-arm trial using hepatitis C donors whose lungs were transplanted into hepatitis

Table 2 Indications for EVLP	
Common Indications	**Other Indications**
Pao$_2$<300 mm Hg	Pulmonary embolism
Declining Pao$_2$/Fio$_2$ ratio	Clinical trial
Concerning bronchoscopic findings	Procurement by unknown surgeon
DCD procurement	Logistics
Concern for pulmonary edema or pneumonia	
High risk donor	

Table 3 Hepatitis C status and implications[51]		
NAT	Antibody	Infection Status and Treatment Plan
+	+	Active infection, needs treatment if used for implantation
+	-	Possible active infection, needs treatment if used for implantation
-	+	Recent exposure, no active infection, no treatment needed
-	-	No active infection, no treatment needed

C–negative recipients with 8 weeks postimplant treatment of glecaprevir-pibrentasvir led to equivalent outcomes at 1 year.[11] In Toronto, treatment of NAT+ donor lungs begins before implantation, where the recipient receives ezetimibe in combination with glecaprevir-pibrentasvir on the day of transplant and is continued postimplant for only 7 days.[53] In many other programs, the recipients are evaluated with frequent blood tests to document hepatitis C virus positivity and genomic viral classification before starting therapy with DAA. Using this protocol, no recipient infection was observed thus far in more than 50 patients. The landscape of hepatitis C–positive donor lungs is changing, and examination of the UNOS database demonstrated that 189 patients have been transplanted with hepatitis C NAT+ lungs from 2016 to 2019 with no difference in short-term survival or outcomes.[54] The ISHLT expert consensus on utilization of hepatitis C donors in cardiothoracic transplant was published in 2020 with important guidelines regarding use, ethics, and treatment of hepatitis C donors.[51] Importantly, although NAT donors do not require treatment, they still require surveillance of hepatitis C, usually at 1 month and 3 months after transplantation. Current guidelines suggest that there is not enough evidence to change immunosuppression regimens while undergoing treatment of hepatitis C, but there is ongoing discussion and opinions about this topic.[51] In addition, there is no consensus on type and duration of treatment, and multiple options have been tested and published. As a community, we need to continue to decrease the stigmata associated with hepatitis C donors, especially in the setting of encouraging survival and graft function results in lung transplantation.

SUMMARY

Lung transplantation continues to grow in part due to expansion of donor lungs and innovative methods of procurement and preservation. The ability to assess and evaluate lungs postprocurement with EVLP to ascertain suitability of transplantation has opened the door to use of extended criteria donors by lowering the associated risk. Currently, controlled DCD procurement for lung transplant is an underutilized resource of good donor lungs in the United States. As we adopt this method of procurement into becoming mainstream, we will continue to push the boundaries on lung preservation (time and temperature),[48] advancing new treatment strategies to transform nontransplantable lungs and expand the indications of donor lungs; this is certainly an exciting time to be part of the lung transplant field.

DISCLOSURE

The authors have nothing to disclose.

REFERENCES

1. Chiu S, Mills SE, Bharat A. Expanding the lung donor pool and improving outcomes. JAMA Surg 2019;154(12):1151.
2. Aigner C, Winkler G, Jaksch P, et al. Extended donor criteria for lung transplantation-a clinical reality. Eur J Cardiothorac Surg 2005;27:757–61.
3. Dominguez-Gil B, Ascher N, Capron AM, et al. Expanding controlled donation after the- circulatory determination of death: statement from an international collaborative. Intensive Care Med 2021; 47(3):265–81.
4. Holm AM, Courtwright A, Olland A, et al. ISHLT position paper on thoracic organ transplantation in controlled donation after circulatory determination of death (cDCD). J Heart Lung Transplant 2022; 41(6):671–7.
5. Divithotawela C, Cypel M, Martinu T, et al. Long-term outcomes of lung transplant with ex vivo lung perfusion. JAMA Surg 2019;154(12):1143–50.
6. Cypel M, Keshavjee S, Ex Vivo Lung Perfusion. Operative techniques in thoracic and cardiovascular surgery 2004;19(14):433–42.
7. Halpern SE, Kesseli SJ, Au S, et al. Lung Transplantation after Ex Vivo Lung Perfusion versus static cold storage: an institutional cost analysis. Am J Transpl 2021;22(2):552–64. online PMID: 34379885.
8. Nakajima D, Date H. Ex vivo lung perfusion in lung transplantation. Gen Thorac Cardiovasc Surg 2021;69(4):625–30.
9. Cypel M, Keshavjee S. Extracorporeal lung perfusion. Curr Opin Organ Transpl 2011;16(5):469–75.

10. Cypel M, Keshavjee S. Strategies for safe donor expansion: donor management, donations after cardiac death, ex-vivo lung perfusion. Curr Opin Organ Transpl 2013;18(5):513–7.

11. Lewis TC, Lesko M, Rudym D, et al. One-year immunologic outcomes of lung transplantation utilizing hepatitis C-viremic donors. Clinical Transpl 2022;36(8):e14749.

12. Bobba CM, Whitson BA, Henn MC, et al. Trends in donation after circulatory death in lung transplanation in the United States: impack of era. Transpl Int 2022;35:10172.

13. Lindermann J, Dageforde LA, Vachharajani N, et al. Cost evaluation of a donation after cardiac death program: how cost per organ compares to other donor types. J Am Coll Surg 2018;226:909–16.

14. Levvey B, Keshavjee S, Cypel M, et al. Influence of lung donor agonal and warm ischemic times on early mortality: analyses from the ISHLT DCD Lung Transplant Registry. J Heart Lung Transpl 2019;38(1):26–34.

15. Qaqish R, Watanabe Y, Hoetzenecker K, et al. Impact of donor time to cardiac arrest in lung donation after circulatory death. J Thorac Cardiovasc Surg 2021;161:1546–55.

16. Cypel M, Levvey B, Van Raemdonck D, et al. Lung transplantation using controlled donation after circulatory death donors: trials and tribulations. J Heart Lung Transpl 2016;35(1):146–7.

17. Cypel M, Levvey B, Van Raemdonck D, et al. International society for heart and lung transplantation donation after circulatory death Registry report. J Heart Lung Transpl 2015;34(10):1278–82.

18. Raemdonck DV, Keshavjee S, Levvey B, et al. Donation after circulatory death in lung transplantation-five-year follow-up from ISHLT Registry. J Heart Lung Transpl 2019;38(12):1235–45.

19. Thuong A, Ruiz A, Evrard P, et al. New classification of donation after circulatory death donors definitions and terminology. Transpl Int 2016;29:749–59.

20. Krutsinger D, Reed RM, Blevins A, et al. Lung Transplantation from donation after cardiocirculatory death: a systematic review and meta-analysis. J Heart Lung Transpl 2015;34:675–84.

21. Inci I, Hillinger S, Schneiter D, et al. Lung transplantation with controlled donation after circulatory death donors. Ann Thorac Cardiovasc Surg 2018;24:296–302.

22. De Oliveira NC, Osaki S, Maloney JD, et al. Lung Transplantation with donation after cardiac death donors: long-term follow-up in a single center. J Thorac Cardiovasc Surg 2010;139:1306–15.

23. Egan T, Blackwell J, Birchard K, et al. Assessment of lungs for transplant recovered from uncontrolled donation after circulatory determination of death donors. Ann Am Thorac Soc 2017;14:S251.

24. Healey A, Watanabe Y, Mills C, et al. Initial lung transplantation experience with uncontrolled donation after cardiac death in North America. Am J Transpl 2020;20:1574–81.

25. de Antonio DG, Marcos R, Laporta R, et al. Results of clinical lung transplant from uncontrolled non-heart-beating donors. J Heart Lung Transpl 2007;26:529–34.

26. Suberviola B, Mons R, Ballesteros MA, et al. Excellent long-term outcome with lungs obtained from uncontrolled donation after circulatory death. Am J Transpl 2019;19:1195–201.

27. Watanabe T, Kawashima M, Kohno M, et al. Outcomes of lung transplantation from organ donation after medical assistance in dying: first North American Experience. Am J Transpl 2022;22(6):1637–45.

28. Ceulemans LJ, Vanluyten C, Monbaliu D, et al. Lung transplant outcome following donation after euthanasia. J Heart Lung Transpl 2022;41(6):745–54.

29. Reeb J, Keshavjee S, Cypel M. Expanding the lung donor pool: advancements and emerging pathways. Curr Opin Organ Transpl 2015;20(5):498–505.

30. Okahara S, Levvey B, McDonald M, et al. An audit of lung donor pool: optimal current donation strategies and the potential of novel time-extended donation after circulatory death donation. Heart Lung Circ 2021;S1443-9506(21):00573–4.

31. Suzuki Y, Cantu E, Christie JD. Primary graft dysfunction. Semin Respir Crit Care Med 2013;34(3):305–19.

32. Tane S, Noda K, Shigemura N. Ex Vivo Lung Perfusion: a key tool for translational science in the lungs. Chest 2017;151(6):1220–8.

33. Valenza F, Rosso L, Coppola S, et al. Ex vivo lung perfusion to improve donor lung function and increase the number of organs available for transplantation. Transpl Int 2014;27(6):553–61.

34. Munshi L, Keshavjee S, Cypel M. Donor management and lung preservation for lung transplantation. Lancet Repir Med 2013;1(4):318–28.

35. Cypel M, Yeung JC, Liu M, et al. Normothermic ex vivo lung perfusion in clinical lung transplantation. N Engl J Med 2011;364(15):1431–40.

36. Sanchez PG, Davis RD, D'Ovidio F, et al. The NOVEL lung trial one-year outcomes. JHLT 2014;33(4):S71–2.

37. Loor G, Warnecke G, Villavicencio M, et al. Portable normothermic ex-vivo lung perfusion, ventilation, and functional assessment with the Organ Care System on donor lung use for transplantation from extended-criteria donors (EXPAND): a single-arm, pivotal trial. Lancet 2019;7(11):P975–84.

38. Bery A, Ali A, Cypel M, Kreisel. Centralized Organ Recovery and Reconditioning Centers. Thorac Surg Clin 2022;32(2):167–74.

39. Yeung JC, Krueger T, Yasufuku K, et al. Outcomes after transplantation of lungs preserved for more than 12 hrs. A Retrospective Study Lancet Respir Med 2017;5(2):119–24.

40. Hsin MK, Iskender I, Nakajima D, et al. Extension of donor lung preservation with hypothermic storage after normothermic ex vivo lung perfusion. J Heart Lung Transpl 2016;35(1):130–6.

41. Leiva-Juarez M, Urso A, Tomas EA, et al. Extended post-ex vivo lung perfusion cold preservation predicts primary graft dysfunction and mortality: results from a multicentric study. J Heart Lung Transpl 2020; 39(9):954–61.

42. Nakajima D, Cypel M, Bonato R, et al. Ex vivo perfusion treatment of infection in human donor lungs. Am J Transpl 2016;16(4):1229–37.

43. Andreasson A, Karamanou DM, Perry JD, et al. The effect of ex vivo lung perfusion on microbial load in human donor lungs. J Heart Lung Transpl 2014; 33(9):910–6.

44. Inci I, Yamada Y, Hillinger S, et al. Successful lung transplantation after donor lung reconditioning with urokinase in ex vivo lung perfusion system. Ann Thorac Surg 2014;98(5):1837–8.

45. Weathington NM, Alvarez D, Sembrat J, et al. Ex vivo lung perfusion as a human platform for preclinical small molecule testing. JCI Insight 2018;3(19): e95515.

46. Galasso M, Feld JJ, Watanabe Y, et al. Inactivating hepatitis C virus in donor lungs using light therapies during normothermic ex vivo lung perfusion. Nat Commun 2019;10(1):481.

47. Machuca TN, Cypel M, Bonato R, et al. Safety and Efficacy of Ex Vivo Donor Lung Adenoviral IL-10 gene therapy in a large animal lung transplant survival model. Hum Gene Ther 2017;28(9):757–65.

48. Ali A, Wang A, Ribeiro RVP, et al. Static lung storage at 10C maintains mitochondrial health and preserves donor organ function. Sci Transl Med 2021; 13(611):eabf7601.

49. Michaelsen VS, Ribeiro RVP, Ali A, et al. Safety of continuous 12-hour delivery of antimicrobial doses of inhaled nitric oxide during ex vivo lung perfusion. J Thorac Cardiovasc Surg 2022;163(3):841–9.

50. Haam S, Lee JG, Paik HC, et al. Hydrogen gas inhalation during ex vivo lung perfusion of donor lungs recovered after cardiac death. J Heart Lung Transpl 2018;37(10):1271–8.

51. Aslam S, Grossi P, Schlendorf KH, et al. Utlizations of hepatitis C virus-infected organ donors in cardiothoracic transplantation: an ISHLT expert consensus statement. J Heart Lung Transpl 2020;39(5):418–32.

52. Woolley AE, Singh SK, Goldberg HJ, et al. Heart and lung transplants from HCV-infected donors to uninfected recipients. N Engl J Med 2019;380:1606–17.

53. Feld JJ, Cypel M, Kumar D, et al. Short-course, direct-acting antivirals and ezetimibe to prevent HCV infection in recipients of organs from HCV-infected donors: a phase 3, single-cetre, open-label study. Lancet Gastroenterol Hepatol 2020;5(7): 649–57.

54. Li SS, Osho A, Moonsamy P, et al. Outomes of lung transplantation from hepatitis C viremic donors. Ann Thorac Surg 2022;113(5):1598–607.

The Highly Sensitized Recipient
Pretransplant and Posttransplant Considerations

Andrew Courtwright, MD, PhD[a], Carl Atkinson, PhD[b], Andres Pelaez, MD[c],*

KEYWORDS

- DSA • HLA • Highly sensitized • Lung transplantation

KEY POINTS

- Lung transplant candidates with anti-HLA antibodies against ≥80% of potential donors are considered highly sensitized. This group is at increased risk for prolonged wait time and waitlist mortality.
- Advances in laboratory methods for characterizing HLA antibodies, including donor-specific antibodies (DSA), have allowed for the development of protocols to risk-stratify pretransplant DSA and to provide more targeted immunosuppression (ie, desensitization) for highly sensitized candidates.
- Desensitization protocols typically include preoperative or perioperative HLA antibody-targeted therapy, such as therapeutic plasma exchange, intravenous immunoglobulin, and B-cell targeting agents.
- Several single-center studies have shown that highly sensitized candidates have similar overall survival and freedom from chronic lung allograft dysfunction as nonsensitized candidates, when appropriate pretransplant DSA risk stratification or desensitization is used.
- Multicenter studies are needed to identify the optimal approach for successful transplantation in highly sensitized candidates, including the ideal time and extent of desensitization.

INTRODUCTION

Lung transplant candidates are considered sensitized if they have one or more HLA antibodies directed against potential donors. Sensitization can occur from a variety of exposures, including prior pregnancy (particularly multiple pregnancies with different fathers), autoimmune disease, prior infections, transfusions, or environmental contacts.[1–5] The extent of sensitization is formally expressed by the calculated panel reactive antibody (cPRA), which ranges from 1% (antibodies against 1% of possible donors) to 100% (antibodies against all possible donors). Although there are important nuances to cPRA (for example,

antibodies against DP antigens are not currently reflected in the US cPRA calculator), most transplant programs use cPRA as a metric of the difficulty of finding an HLA-compatible donor. Unsurprisingly, highly sensitized patients (defined here as having a cPRA ≥ 80%) have reduced access to donor pools and now receive a higher score in the recently implemented continuous allocation system in the United States. Between 2005 and 2019, only 526 lung recipients (or 2.6% of all lung transplants) were highly sensitized.[6] Because there are no national data on patients referred for lung transplants but not listed because of the degree of sensitization, the number of potential candidates in this group is likely significantly higher.

a Hospital of University of Pennsylvania, 3400 Spruce Street, Philadelphia, PA 19104, USA; b University of Florida, 1600 Southwest Archer Road, Gainesville, FL 32608, USA; c Jackson Health System, University of Miami, Miller School of Medicine, Miami Transplant Institute, 1801 Northwest 9th Avenue, Miami, FL 33136, USA
* Corresponding author.
E-mail address: apelaez@med.miami.edu

Clin Chest Med 44 (2023) 85–93
https://doi.org/10.1016/j.ccm.2022.10.007

Multiple single-center and national cohort studies have demonstrated that highly sensitized patients have almost twice the wait time as non-sensitized patients (mean of 294 days vs 143 days).[7] A third of highly sensitized patients wait more than a year for a transplant.[6] Highly sensitized patients are also 52% less likely to receive a lung transplant, and 92% more likely to die on the waitlist than nonsensitized candidates.[8] Unsurprisingly, many transplant programs are thus unwilling to list highly sensitized patients or offer advanced mechanical support, given anticipated difficulties in finding a compatible donor.[4] Sensitization and access to donor pools should be considered an especially pressing concern for the lung transplant community, given health equity implications. Women, particularly black and Hispanic women, are significantly more likely to be highly sensitized than white and non-white men.[6] Sensitization compounds the multiple other barriers to accessing transplantation for these groups.[9]

The central concern regarding transplanting highly sensitized candidates relates to the potential impact of the circulating antibodies on post-transplant outcomes. Several early studies in lung transplantation demonstrated the potential for complications when transplant proceeds in the presence of donor-specific antibodies (DSA). This includes hyperacute rejection as well as early antibody-mediated rejection (AMR).[8,10,11] However, avoiding all DSA at the time of transplant does not guarantee a successful postoperative outcome. Highly sensitized patients are more likely to form de novo DSA, which have been associated with AMR, chronic lung allograft dysfunction (CLAD), and decreased survival.[12–14] Here, the authors focus on strategies to navigate highly sensitized candidates to and through lung transplantation, with an emphasis on individualized HLA antibody profile assessments combined with tailored perioperative immunosuppression protocols.

TRANSPLANTING THE HIGHLY SENSITIZED PATIENT
Antibody Interrogation

Histocompatibility testing in lung transplantation aims to assess candidates for preformed DSA. These antibodies can be directed against class I (A, B, and C) or class II (DQ, DR, and DP) HLA. Advances in laboratory assays have led to increasingly sophisticated methods for characterizing HLA antibodies and stratifying them according to risk of postoperative complications, such as hyperacute rejection, AMR, or CLAD.[15,16] At the time of transplant evaluation, candidate serum is screened for HLA antibodies using solid phase assays that produce a semiquantitative assessment of antibody strength known as mean fluorescence intensity (MFI). MFI can run from 0 to 20,000+ with individual transplant centers assigning an MFI threshold above which an antibody should be considered present (eg, MFI $\geq$ 1000) and above which donors with the corresponding antigen would not be a favorable match (eg, MFI $\geq$ 3000) (**Table 1**).

Although often treated as a present/absent (yes/no) factor, there are many ways to further characterize HLA antibodies. For example, it is possible to risk-stratify individual antibodies (according to their corresponding MFI) when deciding whether and how many to cross.[17,18] Although semiquantitative, MFI can provide a rough guidepost for categorizing patients by risk level, where MFI 1000 to 3000 is often considered lower risk; 3000 to 5000 is often considered intermediate risk; and 5000+ is often considered high risk.[16,18] It is also important to consider the identities of the detected HLA. Low expressivity antigens, such as DP, which potentially carries less immunologic risk than HLA-DQ, may be safer to cross at the time of transplant. In addition, some antibodies may have shared epitopes or broad specificities (for example, Bw4 or Bw6), imparting a higher risk of hyperacute rejection, even at lower MFI.[19] The degree of recipient-donor HLA matching—particularly at the DR locus—may also impact the immunologic risk of pretransplant antibodies and CLAD.[19] Furthermore, high-resolution donor and antibody typing can provide allele-level information on donor-recipient histocompatibility, although these results are rarely available during a donor lung offer.[20]

Clinicians should partner with their institution's tissue typing laboratory to further interrogate the immunologic risk of specific antibodies for highly sensitized candidates. Titration studies, which involve assessing the MFI of HLA antibodies by preparing serial dilutions, can provide further insight into relative antibody strength. For example, an antibody with an MFI below 3000 at a 1:4 dilution titer is less likely to be cytotoxic than one with a 1:16 dilution titer. Complement 1q (C1q) and complement 3d (C3d) assays assess the ability of HLA antibodies to fix C1q and C3d; whereas this test could identify antibodies that will likely induce complement-mediated cytotoxicity (ie, C1q binding), it is not easily available and not routinely performed in the pretransplant setting. Other relevant antibody data include immunoglobulin G (IgG) subclass (IgG1 and IgG3 more effectively activate the complement

Table 1
Risk stratification for crossing anti-human leukocyte antibodies in highly sensitized lung transplant candidates[a]

| Risk Category | Primary Antibody Characteristics | | | Secondary Antibody Characteristics | | |
	Loci	MFI	Dilution Titer MFI <3000	C1q Fixation	Surrogate Cell Flow Crossmatch[a]	CDC Crossmatch[b]
Very low	Any	<1000	1:4	—	—	—
Low	DP, Cw	1000–3000	1:4	Negative	Negative	Negative
Intermediate	A, B, DR	3000-5000	1:16	Negative	Negative/Positive	Negative
High	DR, DQ	5000-10,000	≥1:16	Positive	Positive	Negative
Very high	Any	>10,000	≥1:64	Positive	Positive	Positive

[a] This table provides a broad conceptual guide to risk stratification when deciding whether to cross specific anti-HLAs in highly sensitized patients. Some combinations of primary and secondary antibody characteristics may substantially alter the risk category.
[b] When available.

cascade) and persistence and MFI trajectory over time.[16]

In conjunction with clinical characteristics—such as the extent of pretransplant immunosuppression, candidate age, and eligibility for posttransplant augmented immunosuppression—histocompatibility data can be used to create an individualized risk profile for a highly sensitized candidate. For example, a specialist's decision to accept a donor organ for a recipient in the presence of a DQ5 antibody at MFI 6000 will differ if it is known that the DQ5 antibody has a low titer less than 3000 in a 1:4 dilution and is not C1q binding, and that there are 0 DR mismatches between the donor and recipient. In contrast, if a recipient has a donor-directed A2 antibody at MFI 6000, a 1:16 titer, and C1q binding, the decision to transplant would require a very different strategy to cross, if at all. **Table 1** provides a general summary of primary and secondary HLA antibody characteristics and associated risk profiles. Some combinations of primary and secondary antibody characteristics may substantially alter the risk category, even if only 1 or 2 factors are present.

Crossing Low-Level Antibodies Without Augmented Immunosuppression

Once an individualized antibody risk profile is developed for a highly sensitized candidate, transplant access can be expedited by crossing low-risk antibodies without planned augmented immunosuppression (**Table 2**: Low risk). For example, in a study conducted at the University of Pennsylvania, low-level antibodies (MFI 1000–5000, non-C1q binding) were crossed without augmented immunosuppression, and most preformed antibodies were no longer detected after transplant.[19] There was no increased risk of grade 3 PGD or CLAD-free survival when crossing low-level antibodies. However, several patients with pretransplant DQ7 and DQ8 antibodies developed early AMR and required treatment. Other transplant centers have also reported increased rates of AMR when DQ7 and DQ8 were crossed, even at relatively low pretransplant MFI levels, suggesting that caution should be exercised when crossing DQ7 or DQ8.[25] Protocols for cross low-level antibodies without augmented immunosuppression typically include contingencies to treat early AMR or increasing posttransplant DSA. When crossing low-level pretransplant antibodies without augmented immunosuppression, one should consider candidate's expected ability to tolerate more intensive postoperative therapies, if necessary.

Prospective Physical Crossmatching

Rather than relying solely on virtual crossmatching (VCM) to assess histocompatibility, some centers have developed prospective, physical crossmatching protocols to determine transplant safety across DSA (see **Table 2**: High risk). For example, the Brigham and Women's Hospital Lung Transplant Program implemented a protocol whereby blood samples for all sensitized candidates were sent to local and regional Organ Procurement Organizations (OPOs).[3] At the time of an organ offer, if the tissue-typing laboratory anticipated DSA based on the VCM, a prospective complement-dependent cytotoxicity (CDC) assay was performed. For this test, donor peripheral blood mononuclear cells were mixed with candidate serum along with complement. If a considerable proportion of the cells underwent complement-

Table 2
Approach to donor acceptance and posttransplant immunosuppression management for highly sensitized lung transplant candidates

Risk Category[a]	Recommendation	Immunosuppression Management	References
Very low-risk/HLA compatible donor	Proceed	Standard immunosuppression,[b] DSA monitoring at routine intervals posttransplant	NA
Low risk	Proceed	Consider standard immunosuppression with potential TPE/IVIG based on retrospective flow XM and status of early graft function	Courtwright et al,[21] 2021
Intermediate- or multiple low-risk DSA	Consider	Consider cytolytic induction immunosuppression (starting before graft reperfusion).[c] Plan for perioperative desensitization with TPE/IVIG ± proteosome inhibitors and rituximab based on early graft status	Perioperative desensitization: Tinckam et al,[22] 2015 Aversa et al,[23] 2021
High-risk or multiple intermediate-risk DSA	Consider based on recipient clinical status	Consider prospective CDC crossmatch, cytolytic induction immunosuppression. Plan for perioperative desensitization with TPE, IVIG, proteosome inhibitors and rituximab	Prospective CDC crossmatch: Courtwright et al,[3] 2021 Perioperative desensitization: Nandavaram et al,[24] 2021
Very high risk	Avoid	Not applicable	NA

Abbreviations: NA, not applicable; XM, crossmatch.
[a] See **Table 1** for risk definitions.
[b] Typically corticosteroid plus interleukin 2 receptor antagonist.
[c] Such as ATG or alemtuzumab.

mediated cell death, the offer was not accepted. Following transplantation, no further augmented immunosuppression therapies were administered if the retrospective flow crossmatch was negative. Otherwise, recipients were treated with intravenous immunoglobulin (IVIG) and therapeutic plasma exchange (TPE).

With a median follow-up of 1.4 years, there was no difference in CLAD-free survival outcomes among patients where DSA was and was not crossed. However, the investigators detected an increase in PGD and AMR among recipients where donor-directed HLA antibodies were crossed. It is,

however, important to note that several recipients had a cPRA above 95% and would likely not have had transplant opportunities without crossing DSA. The disadvantages of this approach include the need for sufficient time to conduct a physical crossmatch, logistical challenges in keeping candidate samples updated at local and regional OPOs, and OPO willingness to make donor material available for prospective crossmatching. As with crossing low-level antibodies, this protocol requires that recipients receive augmented immunosuppression if they have early allograft dysfunction or AMR.

Preoperative Desensitization

More common strategies for transplantation in highly sensitized candidates focus on desensitization protocols (**Table 2**: Intermediate risk, High risk). Desensitization protocols typically involve augmented immunosuppression. These protocols can be applied pretransplant to reduce the number or strength of circulating antibodies or perioperatively when a transplant proceeds in the presence of a known DSA. Desensitization can include cytolytic induction agents, such as antithymocyte globulin (ATG) in conjunction with IVIG, TPE, and B-cell or plasma cell–targeting agents.

To date, there is little evidence that pretransplant desensitization therapies lead to improved postoperative outcomes. First, there is no consistent approach to effectively reducing antibody levels using waitlist desensitization strategies. Second, these approaches significantly increase costs, with many patients not proceeding to transplantation.[26] Those who are transplanted appear to have increased posttransplant infection risk. Finally, there is a significant risk for rebound antibodies, including DSA, in the weeks to months following transplant. For example, in a study of renal transplant candidates, highly sensitized (cPRA > 90%) patients treated with rituximab and IVIG did not experience any improvement in their cPRA.[27] In addition, in a highly sensitized cohort of lung transplant candidates, there was no reduction in pretransplant cPRA after a multimodal desensitization protocol that included TPE, steroids, bortezomib, and rituximab given in combination over 19 days followed by IVIG.[28]

Perioperative Desensitization

Given that highly sensitized patients are more likely to die while on the waitlist than nonsensitized candidates, the strategy of avoiding all DSA based on VCM or cell-based crossmatch (CBCM) results may not be reasonable for this group of patients.[8] Unfortunately, protocols for sensitized recipient matching are not standardized, varying substantially among institutions. According to a recent survey examining global waitlist and perioperative management of sensitized lung transplant candidates, only 8 out of 57 international transplant programs allocate donor lungs to sensitized candidates with positive VCM or CBCM results.[4] The survey did not include questions about waitlist mortality of highly sensitized candidates at each program, but presumably programs that do not offer desensitization strategies have a higher waitlist mortality for these patients.

To increase the eligibility of sensitized recipient for transplantation and abrogate HLA antibodies as a barrier to transplantation, the University of Toronto Lung Transplant Program developed a perioperative desensitization protocol.[22] They proceeded with transplant in DSA-positive (cPRA ≥ 30%) recipients who were desensitized with a regimen that included perioperative TPE, IVIG administration (1 g/kg), ATG induction, and mycophenolic acid (MPA). Although desensitization did not eliminate DSA or prevent de novo DSA formation, recipients who underwent the procedure had similar rates of rejection and graft survival as those who did not. In a subsequent follow-up study 13 years after implementing their protocol, the 5- and 10-year survivals among sensitized patients in which DSA was crossed were similar to outcomes in recipients without pretransplant DSA.[23]

The University of Florida Lung Transplant Program also implemented a modified version of the Toronto perioperative desensitization protocol for recipients with a cPRA greater than 30% and positive VCM.[24] These candidates underwent preoperative TPE (1.5 total plasma volume) conducted in the intensive care unit before surgery, intraoperative basiliximab induction, followed by 5 sessions of daily TPE, IVIG (1 g/kg) administration, and ATG induction (dose 3 mg/kg for VCM-positive or 5 mg/kg for retrospective flow crossmatch). Tacrolimus (12–15 ng/mL), mycophenolate, and prednisone were used for maintenance immunosuppression. Twenty-five patients underwent desensitization, of whom 19 were women. Retrospective flow crossmatch was positive in 24% of the patients. The overall survival of this cohort was 96%, with a median follow-up of 17 months (interquartile range, 5–25.5 months). In addition, before and after desensitization implementation, there was a decline in waitlist mortality (11.4% to 7.6%) and 50th percentile median wait times (8.5 months to 1.3 months).

Some protocols implemented, like the one described by Courtwright and colleagues,[3] have different thresholds for candidate sensitization and transplant urgency at which they will accept VCM-positive lung transplants involving DSA, but many programs require a prospective CDC crossmatch to be negative prior to accepting the offer. The Toronto and Florida programs also have varying thresholds, but neither program requires a prospective CDC crossmatch before accepting the offer. In addition, similar perioperative desensitization strategies in heart transplant appear to be successful.[29,30] No prior work, however, has determined the impact of program-specific practices for accepting crossmatch-positive transplants on waitlist outcomes for candidates with high cPRA values. Nor are there data as to whether the development of desensitization and other strategies has increased the number of highly sensitized patients over time or by era. Although growing evidence urges the transplant community to improve access in this population, the safest and most effective approach to managing highly sensitized candidates remains unclear.

Health Policy

Although the primary focus of this review is to guide clinical decision making for highly sensitized candidates, given the limitations of preoperative desensitization therapies, it is also important to revisit how sensitized candidates are prioritized on the waitlist. The most direct mechanism for improving access is to give additional priority in lung allocation scores based on the degree of sensitization that is currently under implementation in the new continuous allocation system in the in the United States.[31] Although this policy change is now in their early days, other broader changes could target improved national data collection regarding sensitized patients at the Organ Procurement and Transplant Network (OPTN) level via the Scientific Registry of Transplant Recipients. OPTN could track detailed information on HLA antibody locus in addition to the recipient's cPRA. OPTN could also resume collecting data on crossmatch results, which would provide national cohort information on outcomes after crossing antibodies among highly sensitized patients.

FUTURE DIRECTIONS

The authors have focused on the current practices used to optimize highly sensitized patients' access to lung transplantation. Current therapeutic protocols use an arsenal of therapeutics and medical interventions that expand on standard immunosuppressive regimens. Although these have shown promise, clinical trials are needed to standardized protocols, and to develop additional perioperative and postoperative therapeutic strategies for highly sensitized patients.

One of the most direct approaches to crossing pretransplant DSA may be therapies that lyse or degrade IgG. For example, imlifidase is a cysteine protease that eliminates Fc-dependent effector functions, such as CDC, and antibody-dependent cellular cytotoxicity by cleaving the heavy chains of human IgG antibodies. This prevents fragment crystallizable region functions, including antibody-dependent cell-mediated cytotoxicity. Imlifidase has been used to cross high-strength DSA in sensitized kidney-transplant recipients, including those with cPRA greater than 99.9%.[32] Most recipients had rebound in DSA MFI within a week of transplant, and 30% developed AMR within 1 month of transplant.[33] However, the majority of these cases were successfully treated, and 3-year survival was 90%.

It is well accepted that many of the DSA that cause posttransplant injury activate the complement system. Few studies, however, have investigated complement therapeutics as protocolized adjuvant therapeutics for the treatment of presensitized lung transplant candidates. For example, eculizumab, a C5 inhibitor, has been used in clinical trials for sensitized patients in kidney transplantation.[34] Its use was associated with favorable outcomes and helped provide access to kidney transplantation for sensitized patients. However, long-term outcomes were not as favorable as those seen in nonsensitized patients.[35,36] In lung transplantation, Eculizumab has been used as a therapeutic for AMR and anecdotally for complications early post–lung transplant in presensitized recipients.[37,38,39]

Eculizumab functions at the level of C5, and, until recently, was the only Food and Drug Administration (FDA) -approved complement therapeutic available for use. Several new complement therapeutics have recently been FDA-approved or are under rapid clinical development. For example, C1-esterase inhibitor, which inhibits early stages in the complement activation pathway, has been used in lung transplant recipients with severe AMR.[40] Other potential complement-targeting therapies include pegcetacoplan, a pegylated peptide targeting proximal complement protein C3, which is FDA-approved for the treatment of paroxysmal nocturnal hemoglobinuria.[41] As clinical trials are developed for crossing pretransplant DSA, consideration should be given to the adjuvant use of inhibitors that function early in the complement activation pathway, or act to inhibit the central component of the complement system (ie, C3).

Finally, advances in the control of B cells may also be relevant to preoperative desensitization among highly sensitized candidates.[42–44] B-cell–targeted therapies, including those targeting B-cell–surface antigens (rituximab, ocrelizumab, ofatumumab, obinutuzumab, obexelimab, epratuzumab, daratumumab), B-cell survival factors (belimumab, tabalumab, atacicept, blisibimod), or B-cell intracellular functions (ibrutinib, fenebrutinib, proteasome inhibitors), have been developed and are either clinically available or undergoing clinical trials for the treatment of autoimmunity. With the increasing development of therapeutics that target antibodies, and their effector functions, the potential for improving outcomes in presensitized patients is rapidly evolving. It is plausible that a combination of multiple therapies, including TPE, IVIG, prelung reperfusion thymoglobulin, and early and long-standing B-cell and plasma cell inhibition, will be required to decrease the burden of DSAs and to minimize the risk of future AMR and CLAD.

SUMMARY

Highly sensitized patients, who are often black and Hispanic women, are less likely to be listed for lung transplant or to be considered candidates for mechanical circulatory support. They are also at higher risk for waitlist death. Individual institutions have developed strategies—including perioperative desensitization when crossing intermediate- and high-risk DSA—for improving access to transplant in this population. There is, however, ongoing need for multicenter trials to identify novel therapeutics and to define the optimal perioperative and posttransplant immunosuppressive regimen for successful lung transplant in this population.

DISCLOSURE

The authors of this article have no conflicts of interest to disclose. There are no sources of funding for this article.

CLINICS CARE POINTS

- When carefully selected, highly sensitized patients can safely undergo lung transplantation
- To decrease wait list mortality and increase acces to transplant to highly snesitized patients, the transplant comunity need to embrace both policy change and incorporation of desensitization strategies that have been suscefully used

REFERENCES

1. Shah AS, Nwakanma L, Simpkins C, et al. Pretransplant panel reactive antibodies in human lung transplantation: an analysis of over 10,000 patients. Ann Thorac Surg 2008;85(6):1919–24.
2. Kim I, Jordan S, Vo A. Transplantation in highly HLA-sensitized patients: challenges and solutions. Transpl Res Risk Manag 2014;214(6):99–107.
3. Courtwright AM, Cao S, Wood I, et al. Clinical outcomes of lung transplantation in the presence of donor-specific antibodies. Ann Am Thorac Soc 2019;16(9):1131–7.
4. Aversa M, Darley DR, Hirji A, et al. Approaches to the management of sensitized lung transplant candidates: findings from an international survey. J Heart Lung Transpl 2020;39(4):S315.
5. Young KA, Ali HA, Beermann KJ, et al. Lung transplantation and the era of the sensitized patient. Front Immunol 2021;12:689420.
6. Courtwright AM, Kamoun M, Kearns J, et al. The impact of HLA-DR mismatch status on retransplant-free survival and bronchiolitis obliterans syndrome–free survival among sensitized lung transplant recipients. J Heart Lung Transpl 2020;39(12):1455–62.
7. Barac YD, Mulvihill MS, Jawitz O, et al. Increased cPRA is associated with increased waitlist time and mortality in LTx. Ann Thorac Surg 2020;110(2):414–23.
8. Aversa M, Benvenuto L, Kim H, et al. Effect of calculated panel reactive antibody value on waitlist outcomes for lung transplant candidates. Ann Transpl 2019;24:383–92.
9. Courtwright A, Patel N, Chandraker A, et al. Human leukocyte antigen antibody sensitization, lung transplantation, and health equity. Am J Transplant 2022;22(3):698–704.
10. Frost AE, Jammal CT, Cagle PT. Hyperacute rejection following lung transplantation. Chest 1996;110(2):559–62.
11. Masson E, Stern M, Chabod J, et al. Hyperacute rejection after lung transplantation caused by undetected low-titer anti-HLA antibodies. J Heart Lung Transpl Off Publ Int Soc Heart Transpl 2007;26(6):642–5.
12. Ius F, Sommer W, Tudorache I, et al. Early donor-specific antibodies in lung transplantation: risk factors and impact on survival. J Heart Lung Transpl 2014;33(12):1255–63.
13. Roux A, Bendib Le Lan I, Holifanjaniaina S, et al. Antibody-mediated rejection in lung transplantation: clinical outcomes and donor-specific antibody characteristics. Am J Transpl 2016;16(4):1216–28.
14. Courtwright A, Diamond J, Wood I, et al. Detection and clinical impact of human leukocyte antigen antibodies in lung transplantation: a systematic review and meta-analysis. HLA 2018;91(2):102–11.
15. Chin N, Paraskeva M, Paul E, et al. Comparative analysis of how immune sensitization is defined prior to lung transplantation. Hum Immunol 2015;76(10):711–6.

16. Mangiola M, Marrari M, Xu Q, et al. Approaching the sensitized lung patient: risk assessment for donor acceptance. J Thorac Dis 2021;13(11): 6725–36.

17. Xu Q, Mangiola M, Zeevi A. Choosing the right patient for lung transplantation: assessment of histocompatibility and sensitization status. In: Bertani A, Vitulo P, Grossi PA, editors. Contemporary lung transplantation. Organ and tissue transplantation. Cham: Springer; 2020. p. 1–12.

18. Smith JD, Ibrahim MW, Newell H, et al. Pre-transplant donor HLA-specific antibodies: characteristics causing detrimental effects on survival after lung transplantation. J Heart Lung Transpl 2014;33(10): 1074–82.

19. Garcia-Sanchez C, Usenko CY, Herrera ND, et al. The shared epitope phenomenon—a potential impediment to virtual crossmatch accuracy. Clin Transplant 2020;34(8):e13906.

20. Zavyalova D, Abraha J, Rao P, et al. Incidence and impact of allele-specific anti-HLA antibodies and high-resolution HLA genotyping on assessing immunologic compatibility. Hum Immunol 2021;82(3): 147–54.

21. Courtwright AM, Kamoun M, Diamond JM, et al. Lung transplantation outcomes after crossing low-level donor specific antibodies without planned augmented immunosuppression. Clin Transpl 2021; 35(11):e14447.

22. Tinckam KJ, Keshavjee S, Chaparro C, et al. Survival in sensitized lung transplant recipients with perioperative desensitization: successful desensitization in lung transplant recipients. Am J Transpl 2015;15(2):417–26.

23. Aversa M, Martinu T, Patriquin C, et al. Long-term outcomes of sensitized lung transplant recipients after peri-operative desensitization. Am J Transpl 2021;21(10):3444–8.

24. Nandavaram S, Shahmohammadi A, Chandrashekaran S, et al. Perioperative desensitization for sensitized lung transplant candidates. J Heart Lung Transpl 2021;40(4):S371.

25. Kayawake H, Chen-Yoshikawa TF, Gochi F, et al. Postoperative outcomes of lung transplant recipients with preformed donor-specific antibodies. Interact Cardiovasc Thorac Surg 2020;32(4): 616–24.

26. Patel J, Everly M, Chang D, et al. Reduction of alloantibodies via proteosome inhibition in cardiac transplantation. J Heart Lung Transpl 2011;30(12): 1320–6.

27. Marfo K, Ling M, Bao Y, et al. Lack of effect in desensitization with intravenous immunoglobulin and rituximab in highly sensitized patients. transplantation 2012;94(4):345–51.

28. Snyder LD, Gray AL, Reynolds JM, et al. Antibody desensitization therapy in highly sensitized lung transplant candidates: antibody desensitization therapy. Am J Transpl 2014;14(4):849–56.

29. Alhussein M, Moayedi Y, Posada JD, et al. Peri-operative desensitization for highly sensitized heart transplant patients. JF Heart Lung Transpl 2018; 37(5):667–70.

30. Plazak ME, Gale SE, Reed BN, et al. Clinical outcomes of perioperative desensitization in heart transplant recipients. Transpl Direct 2021;7(2): e658.

31. Update on the continuous distribution of organs project - OPTN. Available at: https://optn.transplant.hrsa.gov/policies-bylaws/public-comment/update-on-the-continuous-distribution-of-organs-project/. Accessed May 12, 2022.

32. Lonze BE, Tatapudi VS, Weldon EP, et al. IdeS (Imlifidase): a novel agent that cleaves human IgG and permits successful kidney transplantation across high-strength donor-specific antibody. Ann Surg 2018;268(3):488–96.

33. Kjellman C, Maldonado AQ, Sjöholm K, et al. Outcomes at 3 years posttransplant in imlifidase-desensitized kidney transplant patients. Am J Transplant 2021;21(12):3907–18.

34. Marks WH, Mamode N, Montgomery RA, et al. Safety and efficacy of eculizumab in the prevention of antibody-mediated rejection in living-donor kidney transplant recipients requiring desensitization therapy: a randomized trial. Am J Transplant 2019; 19(10):2876–88.

35. Schinstock CA, Bentall AJ, Smith BH, et al. Long-term outcomes of eculizumab-treated positive crossmatch recipients: allograft survival, histologic findings, and natural history of the donor-specific antibodies. Am J Transplant 2018;19(6): 1671–83.

36. Stegall D, Diwan T, Raghavaiah S, et al. Terminal complement inhibition decreases antibody-mediated rejection in sensitized renal transplant recipients 2011M. Am J Transpl 2013;13(1):241.

37. Stegall MD, Diwan T, Raghavaiah S, et al. Terminal complement inhibition decreases antibody-mediated rejection in sensitized renal transplant recipients. Am J Transplant 2011;11(11):2405–13.

38. Muller YD, Aubert JD, Vionnet J, et al. Acute antibody-mediated rejection 1 week after lung transplantation successfully treated with eculizumab, intravenous immunoglobulins, and rituximab. Transplantation 2018b;102(6):e301–3.

39. Dawson KL, Parulekar A, Seethamraju H. Treatment of hyperacute antibody-mediated lung allograft rejection with eculizumab. J Heart Lung Transplant 2012;31(12):1325–6.

40. Sommer W, Tudorache I, Kühn C, et al. C1-Esterase-Inhibitor counteracts severe primary graft dysfunction in lung transplantation. J Heart Lung Transplant 2013;32(4):S222.

41. Hillmen Peter, Szer Jeff, Weitz Hene, et al. Pegceta-coplan versus eculizumab in paroxysmal nocturnal hemoglobinuria. N Engl J Med 2021 Mar 18; 384(11):1028–37.

42. Wemlinger SM, Parker Harp CR, Yu B, et al. Preclin-ical analysis of candidate anti-human CD79 thera-peutic antibodies using a humanized CD79 mouse model. J Immunol 2022;208(7):1566–84.

43. Bag-Ozbek A, Hui-Yuen JS. Emerging B-Cell thera-pies in systemic lupus erythematosus. Ther Clin Risk Manag 2021;17:39–54.

44. Furie R, Petri M, Zamani O, et al. A phase III, ran-domized, placebo-controlled study of belimumab, a monoclonal antibody that inhibits B lymphocyte stimulator, in patients with systemic lupus erythema-tosus. Arthritis Rheum 2011;63(12):3918–30.

Antibody-Mediated Rejection
Diagnosis and Treatment

Laura P. Halverson, MD*, Ramsey R. Hachem, MD

KEYWORDS

- Antibody-mediated rejection • Donor-specific antibodies • Chronic lung allograft survival
- Lung transplantation

KEY POINTS

- AMR after lung transplantation is an increasingly recognized form of lung rejection.
- The optimal treatment for AMR after lung transplantation remains unclear.
- Outcomes after AMR are dismal with a high death rate and a high incidence of CLAD.

INTRODUCTION

Despite improvements in surgical techniques and overall management of lung transplant recipients, outcomes lag other solid-organ transplants, with an overall and conditional survival of 1-year post-transplant median survival of 6.7 years and 8.9 years, respectively.[1] Graft failure in the form of chronic lung allograft dysfunction (CLAD) is the leading cause of death beyond the first year after transplant.[2,3] The development of humoral immunity in the form of antibody-mediated rejection (AMR) is now well established as an important cause of graft-failure and CLAD, with an associated high level of mortality.[4–8] Unfortunately, although we now recognize its clinical importance, AMR remains a challenging diagnosis to make, and there is not yet a standardized approach to treatment. This review will aim to summarize both our current approach and emerging areas in the diagnosis and treatment of AMR.

Mechanism and Pathogenesis

AMR occurs with the development of antibodies against mismatched human leukocyte antigens (HLA) expressed on the donor lung, leading to endothelial cell injury and graft dysfunction. More specifically, AMR involves activation of allospecific B-cells and plasma cells leading to the formation of donor-specific antibodies (DSA), usually against either class I or class II HLA (**Table 1**).[9] Class I antigens (HLA-A, HLA-B, or HLA-C) present proteins that have been processed within the cell cytoplasm and are present on nearly every nucleated cell. Class II antigens (HLA-DQ, HLA-DR, and HLA-DP) present exogenous material on antigen-presenting cells (eg, macrophages and dendritic cells).[9] When antibodies bind to HLA on the endothelium of the allograft, the complement cascade is activated resulting in endothelial cell necrosis and acute lung injury.[10]

This mechanism was originally worked out in the context of hyperacute rejection, which often caused fulminant graft failure intraoperatively or in the immediate posttransplant period.[11] In this context, both circulating DSA and pathologic evidence of antigen–antibody complex deposition in capillaries were observed, leading to the conclusion that humoral immunity was capable of

Disclosure Statement: R.R. Hachem has received grant funding from Bristol Myers Squibb, United States and Mallinckrodt Pharmaceuticals, Canada and is a consultant for Transmedics, CareDx, and Natera. This work was funded in part by NHLBI, United States grant HL138186. L.P. Halverson has no financial relationships to disclose.
Funded by: WUSL.
Division of Pulmonary & Critical Care, Washington University School of Medicine, 660 South Euclid Avenue, Campus Box 8052, Saint Louis, MO 63108, USA
* Corresponding author.
E-mail address: laura.halverson@wustl.edu

Clin Chest Med 44 (2023) 95–103
https://doi.org/10.1016/j.ccm.2022.10.008
0272-5231/23/© 2022 Elsevier Inc. All rights reserved.

chestmed.theclinics.com

Table 1
Description of antibodies involved in antibody-mediated rejection

Antibody	Category of Antigen	Comments
HLA-A HLA-B HLA-C	Human leukocyte antigens class I	Donor-recipient mismatch does not predict CLAD
HLA-DQ (A1, B1) HLA-DR (A1, B1) HLA-DP (A1, B1)	Human leukocyte antigens class II	Much more closely associated with development of CLAD and increased mortality, particularly the HLA-DQ
Kα 1 Tubulin Collagen V	Lung-associated tissue-restricted self-antigens	Failure to clear self-antigens associated with independent risk of CLAD/BOS

fulminant graft failure.[10] The advent of solid-phase assays enhanced the detection of HLA antibodies before transplantation with greater sensitivity and specificity.[12] This allowed the use of the virtual cross-match to select potential donors for allosensitized patients, which made hyperacute rejection after lung transplantation rare. However, clinicians began to identify cases of graft dysfunction occurring at later time points with pathologic findings similar to those seen in hyperacute rejection and circulating DSA.[13,14] This clinical experience has since led to our current acceptance of AMR as an important form of graft rejection beyond the immediate posttransplant setting.

Donor-Specific Antibodies

Pretransplant allosensitization: The number of pre-existing HLA antibodies indicates the degree of allosensitization before transplant, and the risk for hyperacute rejection and early graft failure if the reactive HLA are not avoided in a potential donor. Exposure to foreign HLA can result in allosensitization, and commonly sensitizing events include pregnancy, blood product transfusion, organ transplantation, or human tissue implantation.[15] However, some allosensitized patients have never had an obvious sensitizing event. This may be due to infection, vaccination, or some other proinflammatory event that is not recognized as a sensitizing event.[16] Although such preformed antibodies were initially linked to hyperacute rejection, they have also been associated with an increased risk of CLAD and death especially if they were class II or complement-activating.[17,18] In particular, DSA to HLA-DQ has been identified as a predictor of AMR.[8,19] While avoiding the reactive HLA in a prospective donor prevents hyperacute rejection and may decrease the risk of CLAD and death, this approach prolongs waitlist time, decreasing the likelihood of transplantation, and increasing waitlist mortality.[20,21] This has led to the development of protocols to distinguish high-risk DSA from acceptable allosensitization, using various DSA characteristics including the mean fluorescence intensity (MFI) titer, and the antibody's ability to activate complement.[22] Regardless, several studies suggest that a high PRA is associated with decreased survival, increased acute rejection, prolonged duration of mechanical ventilation after transplant, as well as an increased risk of AMR and CLAD.[18,23]

Posttransplant de novo donor-specific antibodies: DSA may also develop de novo after transplantation, most commonly directed at class II HLA.[24–26] A leading theory for its development is that recurrent episodes of lung inflammation or injury increase HLA expression in the graft along with leukocyte infiltration resulting in increased immunogenicity of the graft. This is supported by evidence of de novo DSA development seen after acute cellular rejection (ACR) and some respiratory infections. In a prospective multicenter study in the United States, 36% of patients developed DSA within 120 days of transplantation, and previous single-center studies reported an incidence of approximately 50% with longer term follow-up.[26,27] This study also noted an MFI cutoff of 3000 as predicting acute rejection.[26] DSA are typically identified early after transplantation, with most patients developing DSA within the first 90 days.[26,28] This evidence of DSA as an early posttransplant phenomenon led to research hypothesizing that the choice of induction immunosuppression may affect the development of DSA. In one example, a recent study of patients treated with alemtuzumab demonstrated an incidence of 13% compared with a previously cited incidence of 30% to 50% in patients treated with basiliximab.[25] Of note, there is evidence that the highest risk associated with de novo DSA is in patients who have persistent DSA. In one retrospective study, patients with persistent DSA in the first year after transplantation had a significantly higher mortality, with 60% of these patients dying within the first year.[29]

Non-HLA antibodies: There is mounting evidence that the development of antibodies to lung-restricted self-antigens also plays an important role in the development of AMR and CLAD.[30] This autoimmunity occurs when graft injury exposes normally sequestered self-antigens (SAgs), followed by the loss of peripheral tolerance, and the development of antibodies to self-antigens. Collagen V, an extracellular matrix protein, and K-alpha-1 tubulin, a gap junction protein, are both expressed on airway epithelial cells. While the literature has focused on these 2 SAgs, there is evidence of antibodies to several other SAgs.[30–34] Similar to HLA antibodies, these can exist before transplant or develop *de novo* after transplant. A candidate's underlying lung disease may affect the prevalence of pretransplant antibodies to SAgs, with one study demonstrating that a third of patients with pulmonary fibrosis and cystic fibrosis had antibodies to SAgs compared with only 18% of patients with COPD.[33] An estimated 70% of lung transplant recipients may ultimately develop antibodies to Sags, and there is a strong relationship between the development of DSA and antibodies to SAgs.[34] To date, there has been no commercially available assay to screen for antibodies to SAgs but research in this area is ongoing, given the mounting evidence that the presence of antibodies to SAgs has important clinical consequences independent of HLA antibodies.[34]

Diagnosis

In the most recent consensus definition for AMR, the International Society for Heart and Lung Transplantation (ISHLT) identified 5 criteria that lead to possible, probable or definite AMR depending on the number of criteria present.[35] The 5 criteria include (1) clinically apparent graft dysfunction, (2) lung injury pathology, (3) capillary C4d deposition, (4) circulating DSA, and (5) clinical exclusion of other possible causes of allograft dysfunction.[35] Despite this framework, however, within each category of the definition, there remains a great deal of variability, and the diagnosis remains one that requires a high index of suspicion on the part of the clinician. Below, we explore each of the criteria in greater depth to briefly underscore the current diagnostic challenges.

Graft dysfunction: Graft dysfunction in AMR has a range of presentations from asymptomatic decline in spirometry to mild dyspnea, or fulminant hypoxemic respiratory failure.[33] Dysfunction of pulmonary physiology, even asymptomatic, is the key distinction between clinical and subclinical AMR, which is defined as definitive changes of AMR found on surveillance transbronchial biopsies in the absence of graft dysfunction. Further categorization of AMR into distinct clinical phenotypes is also an ongoing area of study. While historically, time from transplant has been used to distinguish hyperacute (within 24 hours of transplant surgery) from acute (>24 hours from surgery) AMR, emerging evidence supports the presence of chronic AMR although this remains poorly characterized although it is well-established in other solid-organ transplants.

Circulating antibody: Considered most central to the diagnosis, DSA also has significant variability. Although technology using solid-phase assays has significantly improved the overall sensitivity and specificity for antibody detection, there is variability in thresholds to define positivity at different centers.[36–38] Consequently, it is possible that centers using a higher MFI cutoff may miss some DSA and some cases of AMR. For example, a retrospective cohort study found that patients with an MFI 3000 or greater had significantly higher incidence of AMR compared with those with MFI less than 3000, such that the use of a higher cutoff would miss many cases of potentially pathogenic antibodies.[23,39] Finally, although it is required for the definite diagnosis of AMR, there are patients who meet all other criteria for AMR but never have detectable DSA.[40,41] It is also important to note that only a proportion of patients who have DSA go on to develop AMR.[4]

Complement deposition: The complement cascade produces the split-product C4d, which covalently binds to the capillary endothelium allowing it to be detected for many days. Its presence on histopathology is another diagnostic criteria, often thought of as the most conclusive evidence for AMR. Unfortunately, although C4d deposition can be a marker of complement activation and serve to confirm antibody-mediated damage, it has several notable limitations. First, interreader reliability of C4d staining is poor, and while the ISHLT pathology council recommends greater than 50% positivity be considered significant, every center has developed its own experience, expertise, and thresholds for positivity.[10,42] Further complicating its interpretation, there has been demonstrated C4d deposition in the absence of DSA because of ischemia-reperfusion injury, infection, or ACR, which undermines its specificity.[43] A recent study emphasized this lack of specificity by comparing C4d levels in BAL samples in patients with a variety of posttransplant complications.[44] Levels were increased in all acute events including acute rejection, lymphocytic bronchiolitis, AMR, and infections, with the highest levels noted in the infection group.[44] Finally, many cases of probable AMR are C4d negative.[19,39] Although C4d negative AMR may be explained by variation in the methodology of staining and interpretation of C4d, there is evidence of complement independent pathways that lead to AMR.[45–47] Evidence from renal transplantation has established a distinct C4d-negative AMR phenotype that results from natural killer cells and macrophage interactions with HLA antibodies.[48,49] A similar complement-independent phenotype of AMR in lung transplantation has been hypothesized but evidence supporting this paradigm remains limited.[19] Nevertheless, this suggests that while C4d is a key component of AMR diagnosis, its absence is not exculpatory.

Tissue histopathology: In keeping with the significant variety of graft dysfunction seen in individual AMR presentations, the histologic findings of AMR include various nonspecific patterns of lung injury.[10,50] This includes acute lung injury, organizing lung injury, pneumonitis, diffuse alveolar damage, and capillaritis. Although a pattern of neutrophilic capillaritis raises the index of suspicion for AMR, it too is nonspecific, and requires distinction from neutrophilic margination or congestion. Capillaritis can also be obscured by acute lung injury and is not seen in most cases of confirmed AMR.[8] Recent study in electron microscopy (EM) has demonstrated significant differences between AMR and other forms of graft injury, with prominent endothelial swelling, endothelial vacuolization, and neutrophilic margination occurring in both clinical and subclinical AMR.[51] These differences are enhanced by the finding that EM identification of endothelial swelling correlated with the presence of circulating DSA, and the severity of injury was more prominent in cases with DSA.[51] EM may represent a future method for enhanced diagnostic accuracy in the histopathology of AMR.

Emerging Diagnostics

Table 2 summarizes the current consensus definition of AMR, emphasizing the significant variety of scenarios present particularly in possible AMR. For example, for a patient with histopathology of acute lung injury and allograft dysfunction in whom other causes have been excluded can be considered to have possible AMR in the absence of DSA and C4d deposition. Although this is not the most common scenario, it underscores how challenging it can be to study AMR on a broader scale, when such clinical heterogeneity exists even within its definition. Further, the diagnosis in all instances hinges on the presence of allograft function, underscoring that our current standards of diagnosis do not allow for the detection of the process before graft damage. These limitations have led to ongoing research into novel ways to more accurately identify AMR even before allograft damage has occurred. Next, we discuss 2 of the more promising advances in diagnostics.

Cell free DNA: An area of increasing research and clinical utilization in the diagnosis of all forms of rejection including AMR is donor-derived cell free DNA (ddcfDNA). After transplantation, when donor allograft cells are damaged, ddcfDNA is released into circulation. The percent of plasma ddcfDNA can be quantified and followed over time, with higher percentages correlating with allograft injury, including during acute cellular or AMR.[52,53] In addition to its high sensitivity, ddcfDNA has the great advantage of being a noninvasive test available to screen for allograft injury, able to be used in cases when bronchoscopy and/or transbronchial biopsies are too risky or contraindicated. Its major limitation is that any process that results in donor cell damage—infection, ischemia, or immune-mediated injury—will increase its detected level. However, although ddcfDNA alone has poor specificity, when combined with DSA testing, one group showed improvement in the specificity for AMR with cell-free donor DNA from 35% to 90%, coupled with near 100% sensitivity.[52] However, perhaps most importantly, ddcfDNA levels have been noted to be elevated approximately 3 months before the onset of clinically apparent allograft dysfunction, making ddcfDNA a particularly impactful advancement in early detection and possible prevention of clinical AMR.[52,54] One multicenter cohort study following 148 patients postlung transplant with serial levels of percent ddcfDNA examined its performance with respect to changes seen in histologically confirmed episodes of ACR, AMR, and infections.[54] They found a 2-fold higher level of ddcfDNA in AMR compared with ACR, and a significant increase in ddcfDNA preceding the confirmed tissue diagnosis was also more common in AMR compared with ACR (82% of AMR episodes had an increase of greater than 1% a month before diagnosis compared with only 18%).[54]

Donor-Derived Exosomes: Exosomes, small extracellular vesicles shed by cells, carry various nucleic acids (ranging from DNA to microRNA), proteins, and metabolites but can also carry various antigen-presenting proteins and HLA class I and class II.[55] If these vesicles express both donor HLA and non-HLA SAgs, they can activate antigen-presenting cells and lead to immune responses and the development of antibodies to both donor HLA and non-HLA tissue-associated antigens.[55,56] This mechanism illustrates the role exosomes may play in AMR. Donor-derived

Table 2
Definition of antibody-mediated rejection

Diagnostic Criteria	Definite AMR	Probable AMR (Dysfunction Plus Any 4 Criteria Met)	Possible AMR (Dysfunction Plus Any 3 Criteria Met)
Allograft dysfunction	+	+	+
Circulating DSA	+	+/−	+/−
C4d deposition	+	+/−	+/−
Lung injury histopathology	+	+/−	+/−
Exclusion of other causes	+	+/−	+/−

exosomes could therefore serve both as a biomarker for allograft rejection, one that could be detected before antibody development and subsequent allograft damage.[55,56] Ongoing study in donor-derived exosomes is another important focus in the future of AMR diagnosis and prevention.

Treatment

The goals of AMR treatment are 3-fold: deplete circulating DSA, stop additional DSA formation, and prevent (further) allograft injury. It follows then, that no single medication can accomplish all of these goals, leading to the necessity of multidrug regimens. These therapies are derived from treatment regimens developed for other antibody-based disease processes and evidence from other solid-organ transplants, primarily renal. Unfortunately, no randomized controlled trials or head-to-head comparisons in lung transplantation have been feasible to date, leading to treatment choices that are driven by individual center protocols and patient factors. In practice, multiple treatments are usually given simultaneously to bring maximal effect rapidly, further limiting the assessment of any single therapy's efficacy. Although the establishment of an optimal regimen remains to be determined, observational studies have demonstrated improvement in allograft function after several described therapies, suggesting AMR is potentially reversible if identified and treated early.[8] **Table 3** summarizes current treatment options, their mechanism of action, and important considerations when choosing therapies.

Novel Therapeutic Targets

New treatment possibilities for AMR continue to emerge. There is ongoing research in solid organ transplant AMR investigating the role of IL-6 inhibition (tocilizumab), CTLA4-Ig (belatacept), B-cell-activating factor antagonists (belimumab,

tabalumab, atacicept), and JAK inhibitors (tofacitinib).[57,58] All these therapies are mechanistically designed to reduce alloantibody production and would be novel additions to the AMR regimen. One particularly important area of focus involves understanding the role regulatory T cells (Tregs) play in the pathophysiology of AMR. Best understood as regulators of self-tolerance, Tregs suppress production of inflammatory cytokines, cytotoxic T cells, and APCs.[59] The loss of Tregs is associated with a loss of tolerance and has been recently demonstrated in a mouse model of lung transplant to play a significant role in the development of DSA and AMR.[59]

Investigators demonstrated that the depletion of resident lung allograft Foxp3+ T regulatory cells allowed prolonged B and T cell interactions that resulted in the production of DSA and subsequent antibody-mediated destruction of the graft. The interaction was dependent on a CXCL13 ligand-mediated chemokinesis, which when neutralized, was shown to prevent the development of DSA.[59] Investigators then analyzed the expression of genes known to play a role in B cell activation by T cell interaction and found significant elevation of ICOS, ICOS ligand, CD40, and CD40 ligand. When specific antibodies blocked these ligands, it also prevented DSA generation and graft injury.[59] This study represents an important paradigm shift in considering the lung allograft as a secondary lymphoid organ where tolerance is maintained or impaired on a local level. This argument is made more compelling considered in conjunction with evidence that respiratory infections, a well-demonstrated predisposing factor in the development of DSA, are associated with disruption in Treg function.[60] Considered together, this graft-resident T lymphocyte-dependent mechanism for the suppression or activation of the humoral response represents a significant advance in the understanding of 2 future potential therapeutic targets—those designed to preserve and augment

Table 3
Summary of common therapeutic options for antibody-mediated rejection

Category	Example	Mechanism of Action	Effect	Dosing	Considerations
Corticosteroids	IV methylprednisolone	Suppression of leukocyte transcription factors	Decrease allograft injury	500–1000 mg daily for 3–5 d	Insufficient as monotherapy
Plasma exchange	N/A	Depletion of circulating antibodies, decrease deposition of complement split products	Decrease allograft injury, clear existing antibodies	No consensus on duration or number of sessions Range from 5–20 sessions	Will deplete therapeutic antibodies so should be done before IVIG administration
Intravenous immunoglobulin (IVIG)	Pooled serum from thousands of donors	DSA neutralization, complement inhibition, B-cell downregulation	Clear existing antibodies	500–2000 mg/kg (Reduced to 100 mg/kg if given with plasma exchange)	Primary therapy for DSA, should be continued after AMR therapy as maintenance
Antithymocyte globulin, rabbit or equine	Thymoglobulin	Deplete cytotoxic T-cells; also inhibits memory T-cells; broader immunomodulatory effects may also lead to loss of CD138+ plasma cells	Decrease allograft injury and antibody production	Goal of 5–7 mg/kg delivered over 3–4 doses	Adjuvant therapy. Also used for immunosuppression induction and treatment of CLAD
Anti-CD20 antibody	Rituximab	Deplete B-cells by inducing apoptosis of pre-B and mature B-lymphocytes	Decrease antibody production	375 mg/m^2 once	No effect on plasma cells already producing antibodies
Proteosome inhibitors	Bortezomib (26S) Carfilzomib (20S)	Inactivate proteasome, leading to plasma cell apoptosis	Decrease antibody production	20 mg/kg for 6 doses spaced over 3 wk	Observational study evidence for allograft recovery in AMR
Complement inhibition	Eculizumab (C5)	Prevents membrane-attack complex (MAC) formation required for complement-mediated endothelial injury	Decrease allograft injury	1200 mg IV once followed by 900 mg weekly	Requires meningococcal prophylaxis during therapy

Treg presence in the graft and those designed to block the costimulatory or chemotactic pathways responsible for the activation of B lymphocytes by T cells.

Outcomes

Unfortunately, the diagnosis of AMR remains associated with poor short-term and long-term prognosis. There is both increased mortality and incidence of CLAD among survivors.[8,19,23,61] In one example case series, 1-year survival was profoundly impacted (mortality of 47% with 29% dying of refractory AMR), and of those who survived past 1 year, 93% went on to develop CLAD.[8] The largest single-center retrospective study of 55 patients treated for AMR demonstrated similarly dire long-term outcomes, with a 38% 1-year mortality.[61] These results have been replicated in various case series and underscore that although the acute allograft dysfunction associated with AMR may be reversible with early and intensive therapy, there remains a high risk of CLAD with poor long-term survival. Altogether, this emphasizes the need for earlier identification and prevention to improve longitudinal patient outcomes with AMR.

SUMMARY

Long after its establishment as an important form of lung allograft rejection, AMR remains a formidable clinical challenge to diagnose, limited by its diverse presentation, nonspecific diagnostic features, and the variable relationship between antibody formation and graft dysfunction. Even in the setting of a confirmed diagnosis, treatment regimens borrow nearly exclusively from other solid-organ transplants because AMR's diagnostic variability continues to limit the ability to conduct broad, multicenter trials required to establish true evidence-based protocols. However, as our understanding of the pathophysiology of AMR continues to expand, more specific diagnostic methods are emerging, with both cfDNA and exosome analysis offering hope for an earlier diagnosis before the onset of graft injury. Similarly, novel treatment options are being evaluated, and the focus on understanding the inflammatory milieu that leads to antibody development offers the exciting prospect of preventative strategies rather than reactive therapies. Looking forward, the focus in AMR should remain on the development of accurate and reproducible diagnostic methods with the subsequent ability to design and conduct prospective, multicenter treatment trials.

CLINICS CARE POINTS

- AMR is a common but underrecognized form of lung rejection
- Optimal treatment for AMR is uncertain
- Outcomes after AMR are very poor

REFERENCES

1. Chambers DC, Cherikh WS, Harhay MO, et al. International Society for heart and lung transplantation. The International Thoracic organ transplant Registry of the International Society for heart and lung transplantation: Thirty-sixth adult lung and heart-lung transplantation report-2019; focus theme: donor and recipient size match. J Heart Lung Transpl 2019 Oct;38(10):1042–55. https://doi.org/10.1016/j.healun.2019.08.001. Epub 2019 Aug 8. PMID: 31548030.

2. Chambers DC, Cherikh WS, Goldfarb SB, et al. The International Thoracic organ transplant Registry of the International Society for heart and lung transplantation: Thirty-fifth adult lung and heart-lung transplant report-2018; focus theme: Multiorgan transplantation. J Heart Lung Transpl 2018;37: 1169–83.

3. Cohen DG, Christie JD, Anderson BJ, et al. Cognitive function, mental health, and health-related quality of life after lung transplantation. Ann Am Thorac Soc 2014;11:522–30.

4. Hachem R. Antibody-mediated lung transplant rejection. Curr Respir Care Rep 2012;1:157–61.

5. Westall GP, Snell GI. Antibody-mediated rejection in lung transplantation. Transplantation 2014;98: 927–30.

6. Daoud AH, Betensley AD. Diagnosis and treatment of antibody mediated rejection in lung transplantation: a retrospective case series. Transpl Immunol 2013;28:1–5.

7. DeNicola MM, Weigt SS, Belperio JA, et al. Pathologic findings in lung allografts with anti-HLA antibodies. J Heart Lung Transpl 2013;32:326–32.

8. Witt CA, Gaut JP, Yusen RD, et al. Acute antibody-mediated rejection after lung transplantation. J Heart Lung Transpl 2013;32:1034–40.

9. Angaswamy N, Tiriveedhi V, Sarma NJ, et al. Interplay between immune responses to HLA and non-HLA self-antigens in allograft rejection. Hum Immunol 2013;74:1478–85.

10. Berry G, Burke M, Andersen C, et al. Pathology of pulmonary antibody-mediated rejection: 2012 update from the Pathology Council of the ISHLT. J Heart Lung Transpl 2013;32:14–21.

11. Zander DS, Baz MA, Visner GA, et al. Analysis of early deaths after isolated lung transplantation. Chest 2001;120:225–32.

12. Tait BD. Detection of HLA antibodies in organ transplant recipients – Triumphs and challenges of the solid phase bead assay. Front Immunol 2016;7:570.

13. Badesch DB, Zamora M, Fullerton D, et al. Pulmonary capillaritis: a possible histologic form of acute pulmonary allograft rejection. J Heart Lung Transpl 1998;17:415–22.

14. Saint Martin GA, Reddy VB, Garrity ER, et al. Humoral (antibody-mediated) rejection in lung transplantation. J Heart Lung Transpl 1996;15:1217–22.

15. Colvin MM, Cook JL, Chang PP, et al. Sensitization in heart transplantation: emerging knowledge: a scientific statement from the American Heart Association. Circulation 2019;139(12):e553–78.

16. Rees L, Kim JJ. HLA sensitization: can it be prevented? Pediatr Nephrol 2015;30(4):577–87.

17. Smith JD, Ibrahim MW, Newell H, et al. Pre-transplant donor HLA-specific antibodies: characteristics causing detrimental effects on survival after lung transplantation. J Heart Lung Transpl 2014;33:1074–82.

18. Brugière O, Suberbielle C, Thabut G, et al. Lung transplantation in patients with pretransplantation donor-specific antibodies detected by Luminex assay. Transplantation 2013;95:761–5.

19. Aguilar PR, Carpenter D, Ritter J, et al. The role of C4d deposition in the diagnosis of antibody-mediated rejection after lung transplantation. Am J Transpl 2018;18:936–44.

20. Bosanquet JP, Witt CA, Bemiss BC, et al. The Impact of pre-transplant allosensitization on outcomes after lung transplantation. J Heart Lung Transpl 2015;34:1415–22.

21. Tague LK, Witt CA, Byers DE, et al. Association between allosensitization and waiting list outcomes among adult lung transplant candidates in the United States. Ann Am Thorac Soc 2019;16(7):846–52.

22. Hachem RR. Donor-specific antibodies in lung transplantation. Curr Opin Organ Transpl 2020 Dec;25(6):563–7.

23. Kim M, Townsend KR, Wood IG, et al. Impact of pre-transplant anti-HLA antibodies on outcomes in lung transplant candidates. Am J Respir Crit Care Med 2014;189:1234–9.

24. Tinckam KJ, Keshavjee S, Chaparro C, et al. Survival in sensitized lung transplant recipients with perioperative desensitization. Am J Transpl 2015;15:417–26. https://doi.org/10.1111/ajt.13076.

25. Morrell MR, Pilewski JM, Gries CJ, et al. De novo donor-specific HLA antibodies are associated with early and high-grade bronchiolitis obliterans syndrome and death after lung transplantation. J Heart Lung Transpl 2014;33:1288–94.

26. Hachem RR, Kamoun M, Budev MM, et al. Human leukocyte antigens antibodies after lung transplantation: primary results of the HALT study. Am J Transpl 2018;18(9):2285–94.

27. Hachem RR, Yusen RD, Meyers BF, et al. Anti-human leukocyte antigen antibodies and preemptive antibody-directed therapy after lung transplantation. J Heart Lung Transpl 2010;29:973–80.

28. Tikkanen JM, Singer LG, Kim SJ, et al. De novo DQ donor-specific antibodies are associated with chronic lung allograft dysfunction after lung transplantation. Am J Respir Crit Care Med 2016;194(5):596–606.

29. Schmitzer M, Winter H, Kneidinger N, et al. Persistence of de novo donor specific HLA-Antibodies after lung transplantation: a potential marker of decreased patient survival. HLA 2018;92(1):24–32.

30. Wilkes DS. Autoantibody formation in human and rat studies of chronic rejection and primary graft dysfunction. Semin Immunol 2012 Apr;24(2):131–5.

31. Reinsmoen NL, Mirocha J, Ensor CR, et al. A 3-center study Reveals New Insights into the impact of non-HLA antibodies on lung transplantation outcome. Transplantation 2017;101(6):1215–21.

32. Hagedorn PH, Burton CM, Sahar E, et al. Integrative analysis correlates donor transcripts to recipient autoantibodies in primary graft dysfunction after lung transplantation. Immunology 2011;132(3):394–400.

33. Tiriveedhi V, Gautam B, Sarma NJ, et al. Pre-transplant antibodies to Kα1 tubulin and collagen-V in lung transplantation: clinical correlations. J Heart Lung Transpl 2013;32(8):807–14.

34. Hachem RR, Tiriveedhi V, Patterson GA, et al. Antibodies to K-α 1 tubulin and collagen V are associated with chronic rejection after lung transplantation. Am J Transpl 2012;12(8):2164–71.

35. Levine DJ, Glanville AR, Aboyoun C, et al. Antibody-mediated rejection of the lung: a consensus report of the International Society for heart and lung transplantation. J Heart Lung Transpl 2016;35:397–406.

36. Patel JK, Kobashigawa JA. Thoracic organ transplantation: laboratory methods. Methods Mol Biol 2013;1034:127–43.

37. Pajaro OE, George JF. On solid-phase antibody assays. J Heart Lung Transpl 2010;29(11):1207–9.

38. Tambur AR, Herrera ND, Haarberg KM, et al. Assessing antibody Strength: Comparison of MFI, C1q, and titer Information. Am J Transpl 2015;15:2421–30.

39. Otani S, Davis AK, Cantwell L, et al. Evolving experience of treating antibody-mediated rejection following lung transplantation. Transpl Immunol 2014;31:75–80.

40. Djamali A, Kaufman DB, Ellis TM, et al. Diagnosis and management of antibody-mediated rejection: current status and novel approaches. Am J Transpl 2014;14:255–71.

41. Girnita AL, McCurry KR, Iacono AT, et al. HLA-specific antibodies are associated with high-grade and persistent-recurrent lung allograft acute rejection. J Heart Lung Transpl 2004;23:1135–41.

42. Roden AC, Maleszewski JJ, Yi ES, et al. Reproducibility of Complement 4d deposition by immunofluorescence and immunohistochemistry in lung allograft biopsies. J Heart Lung Transpl 2014;33:1223–32.

43. Wallace WD, Weigt SS, Farver CF. Update on pathology of antibody-mediated rejection in the lung allograft. Curr Opin Organ Transpl 2014;19:303–8.

44. Heigl T, Saez-Gimenez B, Van Herck A, et al. Free airway C4d after lung transplantation - a Quantitative analysis of Bronchoalveolar Lavage Fluid. Transpl Immunol 2020;64:101352.

45. Haas M, Sis B, Racusen LC, et al. Banff 2013 meeting report: inclusion of c4d-negative antibody-mediated rejection and antibody-associated arterial lesions. Am J Transpl 2014;14:272–83.

46. Valenzuela NM, McNamara JT, Reed EF. Antibody-mediated graft injury: complement-dependent and complement-independent mechanisms. Curr Opin Organ Transpl 2014;19:33–40.

47. Sellarés J, Reeve J, Loupy A, et al. Molecular diagnosis of antibody-mediated rejection in human kidney transplants. Am J Transpl 2013;13(4):971–83.

48. Hidalgo LG, Sis B, Sellares J, et al. NK cell transcripts and NK cells in kidney biopsies from patients with donor-specific antibodies: evidence for NK cell involvement in antibody-mediated rejection. Am J Transpl 2010;10:1812–22.

49. Orandi BJ, Alachkar N, Kraus ES, et al. Presentation and outcomes of C4d-negative antibody-mediated rejection after kidney transplantation. Am J Transpl 2016;16(1):213–20.

50. Takemoto SK, Zeevi A, Feng S, et al. National conference to assess antibody-mediated rejection in solid organ transplantation. Am J Transpl 2004;4:1033–41.

51. Alexander MP, Bentall A, Aleff PCA, et al. Ultrastructural changes in pulmonary allografts with antibody-mediated rejection. J Heart Lung Transpl 2020;39(2):165–75.

52. Agbor-Enoh S, Jackson AM, Tunc I, et al. Late manifestation of alloantibody-associated injury and clinical pulmonary antibody-mediated rejection: evidence from cell-free DNA analysis. J Heart Lung Transpl 2018;37:925–32.

53. Agbor-Enoh S, Wang Y, Tunc I, et al. Donor-derived cell-free DNA predicts allograft failure and mortality after lung transplantation. EBioMedicine 2019;40:541–53.

54. Jang MK, Tunc I, Berry GJ, et al. Donor-derived cell-free DNA accurately detects acute rejection in lung transplant patients, a multicenter cohort study. J Heart Lung Transplant 2021;40:822–30.

55. Ravichandran R, Bansal S, Rahman M, et al. Extracellular vesicles mediate immune responses to tissue-associated self-antigens: role in solid organ transplantation. Front Immunol 2022;13:1–15.

56. Ravichandran R, Bansal S, Rahman M, et al. The role of donor derived exosomes in lung allograft rejection. Hum Immunol 2019;80(8):588–94.

57. Lavacca A, Presta R, Gai C, et al. Early effects of first-line treatment with anti-interleukin-6 receptor antibody tocilizumab for chronic active antibody-mediated rejection in kidney transplantation. Clin Transplantion 2020;34(8):e13908.

58. Jordan SC, Ammerman N, Choi J, et al. Novel therapeutic approaches to allosensitization and antibody-mediated rejection. Transplantation 2018;103:262–72.

59. Li W, Gauthier JM, Higashikubo R, et al. Bronchus-associated lymphoid tissue-resident Foxp3+ T lymphocytes prevent antibody-mediated lung rejection. J Clin Invest 2019;129(2):556–68.

60. Chiu S, Fernandez R, Subramanian V, et al. Lung injury combined with loss of regulatory T cells leads to de novo lung-restricted autoimmunity. J Immunol 2016;197(1):51–7.

61. Neuhaus K, Hohlfelder B, Bollinger J, et al. Antibody-mediated rejection management following lung transplantation. Ann Pharmacother 2022;56(1):60–4.

Critical Care Management of the Lung Transplant Recipient

Jake G. Natalini, MD, MSCE[a],*, Emily S. Clausen, MD[b]

KEYWORDS

- Critical care • Lung transplantation • Primary graft dysfunction • Acute rejection
- Extracorporeal membrane oxygenation

KEY POINTS

- Extracorporeal membrane oxygenation can be successfully used as a supportive means to bridge critically ill patients to lung transplantation, either without or in conjunction with mechanical ventilation.
- Graft failure (including primary graft dysfunction and acute rejection) and non-cytomegalovirus infection are the most common causes of mortality in the first year after lung transplantation, whereas bronchiolitis obliterans syndrome, a subtype of chronic lung allograft dysfunction, is the most common cause of death among lung transplant recipients who survive beyond 1 year.
- Primary graft dysfunction is a form of acute allograft ischemia-reperfusion injury characterized by hypoxemia and radiographic alveolar infiltrates that develop within 72 h after lung transplantation.
- Anastomotic complications such as ischemia and necrosis, bronchial dehiscence, bronchial infections, and bronchial stenosis are common in the first few weeks to months after lung transplantation, in part because of a lack of revascularization of the bronchial circulation.
- The three types of allograft rejection, categorized according to the timing of onset after lung transplantation and distinct histopathologic features, are antibody-mediated rejection, which can rarely appear as a form of hyperacute rejection, acute cellular rejection, and chronic lung allograft dysfunction, which can present as bronchiolitis obliterans syndrome and/or restrictive allograft syndrome.

INTRODUCTION

Lung transplantation has become an increasingly utilized therapeutic intervention for patients with end-stage lung diseases.[1] Since the first successful lung transplant was performed in 1983, survival outcomes have steadily improved, likely because of a multitude of factors including better donor and recipient selection, systematic changes in organ allocation, surgical advancements, modifications to immunosuppression, and evolving practices in managing postoperative illnesses such as primary graft dysfunction (PGD), acute rejection, and infections.[2] However, lung transplant recipients still experience frequent complications, often requiring treatment in an intensive care environment. In addition, both invasive mechanical ventilatory support and extracorporeal life support (ECLS) are being more frequently utilized as a means of bridging critically ill patients to transplants.[3] As such, lung transplant candidates and recipients have had an ever-growing presence in surgical and medical intensive care units (ICUs) worldwide.

[a] Division of Pulmonary, Critical Care, and Sleep Medicine, Department of Medicine, New York University Grossman School of Medicine, 530 First Avenue, HCC 4A, New York, NY 10016, USA; [b] Division of Pulmonary, Allergy, and Critical Care, Department of Medicine, Perelman School of Medicine at the University of Pennsylvania, Hospital of the University of Pennsylvania, 3400 Spruce Street, 9036 Gates Building, Philadelphia, PA 19104, USA
* Corresponding author.
E-mail address: jake.natalini@nyulangone.org

Clin Chest Med 44 (2023) 105–119
https://doi.org/10.1016/j.ccm.2022.10.010
0272-5231/23/© 2022 Elsevier Inc. All rights reserved.

Bridging to Lung Transplantation in an Intensive Care Setting

In the spring of 2005, the lung donor allocation system was revised to assign priority for lung offers based on a need-based lung allocation score (LAS) rather than accumulated time on the waiting list.[4,5] The LAS aimed to prioritize sicker patients who were more likely to benefit from lung transplantation. Given the high LAS scores for critically ill patients in the ICU and the more likely availability of suitable donors within weeks for these highest LAS patients, there has been an increase in the use of advanced modalities of support such as invasive mechanical ventilation and extracorporeal membrane oxygenation (ECMO) for actively listed patients awaiting transplant.[3] One prior study noted a significant improvement in 1-year post-transplant survival among patients bridged to transplant with ECMO from 25% in the early 2000s to 74% only a decade later.[6] Another United Network for Organ Sharing (UNOS) registry study reported increasing use of ECMO as a bridging strategy to lung transplantation, with similar survival rates relative to those recipients who were bridged with mechanical ventilation (MV).[7] Despite these similarities, recent data suggest that patients who require bridging with either MV or ECMO have worse outcomes in comparison to those patients who do not require any bridging.[7] However, a 2018 single-center study found that patients less than 40 years of age bridged to transplant on ECMO had similar survival rates compared to those recipients who did not require any bridging,[8] suggesting that age may be an important factor in deciding whether a patient is a candidate for ECMO bridging to transplant if clinically necessary.

Expertise in ECMO has increased significantly since the CESAR trial, which studied the use of early ECMO in the management of acute respiratory distress syndrome (ARDS).[9] Determining an appropriate ECMO strategy is based upon the characterization of respiratory failure, degree of right ventricular dysfunction, need for circulatory support, and insertion sites (peripheral vs central). A venovenous (VV) ECMO configuration provides support for both severe hypercapnic and hypoxemic respiratory failure, whereas venoarterial (VA) or hybrid configurations are utilized in the setting of hemodynamic instability, often because of significant pulmonary hypertension with right ventricular dysfunction in patients awaiting or undergoing evaluation for lung transplantation.

Among individuals with isolated severe hypercapnic respiratory failure, often seen in end-stage chronic obstructive pulmonary disease or severe bronchiectasis, lower-flow platforms such as extracorporeal carbon dioxide removal (ECCO$_2$R) may have potential use.[10,11] One case report previously described successful bridging to redo lung transplantation with ECCO$_2$R.[12] However, future studies comparing the use of ECCO$_2$R and VV EMCO as bridging strategies for lung transplantation are needed.

Regardless of a patient's ECMO configuration, there is a growing body of evidence supporting safe ambulation and rehabilitation practices for patients on ECMO, including central VA ECMO platforms and VV and peripheral VA ECMO platforms with femoral cannulation(s).[13–15] Although practices vary, one possible bridging strategy is to preferentially utilize ECMO to support patients awaiting lung transplantation (in the absence of ECMO-related complications) to minimize or fully eliminate the need for MV support. In doing so, patients generally require less sedation and can more easily engage in ongoing rehabilitation while awaiting transplant.

Complications of Extracorporeal Membrane Oxygenation

Potential complications from ECMO are not inconsequential and include bleeding, limb ischemia, infection, renal failure, and stroke, among others. A retrospective study using the Extracorporeal Life Support Organization (ELSO) registry showed that up to 30% of patients on VA ECMO support have bleeding complications, which is a higher overall incidence than VV ECMO, albeit serious gastrointestinal and pulmonary hemorrhage were more common among VV ECMO subjects.[16] Concerning stroke, another ELSO registry study in VV ECMO subjects showed an incidence of 2.8% for intracranial hemorrhage and 1.2% for ischemic stroke.[17]

Acute kidney injury (AKI) is common among the critically ill population. A large, single-center retrospective study of VA ECMO (not specific to lung transplantation) showed a significant survival disadvantage for those subjects who required renal replacement therapy (RRT) either before or after initiation of ECMO support.[18] A recent meta-analysis examining the overall incidence of AKI for those on ECMO support reported the need for RRT because of AKI in over 40% of patients.[19] The UNOS registry data also demonstrated a more than three-fold increased risk for AKI requiring in-hospital dialysis for those transplant recipients bridged with ECMO compared to those not requiring ECMO bridging.[7]

As cardiac output improves, patients with a peripheral VA ECMO configuration must be monitored for north-south (or Harlequin) syndrome, in which poorly oxygenated blood carried through the pulmonary circulation and not through the ECMO circuit is ejected out of the left ventricle and flows anterograde thereby limiting the retrograde flow of oxygenated blood to the upper extremities and brain.[20] Although far more invasive, a central VA ECMO configuration in which the outflow cannula is positioned in the ascending aorta obviates this risk. Alternatively, a second outflow cannula can be placed in the right internal jugular vein or a subclavian vein referred to as a VAV ECMO configuration.[21,22]

Intraoperative Mechanical Circulatory Support

Regardless of the need for advanced bridging strategies, ECMO support or, in some cases, cardiopulmonary bypass (CPB) is often required for patients with pulmonary hypertension but may also be necessary for those who cannot tolerate single-lung ventilation and perfusion because of hypoxemia or hemodynamic instability. There has been an increasing number of cases (nearly 50% at some institutions) performed on ECMO or CPB.[23] However, there are no randomized controlled trials and only a limited number of cohort studies comparing clinical outcomes for lung transplantation performed on ECMO versus CPB. Both intraoperative ECMO and CPB are associated with a higher risk of PGD in the immediate postoperative period.[24,25] The use of ECMO may carry less risk for bleeding complications, acute renal failure, and early mortality in comparison to CPB, although unplanned or prolonged CPB may be a more important risk factor for increased morbidity and mortality than CPB itself.[24] Finally, prolonged CPB time can be complicated by postoperative vasoplegia, often necessitating hemodynamic vasopressor support.[26]

Postoperative Ventilatory Management

After lung transplantation, patients are transitioned to a single-lumen endotracheal tube and transferred to an ICU. Most patients are ventilated in either a volume assist-control mode or a pressure assist-control mode. Low tidal volume ventilation strategies are preferred, ideally targeting volumes between 6 and 8 mL per kg of the donor's ideal body weight (IBW) rather than the recipient's IBW. In a recent international survey on MV practices after lung transplantation, 35% of respondents preferentially used volume assist-control ventilation, whereas 37% of respondents preferred pressure assist-control ventilation. In addition, survey respondents favored limiting

FiO_2 over positive end-expiratory pressure (PEEP) (69% vs. 31%). The median minimum PEEP used was 5 cm H_2O and the median maximum was 11.5 cm H_2O. Tidal volumes were frequently based on recipient and not donor characteristics, and most respondents selected 6 mL per kg of recipient IBW as a target. In the setting of PGD, the plateau pressure limit for adjusting tidal volumes was 30 cm H_2O—[27]likely an extrapolation from ARDS management guidelines.[28]

Certain patient populations require special ventilator management. For example, mechanically ventilated patients with obstructive airway disease can develop auto-PEEP if they have excessive minute ventilation that results in a relatively short expiratory time.[29] Among single-lung transplant recipients, auto-PEEP can lead to native lung dynamic hyperinflation, which in turn can compromise the newly transplanted lung and lead to hypotension and hemodynamic instability. This problem is magnified among patients who develop PGD or pneumonia in the newly transplanted allograft, thus, decreasing its compliance. In such cases, increased minute ventilation may be required for more effective CO_2 removal, along with higher PEEP to promote improved oxygenation. Consequentially, the more compliant emphysematous lung becomes overexpanded and can herniate toward the contralateral hemithorax.[30] Attempts to prevent or manage this possible complication by using selective independent ventilation with a double-lumen endotracheal tube have been tried, although modern-day practices generally favor the use of ECMO to address this complication.[31,32] Of note, lung hyperinflation is associated with a significantly longer stay in the ICU, a longer duration of MV, and a trend toward higher mortality.[33] For this reason, among others, a bilateral lung transplant is nowadays more commonly recommended for patients with severe emphysema.

Patients further out from lung transplantation who develop chronic lung allograft dysfunction (CLAD), synonymous with chronic rejection, also require special ventilatory considerations. CLAD encompasses two distinct subtypes: bronchiolitis obliterans syndrome (BOS), which is the obstructive and far more common phenotype; and restrictive allograft syndrome (RAS), which is the restrictive, less common phenotype.[34] Strategies for mechanically ventilating a patient with BOS should be aimed at prolonging expiratory time and minimizing risk for dynamic hyperinflation, akin to ventilatory strategies in severe asthma exacerbations or end-stage chronic obstructive pulmonary disease. Conversely, strategies for mechanically ventilating a patient with RAS should prioritize utilizing lower tidal volumes and maintaining acceptable plateau pressures to avoid barotrauma.

Among patients meeting commonly accepted weaning criteria, extubation can be performed as early as 12 to 24 h postoperatively in the absence of any complications, preferably to a high-flow nasal cannula to minimize risk for reintubation.[35]

General Postoperative Management

In cases of prolonged allograft ischemic times where PGD is likely to develop or if the donor lung is oversized, a surgeon may elect to delay chest closure as compression of the mediastinum by the donor allografts can result in hemodynamic compromise. During this time, patients should be kept sedated and maintained on MV. As ischemia-reperfusion injury in PGD subsides, the allografts become less edematous and are more easily accommodated by the closed chest cavity. Similarly, a surgeon may choose to perform a partial or full lobar resection in cases of oversizing.

Chest tubes are inserted intraoperatively into each pleural cavity (usually two per side) and are placed under continuous suction to promote lung reexpansion and continued evacuation of pleural fluid. A clamp trial to assess whether a chest tube can be safely removed is generally performed once there is complete resolution of any air leaks and after chest tube output falls below 100 to 150 mL in 24 h.

Both postural drainage and chest physiotherapy can be routinely employed without concern for mechanical complications at the bronchial anastomoses, and patients should perform incentive spirometry soon after extubation. Many transplant centers utilize devices that simultaneously provide positive pressure, continuous high-frequency oscillations, and aerosol delivery to promote airway clearance and lung expansion,[36] although these devices should be used with caution in patients with air leaks present in their chest tube drainage systems because of concern for pneumothorax.

Prophylactic broad-spectrum antibiotics with activity against both gram-negative and gram-positive bacteria are administered in the first 48 to 72 h after lung transplantation.[37] Donor and recipient sputum, bronchial swab, and/or bronchoalveolar lavage fluid cultures are acquired in the operating room and from bronchoscopies performed in the first 24 to 48 h post-transplant, which can help guide appropriate narrowing of antimicrobial therapies. In addition, most transplant programs administer valganciclovir or ganciclovir for cytomegalovirus (CMV) prophylaxis if either the recipient or the donor CMV IgG serologies are positive before surgery.[38] Finally, most transplant centers routinely administer prophylactic antifungal agents such as inhaled amphotericin B, voriconazole, posaconazole, or isavuconazonium postoperatively, although there is significant variability across transplant centers about specific antifungal regimens and their respective durations.[39]

Post-surgical pain management strategies vary by transplant center and typically require a multimodal approach. Pain is often managed with opioids such as intravenous fentanyl, morphine sulfate, or hydromorphone and/or via an epidural catheter with a patient-regulated pain control system. However, opioid-sparing pain regimens consisting of agents such as acetaminophen, gabapentin, and methocarbamol have been used with success.[40] In addition, intraoperative liposomal bupivacaine intercostal nerve block and intercostal cryoablation have been shown to reduce postoperative pain and opioid use after lung transplantation and other procedures requiring a thoracotomy.[40,41] Lastly, some transplant centers may elect to place either paravertebral or epidural catheters for administration of local anesthetic agents in an effort to minimize postoperative opioid requirements,[42–44] although complicated and often time-sensitive logistical considerations at the time of transplant limit their use.

Overview of Induction and Maintenance Immunosuppression

As part of an induction immunosuppressive regimen, corticosteroids are administered intraoperatively at the time of allograft reperfusion, usually as intravenous methylprednisolone 500 to 1,000 mg. This is often followed by the administration of methylprednisolone 1 to 3 mg per kg daily during the subsequent 3 days and then 0.5 to 0.8 mg per kg daily, which eventually is converted to an equivalent oral prednisone dose that is tapered over the ensuing weeks to months to a maintenance dose of 5 to 10 mg. Along with high-dose methylprednisolone, many centers currently use interleukin-2 receptor blockers (e.g., basiliximab) for induction immunosuppression, given as a fixed dose of 20 mg intraoperatively and again 4 days postoperatively. A retrospective International Society of Heart and Lung Transplantation (ISHLT) registry analysis demonstrated improved survival with the use of IL-2 receptor antagonists in both single and bilateral lung transplant recipients and with the use of anti-thymocyte globulin (ATG), a less commonly used cytolytic induction immunosuppressive agent, in bilateral lung transplant recipients.[45]

Maintenance immunosuppression after lung transplantation most commonly consists of three different agents: a calcineurin inhibitor (either tacrolimus or cyclosporine), a cell cycle inhibitor (either mycophenolate mofetil or azathioprine), and a corticosteroid (initially methylprednisolone and subsequently prednisone, as noted above).[46] Tacrolimus is typically dosed at approximately 0.1 mg per kg orally daily in two divided doses, or as a single dose with the slow-release formulation, and adjusted to maintain serum trough level concentrations of 8 to 15 ng/mL. Cyclosporine is generally dosed at 5 mg per kg orally daily in two divided doses and adjusted to maintain serum trough level concentrations of 250 to 350 ng/mL. Mycophenolate mofetil is dosed at 1 to 3 gm daily in two divided doses and azathioprine is dosed at 1 to 2 mg/kg daily, although lower doses may be required in patients who develop leukopenia as a side effect. The role of mTOR inhibitors such as sirolimus and everolimus after lung transplantation merits further investigation. However, it is recommended that neither agent be used in the early postoperative period (i.e., less than 10 to 12 weeks) because of concerns for impaired wound healing and bronchial anastomosis breakdown.

Several medications interact with calcineurin inhibitors, and levels of tacrolimus and cyclosporine can either increase or decrease depending on the nature of the drug–drug interaction. For example, azoles, particularly voriconazole and posaconazole, cause a significant increase in serum concentrations of tacrolimus and cyclosporine. Cessation of these agents without an appropriate increase in a patient's tacrolimus or cyclosporine dose can cause dangerously low therapeutic concentrations of these drugs. There are other commonly prescribed medications such as calcium channel blockers, macrolide antibiotics, rifampin, anticonvulsants, and gastric motility agents shown to interact with calcineurin inhibitors. Thus, consultation with either a pharmacist or a lung transplant physician may be necessary to ensure immunosuppressive therapies are dosed appropriately. Generally speaking, tacrolimus and cyclosporine levels should be monitored daily in the immediate postoperative period as frequent dosing adjustments may be required.

Early Postoperative Complications

The most frequent causes of mortality among lung transplant recipients are graft failure (including PGD) during the first 30 days following transplantation, non-CMV infection in the first year following transplantation, and chronic rejection in the subsequent years following transplantation.[1] However, there are a multitude of early and late complications that can occur after lung transplantation. Here, we focus on early complications after lung transplantation often necessitating management in a critical care setting.

Primary graft dysfunction

The largest contributor to early mortality after lung transplantation is PGD.[47] PGD is a form of ischemia-reperfusion injury occurring within 72 h after transplant that leads to increased capillary permeability and noncardiogenic pulmonary edema. Several mechanistic pathways have been implicated in the pathogenesis of PGD including endothelial dysfunction, the release of proinflammatory cytokines and chemokines, innate immune dysfunction, and increased oxidative stress.[25,48]

In 2005, the ISHLT proposed a standardized PGD severity grading system based on the radiographic presence or absence of alveolar infiltrates and the degree of gas exchange impairment, quantified using a PaO_2/FiO_2 ratio (**Table 1**).[49] This was subsequently updated in 2017 to also include an alternative grading schema using a ratio of SaO_2/FiO_2 in cases where PaO_2 measurements cannot be obtained, with adjusted cutoffs extracted from prior studies of ARDS (see **Table 1**).[50,51] Of note, both sets of guidelines

Table 1			
Grading classification schema for primary graft dysfunction			
PGD Grade	Pulmonary Edema on Chest Radiograph	PaO_2/FiO_2 Ratio	SpO_2/FiO_2 Ratio[a]
0	No	>300	>315
1	Yes	>300	>315
2	Yes	200–300	235–315
3	Yes	<200	<235

Abbreviations: FiO2, fraction of inspired oxygen; PaO2, partial pressure of arterial oxygen; PGD, primary graft dysfunction; SpO2, peripheral capillary oxygen saturation.
[a] If PaO2 measurements are not available.
Adapted from Christie JD, Carby M, Bag R, et al. Report of the ISHLT Working Group on Primary Lung Graft Dysfunction part II: definition. A consensus statement of the International Society for Heart and Lung Transplantation. J Heart Lung Transplant. 2005;24(10):1454-1459 and Snell GI, Yusen RD, Weill D, et al. Report of the ISHLT Working Group on Primary Lung Graft Dysfunction, part I: Definition and grading-A 2016 Consensus Group statement of the International Society for Heart and Lung Transplantation. J Heart Lung Transplant. 2017;36(10):1097-1103.

emphasize the importance of excluding other disease processes that could look radiographically similar to PGD such as multifocal pneumonia or cardiogenic pulmonary edema.

PGD commonly occurs after lung transplantation and has important prognostic implications. Specifically, grade 3 PGD is associated with significantly longer ICU and hospital lengths of stay as well as increased 90-day and 1-year mortality, compared to absent or lower grades of PGD.[47,51,52] Multiple studies have consistently demonstrated an association between PGD and increased risk for the subsequent development of CLAD.[53–55] Prior studies applying the standardized ISHLT classification system estimate an overall PGD incidence of 30% and a grade 3 PGD incidence of 15 to 20%.[52,56,57]

PGD generally develops within 48 h after lung transplantation, whereas other radiographically similar processes, such as acute rejection and infection, more commonly develop beyond the first 48 h after transplant. Pulmonary venous anastomotic complications (e.g., venous thrombosis, kinking, or external compression) can present similarly, although these diagnoses can be excluded by transesophageal echocardiography. Multiple risk factors have been associated with the development of PGD and can be subdivided into recipient-related, donor-related, perioperative, and postoperative risk factors (**Table 2**).[47,51,52,56,58–62]

Typical radiographic findings include perihilar haziness, patchy alveolar consolidations, and, in its most severe form, dense perihilar and basilar alveolar consolidations with air bronchograms (**Fig. 1**). In addition, PGD can lead to a decrease in compliance and an increase in pulmonary vascular resistance. On histopathology, PGD can appear as diffuse alveolar damage based on reports from biopsy specimens, autopsies, and lung explants removed during re-transplantation; however, a biopsy is rarely necessary to establish the diagnosis. PGD usually stabilizes within 2 to 4 days of onset and subsequently resolves, although in some cases PGD can persist to varying degrees for days to weeks after lung transplantation.

Treatment of PGD is primarily supportive, and clinical management strategies have been mostly extrapolated from existing ARDS literature. Therapies with demonstrated benefits include lung-protective mechanical ventilation, diuretics, inhaled nitric oxide (iNO), and, in more severe cases, VV ECMO.[47] Although low tidal volume ventilation strategies are frequently utilized, set tidal volumes often only take into consideration recipient characteristics and not donor characteristics.[27,63] Use of iNO has been described for both the prevention and treatment of PGD.[64–67] In one randomized placebo-controlled trial, prophylactic iNO initiated 10 min after reperfusion and continued for a minimum of 6 h was not associated with improved clinical outcomes.[64] In cases of refractory hypoxemia because of severe PGD, however, iNO is an effective salvage therapy.[65–67] VV ECMO is being increasingly utilized to support patients who develop severe PGD after lung transplantation, with better outcomes reported if ECMO is initiated early (ideally within the first 24 h after transplantation).[68–70] The rationale for starting earlier ECMO support is to prevent or minimize injury to the newly transplanted lung(s) from a combination of high plateau pressures and excess PEEP and oxygen concentrations. In a 2007 ELSO registry study, only 42% of patients with PGD requiring ECMO support survived to hospital discharge with death most commonly attributed to multiorgan failure,[69] although outcomes have likely improved since then given clinical advances in ECLS. Lastly, re-transplantation in cases of very severe PGD is generally not advised because of poor survival outcomes.[71]

Airway complications

Anastomotic complications including ischemia and necrosis (**Fig. 2**A), dehiscence (**Fig. 2**B), stenosis, and bronchial infection are common in the first few weeks to months after lung transplantation, due in part to the lack or revascularization of the bronchial circulation.[72,73] One 2009 study reported anastomotic complications in 7 to 18% of lung transplant recipients with an associated mortality of 2 to 4%.[74] However, the incidence of anastomotic complications has likely decreased as surgical techniques have improved.

Established risk factors for anastomotic complications after lung transplantation include peri- or postoperative hypotension, certain anastomotic surgical techniques, right-sided anastomoses (which are more than twice as likely to develop airway complications compared to left-sided anastomoses), length of the donor bronchus, PGD, acute cellular rejection, and microbiologic contamination, particularly with *Aspergillus*, *Candida*, *Rhizopus*, and *Mucor* species.[73] Among many but not all of these risk factors, reduced blood flow to the anastomosis is predominantly what compromises its integrity.

Early anastomotic complications generally occur within 4 to 12 weeks after lung transplantation and include partial or complete ischemia or necrosis, bronchial dehiscence, and fungal and bacterial (usually *Staphylococcus* or *Pseudomonas* species) infections. Bronchial dehiscence should be suspected in patients with prolonged

Table 2
Clinical risk factors for the development of primary graft dysfunction

Category	Risk Factor
Recipient-related risk factors[52,56,58,59]	Body mass index >25 kg/mg^2 Diagnoses of IPF, PAH, and sarcoidosis Elevated pulmonary artery pressure at time of transplant Female sex Left ventricular diastolic dysfunction
Donor-related risk factors[52,56,60–62]	Donor age extremes (i.e., pediatric donors and age >55 years old) African American race Smoking history Alcohol use Head trauma Chest trauma or lung contusion Inhalation smoke exposure Prolonged MV Hemodynamic instability after brain death Massive donor blood transfusion
Perioperative risk factors[47,52]	FiO$_2$ >0.40 during allograft reperfusion Single-lung transplantation Intraoperative CPB Use of Euro-Collins preservation solution Prolonged ischemic time Transfusion volume >1 liter Delayed chest closure
Post-transplant risk factors[51]	Aspiration Volume overload Arterial and venous anastomotic complications Hemodynamic instability MV with large tidal volumes Pneumonia

Abbreviations: FiO$_2$, fraction of inspired oxygen; IPF, idiopathic pulmonary fibrosis; PAH, pulmonary arterial hypertension.
Adapted from refs [25,101]

chest tube air leaks in the early post-transplant period. Bronchial dehiscence can predispose patients to serious infectious complications such as empyema, mediastinitis, or the formation of a peribronchial abscess or fistula.

The appearance of extraluminal air on chest CT is very sensitive and specific for the diagnosis of anastomotic dehiscence.[73] However, chest CT cannot reliably detect other early anastomotic complications such as ischemic, necrosis, and infection. Rather, bronchoscopy is the preferred method for comprehensively evaluating bronchial anastomosis. It is often performed before post-transplant extubation, bearing in mind that ischemic changes can take several days to weeks to develop, and again before hospital discharge. Subsequent anastomotic complications are generally monitored during routine surveillance bronchoscopies that occur in the first year after lung transplantation.

Bronchoscopic evaluation of anastomoses should assess for four main elements, per the recently proposed ISHLT consensus guidelines: ischemia and necrosis, dehiscence, stenosis, and malacia.[73] Standardized reporting of airway complications allows clinicians to more easily track evolutionary changes over time in addition to providing better uniformity in research studies. During bronchoscopy, specimens from a bronchial wash or brush should be sent for culture and cytologic examination. If there is any evidence of infection, appropriate antimicrobial therapies should be initiated based on culture results.

Early anastomotic complications can predispose patients to later complications such as bronchial stenosis, bronchomalacia, and the development of exophytic granulation tissue. These conditions can manifest symptomatically as dyspnea at rest or on exertion, wheezing, cough, and/or worsening obstruction as

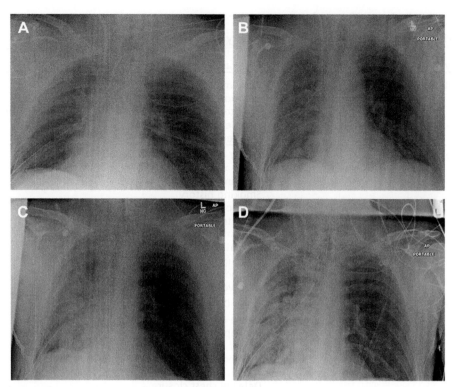

Fig. 1. Evolution of severe primary graft dysfunction following a right single-lung transplant for chronic obstructive pulmonary disease. Chest radiographs are shown at (*A*) baseline (i.e., immediately postoperatively), (*B*) 24 h, (*C*) 48 h, and (*D*) 72 h after transplant. (*From* Lee JC, Christie JD. Primary graft dysfunction. Clin Chest Med. 2011;32(2):279-293.)[100]

documented by pulmonary function testing. Therapeutic options for anastomotic complications include balloon dilation of a stricture, stent placement, cryotherapy, argon beam coagulation, laser procedures, and rarely surgery. Among lung transplant recipients who develop respiratory failure requiring intubation and mechanical ventilation, treating physicians should be aware of any

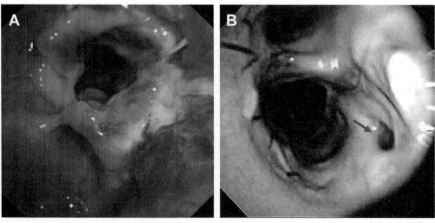

Fig. 2. Two examples of anastomotic complications following lung transplantation. (*A*) Circumferential airway anastomotic necrosis extending >1 cm from the anastomosis to the bronchus intermedius. (*B*) Airway anastomotic necrosis along the membranous wall with a small area of dehiscence (indicated by the *red arrow*). (Crespo MM, McCarthy DP, Hopkins PM, et al. ISHLT Consensus Statement on adult and pediatric airway complications after lung transplantation: Definitions, grading system, and therapeutics. J Heart Lung Transplant 2018;37(5):548-563.)

anastomotic issues as these may alter diagnostic considerations and influence ventilatory management.

Acute allograft rejection

The three types of allograft rejection, categorized according to the timing of onset after lung transplantation and distinct histopathologic features, are antibody-mediated rejection (AMR), which can rarely appear as a form of hyperacute rejection, acute cellular rejection (ACR), and CLAD, which can manifest as BOS and/or RAS.

Hyperacute rejection is a type of rapid-onset AMR that generally occurs intraoperatively after allograft reperfusion. It is caused by preexisting anti-human leukocyte antigen (HLA) antibodies that bind to the donor vascular epithelium leading to activation of complement, vessel thrombosis, and allograft failure. Significant advancements in HLA antibody testing have led to a dramatic reduction in the incidence of hyperacute rejection, which now rarely occurs.

AMR occurs as a result of allospecific B cell and plasma cell production of antibodies directed against donor lung antigens. Antigen–antibody complex formation leads to the activation of both complement-dependent and complement-independent pathways, resulting in acute allograft dysfunction. Despite recently proposed diagnostic criteria,[75] establishing a clinical diagnosis of AMR can still be challenging, especially given that donor-specific antibodies may not always be serologically present. Treatment of AMR includes a combination of plasmapheresis, intravenous immunoglobulin, proteasome inhibitors such as bortezomib and carfilzomib, and/or rituximab, a monoclonal antibody against the CD20 antigen. Of note, AMR is a well-described risk factor for CLAD.[76]

ACR is the far more common type of acute allograft rejection, characterized by the presence of perivascular and interstitial mononuclear cell infiltrates that develop as a result of T lymphocyte recognition of foreign major histocompatibility complexes or other antigens.[77] Approximately half of lung transplant recipients will develop some degree of ACR during the early months after transplant, and as many as 90% of patients will experience at least one episode of ACR within the first year.[78]

Notably, both ACR and AMR can present with varying degrees of severity. More severe cases can be complicated by acute hypoxemic respiratory failure requiring mechanical ventilation or even ECMO support. Both entities, however, are highly treatable, and ECMO should be considered early in cases of rapidly escalating ventilatory requirements to avoid ventilator-induced injury to the allograft(s).

Bleeding and vascular complications

Another complication of lung transplantation is postoperative hemorrhage often requiring chest re-exploration and washout. Early clues to this diagnosis include radiographic evidence of a hemothorax (usually white-out of the hemithorax) or a large volume of blood draining from the thoracostomy tubes. Risk factors include perioperative CPB, postoperative anticoagulation, and the presence of pleural adhesions from prior thoracic surgeries or pleurodesis performed before lung transplantation.[79]

The start of postoperative hemorrhage is frequently observed intraoperatively or in the first 12 to 24 h after arrival to the ICU. The management should focus on adequate resuscitation, correcting any associated coagulopathies, and transfusing as indicated. However, if active bleeding continues despite these measures, particularly if bleeding results in hemodynamic instability and/or multiple blood transfusion requirements, it is imperative to take the patient back to the operating room for better source control to avoid complications associated with hemorrhagic shock or pulmonary complications related to excess blood products.

In addition to the bronchial anastomotic complications discussed earlier, vascular anastomotic complications can occur. Stenosis at the venous anastomosis is suggested by new radiographic evidence of pulmonary edema and/or infiltrates. This condition can be confused with PGD and is usually diagnosed by transesophageal echocardiography (TEE). Stenosis at the arterial anastomosis is suggested by unexplained gas exchange abnormalities and/or new or worsening pulmonary hypertension.[80] To minimize this complication, the anesthesiologist and transplant surgeon should review the intraoperatively TEE to assess the gradients and flow turbulence through each one of the venous anastomoses before chest closure. If turbulent flows or elevated peak systolic velocities are noted on TEE, surgical revision may be necessary.

Infectious complications

Bacterial pneumonia is the most common life-threatening infection that develops during the early postoperative period with an estimated incidence as high as 35%.[81–84] CMV is the most common type of viral infection seen with a 50% cumulative incidence of viremia and/or tissue-invasive disease.[83–85] CMV can cause a wide spectrum of diseases, ranging from localized bronchial shedding or low-level viremia to widespread dissemination. The most common presentation of tissue-invasive CMV infection in lung transplant recipients is pneumonitis, but it can also present as gastroenteritis, hepatitis, or colitis. Other viruses that affect lung transplant recipients include herpes simplex virus (especially early after transplant) and community-acquired respiratory viruses such as respiratory syncytial virus, parainfluenza, influenza, human metapneumovirus, and adenovirus.[86] Lastly, invasive fungal infections are more common among lung transplant recipients compared to other solid organ transplant recipients, with an overall incidence of 15 to 35.[87,88] Such infections usually develop during the first few months after transplant and are associated with significant morbidity and increased risk for mortality.

Other early postoperative complications

Diaphragmatic paralysis because of phrenic nerve injury, which can occur in conjunction with other types of cardiothoracic surgery, is seen in 3 to 9% of lung transplant recipients and is associated with prolonged mechanical ventilation, increased ICU length of stay, and higher rates of tracheostomy tube placement.[89] An inability to wean a patient from mechanical ventilation may be indicative of phrenic nerve dysfunction, particularly in patients who underwent single-lung transplantation. The diagnosis can be confirmed by phrenic nerve conduction studies in mechanically ventilated patients or by fluoroscopic sniff test and/or point-of-care ultrasound of the diaphragm in non-mechanically ventilated patients. If the injury is a result of traumatic stretching of the phrenic nerve but the nerve is not completely transected, a slow recovery can be anticipated. Complete transection is rare, but the damage is permanent. In those cases, diaphragmatic plication or pacing may be warranted.

Pleural effusions also commonly develop and/or persist after lung transplantation. These effusions are usually lymphocyte-predominant exudates and can be associated early on with rejection, infection, or severing of the lymphatics (i.e., chylous effusion). Other causes of pleural effusions include heart failure, pulmonary embolism, and trapped lung. Rarely pleurodesis or decortication may be required.

Patients undergoing lung transplantation are also at risk for gastrointestinal complications. Specifically, lung transplant recipients experience higher rates of gastroparesis and severe gastroesophageal reflux disease, resulting in an increased risk for aspiration pneumonia. In addition, there is a higher incidence of gastrointestinal emergencies such as colonic perforation, small bowel obstruction, diverticulitis, CMV colitis, megacolon, prolonged ileus, ischemic bowel, and pancreatitis.[90]

Cardiac arrhythmias, particularly atrial arrhythmias such as atrial fibrillation, are seen in 16 to 46% of lung transplant recipients and are associated with an increase in hospital length of stay and increased 1-year mortality.[91,92] Risk factors include older age, right ventricular dysfunction or enlargement, elevated right atrial pressure, diastolic dysfunction, left atrial enlargement, and coronary artery disease.[92] One study demonstrated a 35% incidence of atrial fibrillation, which was associated with older age and CPB, with a resultant increase in hospital length of stay but no increase in mortality, ICU length of stay, or days on MV.[93] Early prophylactic administration of beta blockers is common practice across many transplant centers.

The hyperammonemia syndrome after lung transplantation is a rare but potentially fatal complication, occurring in 1- to 4% of lung transplant recipients with a 75% risk for mortality.[94,95] Previous reports have hypothesized that hyperammonemia may be caused by an unmasking of a partial urea cycle disorder under the metabolic stress of transplant or may be related to immunosuppressive agents, particularly calcineurin inhibitors, although its underlying pathophysiology remains poorly understood. Infections because of *Mycoplasma hominis* or *Ureaplasma* species, often donor-acquired, have also been implicated given these pathogens metabolize urea as an energy source and produce ammonia as a byproduct. Early detection is crucial with daily monitoring of ammonia levels in the immediate postoperative period, and management should be individualized based on clinical symptoms and blood ammonia concentrations. Treatment options include bowel decontamination, amino acid supplementation, and, in severe cases, nitrogen scavenger therapy and RRT.

Intensive Care Unit Outcomes

In general, the number of lung transplant recipients who are admitted to the ICU is expected to increase as the number of long-term survivors increase. Early postoperative mortality rates have declined dramatically because of improvements in surgical techniques and perioperative care, with approximately 97% of lung transplant recipients surviving hospital discharge.[96] However, after this immediate post-transplant period, lung transplant recipients are more likely than other solid organ transplant recipients to experience complications such as infection or rejection that necessitate readmission to the ICU.

Nearly 25% of lung transplant recipients require an ICU admission after their initial hospital discharge. The most common admission diagnoses are acute respiratory failure and sepsis.[97,98] The need for MV is common (over 50%), and mortality rates are generally close to 40%. Prognostic factors for mortality include higher acute physiology and chronic health evaluation scores, a reduced FEV1, extrapulmonary organ dysfunction, low serum albumin level, longer duration of MV, and SLT.[97–99] Patients admitted with a diagnosis of BOS who require MV are at particularly high risk for death.[97] Long-term survival among patients who recover from an ICU stay is also compromised[98] highlighting the clinical significance of any ICU readmission in both the immediate and distant future.

SUMMARY

Over the past 40 years, outcomes after lung transplantation have steadily improved likely as a result of better donor and recipient selection and advances in clinical care. Despite this, lung transplant recipients are at risk for numerous complications many of which require management in an intensive care setting. In addition, changes in lung donor allocation have led to an increased number of actively listed patients requiring advanced modalities of support while awaiting transplant. Thus, intensivists should maintain familiarity with core management principals relating to lung transplantation that frequently arise in the critical care setting.

CLINICS CARE POINTS

- ECMO can be used as a bridging strategy to lung transplantation in select patient populations.
- PGD is a leading cause of early morbidity and mortality after lung transplantation and necessitates urgent consideration of ECMO in severe cases.
- Bronchial anastomotic ischemia and necrosis can result in airway dehiscence and thus require close monitoring with serial brochoscopies.

DISCLOSURES

J G. Natalini and E S. Clausen have no relevant conflicts of interest.

REFERENCES

1. Chambers DC, Cherikh WS, Harhay MO, et al. The international thoracic organ transplant registry of the international society for heart and lung transplantation: thirty-sixth adult lung and heart-lung transplantation report-2019; focus theme: donor and recipient size match. J Heart Lung Transplant 2019;38(10):1042–55.
2. Chambers DC, Perch M, Zuckermann A, et al. The international thoracic organ transplant registry of the international society for heart and lung transplantation: thirty-eighth adult lung transplantation report - 2021; focus on recipient characteristics. J Heart Lung Transplant 2021;40(10):1060–72.
3. Chiumello D, Coppola S, Froio S, et al. Extracorporeal life support as bridge to lung transplantation: a systematic review. Crit Care 22 2015;19(1):19.
4. Organ procurement and transplant network. Lung allocation score (LAS) calculator. Available at. http://optn.transplant.hrsa.gov/resources/allocation-calculators/las-calculator/. Accessed April 27, 2021.
5. Davis SQ, Garrity ER Jr. Organ allocation in lung transplant. Chest 2007;132(5):1646–51.
6. Hayanga AJ, Aboagye J, Esper S, et al. Extracorporeal membrane oxygenation as a bridge to lung transplantation in the United States: an evolving strategy in the management of rapidly advancing pulmonary disease. J Thorac Cardiovasc Surg 2015;149(1):291–6.
7. Hayanga JWA, Hayanga HK, Holmes SD, et al. Mechanical ventilation and extracorporeal membrane oxygenation as a bridge to lung transplantation: closing the gap. J Heart Lung Transplant 2019;38(10):1104–11.
8. Hakim AH, Ahmad U, McCurry KR, et al. Contemporary outcomes of extracorporeal membrane oxygenation used as bridge to lung transplantation. Ann Thorac Surg 2018;106(1):192–8.
9. Peek GJ, Mugford M, Tiruvoipati R, et al. Efficacy and economic assessment of conventional ventilatory support versus extracorporeal membrane oxygenation for severe adult respiratory failure (CESAR): a multicentre randomised controlled trial. Lancet 2009;374(9698):1351–63.
10. Burki NK, Mani RK, Herth FJF, et al. A novel extracorporeal CO(2) removal system: results of a pilot study of hypercapnic respiratory failure in patients with COPD. Chest 2013;143(3):678–86.
11. Tiruvoipati R, Buscher H, Winearls J, et al. Early experience of a new extracorporeal carbon dioxide removal device for acute hypercapnic respiratory failure. Crit Care Resusc 2016;18(4):261–9.
12. Bermudez CA, Zaldonis D, Fan MH, et al. Prolonged use of the hemolung respiratory assist system as a bridge to redo lung transplantation. Ann Thorac Surg 2015;100(6):2330–3.

13. Downey P, Ragalie W, Gudzenko V, et al. Ambulatory central veno-arterial extracorporeal membrane oxygenation in lung transplant candidates. J Heart Lung Transplant 2019;38(12):1317–9.

14. Biscotti M, Gannon WD, Agerstrand C, et al. Awake extracorporeal membrane oxygenation as bridge to lung transplantation: a 9-year experience. Ann Thorac Surg 2017;104(2):412–9.

15. Fuehner T, Kuehn C, Hadem J, et al. Extracorporeal membrane oxygenation in awake patients as bridge to lung transplantation. Am J Respir Crit Care Med 2012;185(7):763–8.

16. Willers A, Swol J, Buscher H, et al. Longitudinal trends in bleeding complications on extracorporeal life support over the past two decades-extracorporeal life support organization registry analysis. Crit Care Med 2022. https://doi.org/10.1097/CCM.0000000000005466.

17. Nunez JI, Gosling AF, O'Gara B, et al. Bleeding and thrombotic events in adults supported with venovenous extracorporeal membrane oxygenation: an ELSO registry analysis. Intensive Care Med 2022;48(2):213–24.

18. Levin B, Ortoleva J, Tagliavia A, et al. One-year survival for adult venoarterial extracorporeal membrane oxygenation patients requiring renal-replacement therapy. J Cardiothorac Vasc Anesth 2021. https://doi.org/10.1053/j.jvca.2021.12.027.

19. Thongprayoon C, Cheungpasitporn W, Lertjitbanjong P, et al. Incidence and impact of acute kidney injury in patients receiving extracorporeal membrane oxygenation: a meta-analysis. J Clin Med 2019;8(7). https://doi.org/10.3390/jcm8070981.

20. St-Arnaud C, Thériault MM, Mayette M. North-south syndrome in veno-arterial extra-corporeal membrane oxygenator: the other Harlequin syndrome. Can J Anaesth 2020;67(2):262–3.

21. Falk L, Sallisalmi M, Lindholm JA, et al. Differential hypoxemia during venoarterial extracorporeal membrane oxygenation. Perfusion 2019;34(1_suppl):22–9.

22. Choi JH, Kim SW, Kim YU, et al. Application of veno-arterial-venous extracorporeal membrane oxygenation in differential hypoxia. Multidiscip Respir Med 2014;9(1):55.

23. Hayanga JW, D'Cunha J. The surgical technique of bilateral sequential lung transplantation. J Thorac Dis 2014;6(8):1063–9.

24. Weingarten N, Schraufnagel D, Plitt G, et al. Comparison of mechanical cardiopulmonary support strategies during lung transplantation. Expert Rev Med Devices 2020;17(10):1075–93.

25. Natalini JG, Diamond JM. Primary graft dysfunction. Semin Respir Crit Care Med 2021;42(3):368–79.

26. Ortoleva J, Shapeton A, Vanneman M, et al. Vasoplegia during cardiopulmonary bypass: current literature and rescue therapy options. J Cardiothorac Vasc Anesth 2020;34(10):2766–75.

27. Beer A, Reed RM, Bölükbas S, et al. Mechanical ventilation after lung transplantation. An international survey of practices and preferences. Ann Am Thorac Soc 2014;11(4):546–53.

28. Fan E, Del Sorbo L, Goligher EC, et al. An official American thoracic society/European society of intensive care medicine/society of critical care medicine clinical practice guideline: mechanical ventilation in adult patients with acute respiratory distress syndrome. Am J Respir Crit Care Med 2017;195(9):1253–63.

29. Laghi F, Goyal A. Auto-PEEP in respiratory failure. Minerva Anestesiol 2012;78(2):201–21.

30. Ahya VN, Kawut SM. Noninfectious pulmonary complications after lung transplantation. Clin Chest Med 2005;26(4):613–22, vi.

31. Popple C, Higgins TL, McCarthy P, et al. Unilateral auto-PEEP in the recipient of a single lung transplant. Chest 1993;103(1):297–9.

32. Gavazzeni V, Iapichino G, Mascheroni D, et al. Prolonged independent lung respiratory treatment after single lung transplantation in pulmonary emphysema. Chest 1993;103(1):96–100.

33. Anglès R, Tenorio L, Roman A, et al. Lung transplantation for emphysema. Lung hyperinflation: incidence and outcome. Transpl Int 2005;17(12):810–4.

34. Verleden GM, Glanville AR, Lease ED, et al. Chronic lung allograft dysfunction: definition, diagnostic criteria, and approaches to treatment-A consensus report from the Pulmonary Council of the ISHLT. J Heart Lung Transplant 2019;38(5):493–503.

35. Hernández G, Vaquero C, González P, et al. Effect of postextubation high-flow nasal cannula vs conventional oxygen therapy on reintubation in low-risk patients: a randomized clinical trial. JAMA 2016;315(13):1354–61.

36. Esguerra-Gonzales A, Ilagan-Honorio M, Kehoe P, et al. Effect of high-frequency chest wall oscillation versus chest physiotherapy on lung function after lung transplant. Appl Nurs Res 2014;27(1):59–66.

37. Okamoto K, Santos CAQ. Management and prophylaxis of bacterial and mycobacterial infections among lung transplant recipients. Ann Transl Med 2020;8(6):413.

38. Kotton CN, Kumar D, Caliendo AM, et al. The third international consensus guidelines on the management of cytomegalovirus in solid-organ transplantation. Transplantation 2018;102(6):900–31.

39. Husain S, Camargo JF. Invasive aspergillosis in solid-organ transplant recipients: guidelines from the American society of transplantation infectious diseases community of practice. Clin Transplant 2019;33(9):e13544.

40. Lewis TC, Sureau K, Katz A, et al. Multimodal opioid-sparing pain management after lung transplantation and the impact of liposomal bupivacaine intercostal nerve block. Clin Transplant 2022;36(1): e14512.

41. Yasin J, Thimmappa N, Kaifi JT, et al. CT-guided cryoablation for post-thoracotomy pain syndrome: a retrospective analysis. Diagn Interv Radiol 2020;26(1):53–7.

42. McLean SR, von Homeyer P, Cheng A, et al. Assessing the benefits of preoperative thoracic epidural placement for lung transplantation. J Cardiothorac Vasc Anesth 2018;32(6):2654–61.

43. Hutchins J, Apostolidou I, Shumway S, et al. Paravertebral catheter use for postoperative pain control in patients after lung transplant surgery: a prospective observational study. J Cardiothorac Vasc Anesth 2017;31(1):142–6.

44. Murray AW, Boisen ML, Fritz A, et al. Anesthetic considerations in lung transplantation: past, present and future. J Thorac Dis 2021;13(11): 6550–63.

45. Hachem RR, Edwards LB, Yusen RD, et al. The impact of induction on survival after lung transplantation: an analysis of the International Society for Heart and Lung Transplantation Registry. Clin Transplant 2008;22(5):603–8.

46. Levine SM. A survey of clinical practice of lung transplantation in North America. Chest 2004; 125(4):1224–38.

47. Shah RJ, Diamond JM. Primary graft dysfunction (PGD) following lung transplantation. Semin Respir Crit Care Med 2018;39(2):148–54.

48. Schnickel GT, Ross DJ, Beygui R, et al. Modified reperfusion in clinical lung transplantation: the results of 100 consecutive cases. J Thorac Cardiovasc Surg 2006;131(1):218–23.

49. Christie JD, Carby M, Bag R, et al. Report of the ISHLT working Group on primary lung graft dysfunction, part II: definition — a consensus statement of the international society for heart and lung transplantation. J Heart Lung Transplant 2005; 24(10):1454–9.

50. Rice TW, Wheeler AP, Bernard GR, et al. Comparison of the SpO2/FIO2 ratio and the PaO2/FIO2 ratio in patients with acute lung injury or ARDS. Chest 2007;132(2):410–7.

51. Snell GI, Yusen RD, Weill D, et al. Report of the ISHLT working Group on primary lung graft dysfunction, part I: definition and grading-A 2016 consensus Group statement of the international society for heart and lung transplantation. J Heart Lung Transpl 2017;36(10):1097–103.

52. Diamond JM, Lee JC, Kawut SM, et al. Clinical risk factors for primary graft dysfunction after lung transplantation. Am J Respir Crit Care Med 2013; 187(5):527–34.

53. Daud SA, Yusen RD, Meyers BF, et al. Impact of immediate primary lung allograft dysfunction on bronchiolitis obliterans syndrome. Am J Respir Crit Care Med 2007;175(5):507–13.

54. Fisher AJ, Wardle J, Dark JH, et al. Non-immune acute graft injury after lung transplantation and the risk of subsequent bronchiolitis obliterans syndrome (BOS). J Heart Lung Transplant 2002; 21(11):1206–12.

55. Whitson BA, Prekker ME, Herrington CS, et al. Primary graft dysfunction and long-term pulmonary function after lung transplantation. J Heart Lung Transplant 2007;26(10):1004–11.

56. Diamond JM, Arcasoy S, Kennedy CC, et al. Report of the international society for heart and lung transplantation working Group on primary lung graft dysfunction, part II: epidemiology, risk factors, and outcomes-A 2016 consensus Group statement of the international society for heart and lung transplantation. J Heart Lung Transplant 2017;36(10):1104–13.

57. Christie JD, Bellamy S, Ware LB, et al. Construct validity of the definition of primary graft dysfunction after lung transplantation. J Heart Lung Transplant 2010;29(11):1231–9.

58. Porteous MK, Ky B, Kirkpatrick JN, et al. Diastolic dysfunction increases the risk of primary graft dysfunction after lung transplant. Am J Respir Crit Care Med 2016;193(12):1392–400.

59. Porteous MK, Lee JC, Lederer DJ, et al. Clinical risk factors and prognostic model for primary graft dysfunction after lung transplantation in patients with pulmonary hypertension. Ann Am Thorac Soc 2017;14(10):1514–22.

60. de Perrot M, Bonser RS, Dark J, et al. Report of the ISHLT working Group on primary lung graft dysfunction part III: donor-related risk factors and markers. J Heart Lung Transplant 2005;24(10): 1460–7.

61. Borders CF, Suzuki Y, Lasky J, et al. Massive donor transfusion potentially increases recipient mortality after lung transplantation. J Thorac Cardiovasc Surg 2017;153(5):1197–203.e2.

62. Pelaez A, Mitchell PO, Shah NS, et al. The role of donor chronic alcohol abuse in the development of primary graft dysfunction in lung transplant recipients. Am J Med Sci 2015;349(2):117–23.

63. Currey J, Pilcher DV, Davies A, et al. Implementation of a management guideline aimed at minimizing the severity of primary graft dysfunction after lung transplant. J Thorac Cardiovasc Surg 2010;139(1):154–61.

64. Meade MO, Granton JT, Matte-Martyn A, et al. A randomized trial of inhaled nitric oxide to prevent ischemia-reperfusion injury after lung transplantation. Am J Respir Crit Care Med 2003;167(11): 1483–9.

65. Date H, Triantafillou AN, Trulock EP, et al. Inhaled nitric oxide reduces human lung allograft dysfunction. J Thorac Cardiovasc Surg 1996;111(5):913–9.

66. Adatia I, Lillehei C, Arnold JH, et al. Inhaled nitric oxide in the treatment of postoperative graft dysfunction after lung transplantation. Ann Thorac Surg 1994;57(5):1311–8.

67. Macdonald P, Mundy J, Rogers P, et al. Successful treatment of life-threatening acute reperfusion injury after lung transplantation with inhaled nitric oxide. J Thorac Cardiovasc Surg 1995;110(3):861–3.

68. Wigfield CH, Lindsey JD, Steffens TG, et al. Early institution of extracorporeal membrane oxygenation for primary graft dysfunction after lung transplantation improves outcome. J Heart Lung Transplant 2007;26(4):331–8.

69. Fischer S, Bohn D, Rycus P, et al. Extracorporeal membrane oxygenation for primary graft dysfunction after lung transplantation: analysis of the Extracorporeal Life Support Organization (ELSO) registry. J Heart Lung Transplant 2007;26(5):472–7.

70. Bermudez CA, Adusumilli PS, McCurry KR, et al. Extracorporeal membrane oxygenation for primary graft dysfunction after lung transplantation: long-term survival. Ann Thorac Surg 2009;87(3):854–60.

71. Kawut SM, Lederer DJ, Keshavjee S, et al. Outcomes after lung retransplantation in the modern era. Am J Respir Crit Care Med 2008;177(1):114–20.

72. Machuzak M, Santacruz JF, Gildea T, et al. Airway complications after lung transplantation. Thorac Surg Clin 2015;25(1):55–75.

73. Crespo MM, McCarthy DP, Hopkins PM, et al. ISHLT Consensus Statement on adult and pediatric airway complications after lung transplantation: Definitions, grading system, and therapeutics. J Heart Lung Transplant 2018;37(5):548–63.

74. Santacruz JF, Mehta AC. Airway complications and management after lung transplantation: ischemia, dehiscence, and stenosis. Proc Am Thorac Soc 2009;6(1):79–93.

75. Levine DJ, Glanville AR, Aboyoun C, et al. Antibody-mediated rejection of the lung: a consensus report of the international society for heart and lung transplantation. J Heart Lung Transplant 2016;35(4):397–406.

76. Witt CA, Gaut JP, Yusen RD, et al. Acute antibody-mediated rejection after lung transplantation. J Heart Lung Transplant 2013;32(10):1034–40.

77. Stewart S, Fishbein MC, Snell GI, et al. Revision of the 1996 working formulation for the standardization of nomenclature in the diagnosis of lung rejection. J Heart Lung Transplant 2007;26(12):1229–42.

78. Martinu T, Howell DN, Palmer SM. Acute cellular rejection and humoral sensitization in lung transplant recipients. Semin Respir Crit Care Med 2010;31(2):179–88.

79. Oechslin P, Zalunardo MP, Inci I, et al. Established and potential predictors of blood loss during lung transplant surgery. J Thorac Dis 2018;10(6):3845–8.

80. Siddique A, Bose AK, Özalp F, et al. Vascular anastomotic complications in lung transplantation: a single institution's experience. Interact Cardiovasc Thorac Surg 2013;17(4):625–31.

81. Fishman JA. Infection in solid-organ transplant recipients. N Engl J Med 2007;357(25):2601–14.

82. Lease ED, Zaas DW. Complex bacterial infections pre- and posttransplant. Semin Respir Crit Care Med 2010;31(2):234–42.

83. Burguete SR, Maselli DJ, Fernandez JF, et al. Lung transplant infection. Respirology 2013;18(1):22–38.

84. Remund KF, Best M, Egan JJ. Infections relevant to lung transplantation. Proc Am Thorac Soc 2009;6(1):94–100.

85. Zamora MR, Davis RD, Leonard C. Management of cytomegalovirus infection in lung transplant recipients: evidence-based recommendations. Transplantation 2005;80(2):157–63.

86. Kumar D, Erdman D, Keshavjee S, et al. Clinical impact of community-acquired respiratory viruses on bronchiolitis obliterans after lung transplant. Am J Transplant 2005;5(8):2031–6.

87. Hosseini-Moghaddam SM, Husain S. Fungi and molds following lung transplantation. Semin Respir Crit Care Med 2010;31(2):222–33.

88. Solé A, Salavert M. Fungal infections after lung transplantation. Curr Opin Pulm Med 2009;15(3):243–53.

89. Ferdinande P, Bruyninckx F, Van Raemdonck D, et al. Phrenic nerve dysfunction after heart-lung and lung transplantation. J Heart Lung Transplant 2004;23(1):105–9.

90. Lyu DM, Zamora MR. Medical complications of lung transplantation. Proc Am Thorac Soc 2009;6(1):101–7.

91. Roukoz H, Benditt DG. Atrial arrhythmias after lung transplantation. Trends Cardiovasc Med 2018;28(1):53–61.

92. Orrego CM, Cordero-Reyes AM, Estep JD, et al. Atrial arrhythmias after lung transplant: underlying mechanisms, risk factors, and prognosis. J Heart Lung Transplant 2014;33(7):734–40.

93. Raghavan D, Gao A, Ahn C, et al. Contemporary analysis of incidence of post-operative atrial fibrillation, its predictors, and association with clinical outcomes in lung transplantation. J Heart Lung Transplant 2015;34(4):563–70.

94. Leger RF, Silverman MS, Hauck ES, et al. Hyperammonemia post lung transplantation: a review. Clin Med Insights Circ Respir Pulm Med 2020;14. 1179548420966234.

95. Krutsinger D, Pezzulo A, Blevins AE, et al. Idiopathic hyperammonemia after solid organ transplantation: primarily a lung problem? A single-center experience and systematic review. Clin Transplant 2017;31(5). https://doi.org/10.1111/ctr.12957.

96. Scientific Registry of Transplant Recipients. Patient survival after lung transplantation. Available at: http://www.srtr.org. Accessed December 14, 2015.

97. Cohen J, Singer P, Raviv Y, et al. Outcome of lung transplant recipients requiring readmission to the intensive care unit. J Heart Lung Transplant 2011; 30(1):54–8.

98. Banga A, Sahoo D, Lane CR, et al. Characteristics and outcomes of patients with lung transplantation requiring admission to the medical ICU. Chest 2014;146(3):590–9.

99. Hadjiliadis D, Steele MP, Govert JA, et al. Outcome of lung transplant patients admitted to the medical ICU. Chest 2004;125(3):1040–5.

100. Lee JC, Christie JD. Primary graft dysfunction. Clin Chest Med 2011;32(2):279–93.

101. Porteous MK, Lee JC. Primary graft dysfunction after lung transplantation. Clin Chest Med 2017; 38(4):641–54.

Conventional and Novel Approaches to Immunosuppression in Lung Transplantation

Caroline M. Patterson, BMBS, BMedSci, MD[a], Elaine C. Jolly, MBChB, BSc, PhD[b],
Fay Burrows, BPharm[c], Nicola J. Ronan, MbBCh, PhD[a],
Haifa Lyster, MSc, FRPharmS[d,e,f,*]

KEYWORDS

- Immunosupression • Induction • Maintenance • Immune response assays

KEY POINTS

- Induction immunosuppression with an Interleukin (IL)-2 receptor antagonist is now widespread practice. Registry analyses indicate a beneficial effect on survival with induction, and induction may also contribute to a lower incidence of acute rejection and greater freedom from bronchiolitis obliterans syndrome.
- Unchanged over the past three decades, calcineurin inhibitors remain the foundation of maintenance immunosuppression, alongside antimetabolites and steroids.
- Recognition that calcineurin inhibitors are associated with a significant risk of nephrotoxicity has led to the evaluation of regimens targeting delayed initiation and lower doses of calcineurin inhibitor. Transitioning to a four-agent maintenance regimen, incorporating a mammalian target of rapamycin inhibitor, may preserve renal function without loss of immunosuppression efficacy.
- Better understanding of the intensity of immunosuppression for a given individual will facilitate prediction of opportunistic infection and allograft rejection. Immune response assays are being evaluated as biomarkers of immunosuppression in this regard.
- Allograft tolerance is the holy grail of transplantation. Research is ongoing to evaluate a therapeutic role for immune regulatory cells and to explore whether chimerism can be achieved via concomitant stem cell and solid organ transplantation from the same donor.

INTRODUCTION

The concept of immunosuppression to support allograft longevity was introduced in the early twentieth century, yet most therapeutic advances have occurred over the past few decades. Although modern immunosuppression strategies have been effective in reducing T cell-driven acute cellular rejection (ACR), excess immunosuppression comes at the price of toxicity, opportunistic infection, and malignancy. As our understanding of the immune system and allograft rejection becomes more nuanced, there is an opportunity to evolve immunosuppression protocols to optimize longer

[a] Transplant Continuing Care Unit, Royal Papworth Hospital NHS Foundation Trust, Cambridge, United Kingdom; [b] Division of Renal Medicine, Department of Medicine, University of Cambridge, Cambridge, United Kingdom; [c] Department of Pharmacy, St Vincent's Hospital, Sydney, New South Wales, Australia; [d] Cardiothoracic Transplant Unit, Royal Brompton and Harefield Hospitals, Part of Guy's & St Thomas' NHS Foundation Trust, London, United Kingdom; [e] Kings College, London, United Kingdom; [f] Pharmacy Department, Royal Brompton and Harefield Hospitals, Part of Guy's & St Thomas' NHS Foundation Trust, London, United Kingdom
* Corresponding author.
E-mail address: h.lyster@rbht.nhs.uk

Clin Chest Med 44 (2023) 121–136
https://doi.org/10.1016/j.ccm.2022.10.009

term outcomes while mitigating the deleterious effects of traditional protocols. In this review, the authors consider standard and nonstandard agents and approaches for immunosuppression after lung transplantation, presenting the evidence behind these therapies as well as the reported benefits and risks. The authors also present some of the adjunctive therapies and clinical tools that are being developed to guide better targeted and personalized immunosuppressive therapy.

HISTORY OF IMMUNOSUPPRESSION

Murphy, in his work with tumor homografts during the 1920s, was the first to establish the role of the lymphocyte in graft rejection and to pursue lymphocyte eradication with irradiation, splenectomy, or benzol—the earliest chemical immunosuppressive agent.[1,2]

Thereafter, transplant clinicians looked to oncologists, who were evaluating nitrogen mustard (a chemical warfare agent), 6-mercaptopurine (6-MP), and azathioprine (AZA) as chemotherapeutic agents. Although initial studies suggested that 6-MP extended the survival of dog kidney[3] and human skin homografts,[4] experience of human renal transplant recipients treated with 6-MP and AZA resulted in 90% of recipients dying within 6 months.[5]

Starzl offered hope of enhanced renal allograft survival based on the addition of prednisone to AZA.[6] The Starzl "cocktail" of immunosuppression was the standard of care for solid organ transplantation until the emergence of the calcineurin inhibitor (CNI), cyclosporine,[7] which proved to be more potent than AZA.[8,9] Starzl confirmed that concurrent steroid therapy could also be used to amplify the value of cyclosporine[10] and achieve successful extrarenal transplantation.[11] Thereafter, another CNI, tacrolimus, emerged as an even more effective immunosuppressive agent.[12] With the adoption of maintenance CNIs, survival exceeding 1 year with heart–lung transplantation was achieved in 1982[13] and with lung transplantation in 1987.[14]

Muromonab-CD3 (OKT3), introduced in 1985, was the first monoclonal antibody to be adopted for the treatment of acute rejection, but its use in rejection prevention was limited by concerns regarding life-threatening toxicity, and it is no longer available in the United States or Europe. Today, our armamentarium of monoclonal antibodies used for immunosuppression continues to expand.

Immunosuppression practices in lung transplantation remain largely based on strategies pioneered in other organ transplant groups, and lung-specific regulatory approval does not exist for most agents used. There is increasing recognition that immune responses to lung allografts differ from those of other organs and future immunosuppressive protocols will need to address the unique immunologic features of lungs.[15,16]

ALLORECOGNITION PATHWAYS AND EFFECTOR MECHANISMS

The major histocompatibility complex (MHC) is a family of genes encoding polymorphic human leukocyte antigens (HLAs) that act as an alloreactive trigger for the immune cascade, resulting in rejection. ACR and antibody-mediated rejection (AMR) are risk factors for the subsequent development of chronic lung allograft dysfunction (CLAD), which is the leading cause of late mortality post-lung transplant.

The recipient T cells recognize donor antigens to become activated via direct, indirect, or semi-direct allorecognition pathways.[17] In direct allorecognition, recipient T cells trigger a potent immune response against the allograft through the recognition of intact MHC on donor antigen-presenting cells (APCs).[17,18] Attenuation of direct allorecognition occurs as the donor APCs dwindle due to the elimination of donor-derived passenger leukocytes. In parallel, the risk of acute rejection diminishes posttransplantation.[19]

Via semi-direct allorecognition, recipient APCs can acquire functional, intact donor MHC to activate recipient T cells in the absence of passenger leukocytes. With time, the indirect allorecognition pathway of T-cell activation becomes more prominent. T cells identify donor MHC molecules presented as peptide by self-MHC molecules to trigger a less intense yet still injurious immune response which is believed to contribute to CLAD.[17,18]

The indirect pathway is implicated in both humoral and cytotoxic T-cell alloimmunity. T cells activated in response to persistently presented allopeptide epitopes can acquire a T-helper cell phenotype to induce B-cell responses.[20,21] B cells produce donor-specific antibodies (DSAs) and autoantibodies against pulmonary self-antigens such as collagen V or K-α1 tubulin[19] and act as APCs to initiate T-cell activation. Via memory B cells and the generation of long-lived plasma cells, allograft recipients can develop a persistent anti-donor humoral response.

Regulatory immune cells have been identified which may promote transplant tolerance.[22] Translational research has focused on regulatory T cells (Tregs), which control autoimmunity via absorption of pro-inflammatory IL-2, cytotoxic T-lymphocyte-associated protein 4 (CTLA-4)-mediated masking of CD80 and CD86 co-stimulatory ligands on

APCs, expression of immune-inhibitory molecules (IL-10, IL-35, transforming growth factor-beta [TGF-β]), and granzyme-mediated killing of APCs.[23]

Using genomic tools such as microarray analysis and single-cell sequencing with bioinformatic approaches, the prospect of characterizing immune processes at a cellular level is becoming more tangible.[24,25] For now, molecular understanding of graft rejection remains incomplete, with deficits in our comprehension of graft resident and infiltrating immune cell populations, cell-to-cell interactions, and how to harness these to mitigate or prevent rejection.

INDUCTION IMMUNOSUPPRESSION

Short-term, potent immunosuppression in the peritransplant period is advocated to prevent early acute rejection and/or facilitate the delayed initiation or dose reduction of CNIs. The use of induction immunosuppression has increased over time and more than 80% of adult lung transplant recipients now receive some form of induction.[26]

The most commonly used agents are T-cell antibody preparations—the monoclonal agents (basiliximab and alemtuzumab) and the polyclonal agent anti-thymocyte globulin (ATG). Basiliximab is non-lymphocyte depleting, whereas alemtuzumab and ATG cause T-cell depletion. The use of ATG has declined as basiliximab, an IL-2 receptor (IL-2R) antagonist, has gained favor.[27] More than 70% of lung transplant recipients now receive induction with an IL-2R antagonist vs 5% who receive alemtuzumab and 4% who receive ATG.[28]

Basiliximab

Basiliximab (Simulect) is a chimeric mouse–human monoclonal antibody targeted against α subunit (IL2R α; CD25 antigen) of the IL-2R on activated T cells. Basiliximab competitively inhibits IL-2-mediated proliferation and differentiation of T cells.

Alemtuzumab

Alemtuzumab (Campath) is a humanized monoclonal antibody targeted against the CD52 antigen expressed on T and B cells, NK cells, and a lesser degree monocytes, macrophages, and eosinophils. T-cell levels may be suppressed for up to 3 years after alemtuzumab induction, whereas B-cell levels typically recover over a few months.[29] At 1-year posttransplant, microRNA, and cytokine expression differ between recipients who receive alemtuzumab and those without induction, suggesting a prolonged effect on immune reconstitution and a role in promoting graft tolerance.[26]

Anti-thymocyte Globulin

ATG is a polyclonal agent, prepared by immunizing rabbits (rATG, Thymoglobulin) or horses (equine ATG, Atgam) with human thymocytes. ATGs act through the Fc receptor and other proteins on the T-cell surface to induce apoptosis. Although the primary effect is T-cell depletion, thymoglobulin also contains antibodies against B-cell antigens and is thought to induce apoptosis in B cells, including plasma cells, to modulate both cell-mediated and humoral immunity.[30]

Evidence to support the use of induction agents and to guide which agent to use is limited. In the International Society for Heart and Lung Transplantation (ISHLT) registry analysis of 3,970 lung transplant recipients, survival at 4 years was only marginally better in the IL-2R antagonist (64%) and ATG (60%) groups than the no-induction group (57%), but the use of induction was an independent predictor of survival in multivariable Cox analysis.[31] An analysis of United Network for Organ Sharing (UNOS) data confirmed improved survival with either basiliximab or alemtuzumab induction compared with no induction, and prolonged freedom from bronchiolitis obliterans syndrome (BOS) in those receiving alemtuzumab.[32] Direct comparison studies suggest induction with alemtuzumab or basiliximab may result in improved freedom from ACR and improved survival compared with ATG.[33,34] Despite concerns that alemtuzumab induction may increase the risk of infection and malignancy, this has not been supported by data across solid organ transplant groups.[35,36] Indeed, a 2013 Cochrane review of six randomized controlled studies assessing the use of ATG, IL-2R antagonists, alemtuzumab, or OKT3 found no clear benefits or harms associated with the use of any T-cell antibody induction.[37] Thereafter, an international, randomized controlled study was also unable to demonstrate any benefit of ATG over no induction using a composite endpoint of death, graft loss, or acute rejection.[38]

MAINTENANCE IMMUNOSUPPRESSION

Using a combination of agents, it is possible to target multiple aspects of the alloimmune response. Conventional immunosuppression involves a three-drug regimen, incorporating a CNI, an antimetabolite, and a corticosteroid. The most frequently administered combination is tacrolimus, mycophenolate mofetil (MMF), and prednisone,[27] but patients commonly switch between regimens based on individual tolerability or physiology.

Calcineurin Inhibitors

Both cyclosporine and tacrolimus bind to intracellular proteins known as immunophilins to form a drug-immunophilin complex which interrupts the early phase of T-cell activation and the production of IL-2, to decrease T-cell activation and proliferation.

In a meta-analysis of three randomized controlled trials, including 297 lung transplant recipients, tacrolimus was superior to cyclosporine in mitigating acute rejection, and there was a trend toward a lower risk of BOS but survival was comparable between the two agents.[39] A subsequent multicenter randomized controlled trial reported a cumulative incidence of BOS Grade ≥1 at 3 years of 11.6% (tacrolimus) vs 21.3% (cyclosporine).[40]

Cyclosporine (Sandimmune) is poorly and variably absorbed (10%–89%). Modified generic preparations such as Neoral, Gengraf, and Capimmune have improved pharmacokinetics, but these generic agents are not interchangeable. They are available in capsule, oral solution, and intravenous formulations. Tacrolimus is available in capsule, sachet, and intravenous formulations. Tacrolimus has oral absorption ranging from 17% to 23% and may be administered sublingually to patients who are not eating by mouth or where there are gastrointestinal concerns, noting that the sublingual route bypasses the first-pass metabolism.[41,42] Metabolism of both cyclosporine and tacrolimus occurs via the cytochrome P450 system, forming the basis of important pharmacokinetic drug interactions. Both agents have a narrow therapeutic index. Extended-release tacrolimus (Envarsus) allows once daily dosing, optimizing time in therapeutic range and leading to reduced adverse effects and improved adherence.[43–45]

Antimetabolites

AZA, a pro-drug of 6-MP, blocks the de novo and salvage pathways of purine synthesis to inhibit DNA, RNA, and protein synthesis, leading to suppression of all hematopoietic cell lines. Immunosuppressive activity is achieved via the prevention of T- and B-cell proliferation and blockade of the CD28 co-stimulation pathway.

MMF, a pro-drug of mycophenolic acid (MPA), selectively targets the de novo pathway of guanosine nucleotide synthesis. It has cytostatic effects on T and B cells and has been shown to suppress antibody formation.

Although MMF has been shown to be superior to AZA in reducing the incidence of acute rejection in kidney allograft recipients, an increased risk of tissue invasive CMV disease has been reported.[46] In the lung transplant population, no differences have been shown in the incidence of acute rejection, BOS, or overall survival at 6 months between patients treated with MMF or AZA,[47,48] but MMF is better tolerated.[48] Switching from AZA to MMF is associated with a reduced incidence of cutaneous squamous cell carcinoma and MMF may be preferable as a first-line antimetabolite in transplant recipients at a high risk of skin malignancy.[49]

AZA is available in tablet form and as a powder for solution for injection. It is well absorbed following oral administration. MMF is available in oral suspension, capsule, tablet, and intravenous formulations. MPA is available as an enteric-coated tablet (Myfortic), which may be better tolerated in patients with severe MMF-related gastrointestinal side-effects.[50] A 360 mg of MPA is equivalent to 500 mg of MMF.

Corticosteroids

Corticosteroids, oral prednisolone, prednisone and intravenous methylprednisolone, have anti-inflammatory properties and contribute to immunosuppression via decreased T-cell proliferation, decreased macrophage activation, inhibition of cytokine production, and altered lymphocyte migration.[51] Although oral corticosteroids are rapidly absorbed with 80% to 100% availability, greater than three-fold variability in dose-adjusted exposure in transplant recipients has been reported.[52] The impact of corticosteroid therapy on the disposition of cyclosporine, tacrolimus, and sirolimus and the impact of immunosuppressant combinations on corticosteroid exposure need to be further defined.[52]

Mammalian Target of Rapamycin Inhibitors

Two mammalian target of rapamycin inhibitors (mTORi) are approved for clinical use—sirolimus (Rapamune) and everolimus (Certican). mTORi bind to the cytosolic FK506 binding protein 12, which complexes to the serine–threonine kinase mTOR and blocks its activity to disrupt CD28-mediated T-cell activation, progression of T cells through the cell cycle, and transcription of cytokines including IL-2.[53]

There are no intravenous formulations of either sirolimus or everolimus, with sirolimus available as tablets and oral solution and everolimus as tablets. Both drugs are hepatically metabolized by cytochrome P450-3A and are susceptible to the associated drug interactions.

mTORi are most commonly used in place of antimetabolites, and/or as part of a CNI sparing regimen for renal protection and may have a role in the prevention and stabilization of CLAD. A multicenter randomized controlled trial comparing sirolimus with AZA reported that sirolimus did not reduce the incidence of acute or chronic rejection at 1 year posttransplant;[54] however, in a study of BOS-free lung transplant recipients randomized to receive everolimus or AZA (alongside CNI + steroid), the everolimus group experienced a lower rate of the primary composite endpoint of death, graft loss, decline in lung function or loss to follow-up.[55] Comparing everolimus and MMF (alongside CNI + steroid) in 190 patients over a 2-year period, there were fewer episodes of acute rejection and BOS in the everolimus group but the study was underpowered due to a high dropout rate.[56] The largest cohort analysis of sirolimus versus MMF, based on UNOS data, demonstrated improved patient survival with sirolimus plus tacrolimus compared with MMF plus tacrolimus.[57] Sirolimus has been associated with a reduction in the risk of malignancy in solid organ transplant recipients,[58] and mTORi may have a role in the prevention and management of posttransplant lymphoproliferative disorder.[59]

A detrimental effect of mTORi, relating to suppression of fibroblast proliferation and angiogenesis, is the impairment of wound healing, and cases of catastrophic airway dehiscence have been reported.[60,61] As such, mTORi are generally avoided in the first 3 months posttransplant or until anastomotic healing is complete. Another well-recognized hazard of mTORi is interstitial pneumonitis, which occurs as part of a spectrum of pulmonary side effects.[62] Overall, mTORi have lower tolerability compared with other immunosuppressant agents,[63] and discontinuation rates exceeding 60% are reported in lung transplant recipients.[54]

Based on ISHLT registry data, 5% of lung transplant recipients at 1 year and 6.1% at 5 years posttransplant are maintained on a four-drug immunosuppression regimen including an mTORi (mTORi + CNI + antimetabolite + prednisolone). At 5 years posttransplant, 6% are maintained on three-drug regimen with an mTORi in place of an antimetabolite (mTORi + CNI + prednisolone), and 3% are maintained on a CNI-free regimen (mTORi + antimetabolite + prednisolone).[64] CNI-free regimens are associated with higher acute rejection rates and withdrawal of CNI therapy in favor of an mTORi is not recommended.[65]

ADJUNCTIVE THERAPIES

There are no recommendations for the treatment of CLAD beyond conversion of cyclosporine to tacrolimus and trial of azithromycin.[66] There is some evidence to suggest lung function

stabilization may be achievable using extracorporeal photopheresis (ECP) and there is lower grade evidence to support total lymphoid irradiation (TLI), montelukast, and aerosolized immunosuppression agents.[67]

Azithromycin

The neomacrolide antibiotic, azithromycin, has pleiotropic, anti-inflammatory, and immunomodulatory effects.[68] Evidence for azithromycin as a treatment of CLAD has come from case series, observational studies, and a single randomized controlled trial, with an improvement in forced expiratory volume in one second (FEV1) reported in 18% to 60% of those treated.[66,69–71] Meta-analysis of 10 studies indicates a mean percentage increase in FEV1 of 8.8% in patients with BOS treated with azithromycin[72] and an association has been reported between bronchoalveolar lavage neutrophilia and azithromycin response.[66,71,73] A retrospective cohort study comparing patients who received azithromycin to historical controls suggested a survival benefit with azithromycin started at BOS stage 1 but not at later stages of BOS.[74] Some transplant centers are using it preemptively with the hope that azithromycin may increase BOS-free survival.[75]

Extracorporeal Photopheresis

ECP is a leukapheresis-based therapy, whereby recipient peripheral blood mononuclear cells are exposed to long-wavelength ultraviolet-A light in the presence of 8-methoxypsoralen. Although the precise mechanisms are not fully understood, ECP is believed to induce lymphocyte apoptosis, alter cytokine profiles and upregulate Tregs,[76–78] and may have a role in treating azithromycin-refractory CLAD.[79] Observational studies have reported improvement in FEV1 in 12% to 30% of those treated, attenuation of FEV1 decline, and possible mortality benefit after the initiation of ECP.[80–84] Based on published data, patients with BOS occurring within 3 years of transplant are more likely to respond to ECP,[82] whereas patients with rapid CLAD progression or restrictive allograft syndrome (RAS) are less likely to respond,[85] but further validation is required.

Total Lymphoid Irradiation

Irradiation of lymphoid tissue causes rapid and profound depletion of lymphoid cells and may be used to augment oral immunosuppression.[86] Based on the findings of case series and observational studies in patients with CLAD, treatment with TLI can attenuate or stabilize FEV1 decline[87–91] with results lasting up to 72 weeks.[87]

Patients with rapidly declining FEV1 seem to have the greatest response,[88,90,91] and TLI may buy these individuals time for redo-transplantation.[89,91] In general, TLI is well tolerated but delivery of the therapy can be limited by cytopenia and infection.[87,88] Published protocols advocate cessation of antimetabolites on initiation of TLI, which are only restarted after completion of TLI, and in the absence of leukopenia.[91]

Montelukast

Montelukast is a cysteinyl leukotriene receptor antagonist. A small placebo-controlled trial of montelukast in 30 patients with late-onset (>2 years posttransplant) BOS demonstrated no effect on lung function decline in the overall cohort but attenuation of FEV1 decline in the subgroup with BOS stage 1.[92] Thereafter, a single center, retrospective study of 153 patients with CLAD demonstrated attenuation of FEV1 decline in 81% of patients treated with montelukast[93] and responders had significantly better progression-free and overall survival. By contrast, patients with a rapid deterioration in FEV1 pre-montelukast or an RAS phenotype were less likely to stabilise.[93]

Inhaled Immunosuppression

The theoretic advantage of inhaled immunosuppression is the delivery of high drug concentrations directly to the airways affected by BOS while limiting systemic absorption. Case series have demonstrated lower rates of CLAD progression and a possible mortality benefit with inhaled cyclosporine.[94,95] In a randomized placebo-controlled trial, the addition of inhaled cyclosporine to oral immunosuppression had no effect on the incidence of acute rejection but improved BOS-free and overall survival.[96] A placebo-controlled study of inhaled liposomal cyclosporine in 180 BOS-free lung transplant recipients demonstrated a (nonsignificant) 2-year difference in BOS-free survival of 14.1% in favor of inhaled cyclosporine.[97] In a randomized controlled trial involving 21 patients with BOS, patients receiving inhaled liposomal cyclosporine demonstrated a trend toward improved progression-free survival over 48 weeks (82% with inhaled cyclosporine vs 50% with standard care).[98]

In a murine model, inhaled tacrolimus has also been shown to decrease inflammatory airway epithelium cytokine production and inhibit the activation of inducible transcription factors.[99] Work is ongoing to develop efficacious inhaled formulations of tacrolimus for human use.[100] In a single case report of inhaled tacrolimus used to treat a patient with established BOS, there were improvements in functional capacity and oxygenation.[101]

Statins

Statins have anti-inflammatory and immunomodulatory effects that make them an attractive prospect for the maintenance of lung allograft function[102]; however, in a benchmark study of 130 lung transplant recipients receiving statins for a minimum of 6 months, statin use was not associated with a decreased risk of CLAD or a significant delay in the time to CLAD onset.[103] Statins demonstrated a benefit in patient survival at 3 years, which warrants further evaluation.[103]

Antifibrotic Agents

Pirfenidone has anti-inflammatory and antifibrotic properties and is approved for treatment of idiopathic pulmonary fibrosis (IPF). In a study of 17 single-lung transplant recipients with IPF, the incidence of ACR within 30 days of transplant was lower in patients with previous pirfenidone treatment (0.0% vs 19.2%).[104] Case reports and small case series report stabilization of pulmonary function in BOS[105] and attenuation of pulmonary function decline in patients with RAS treated with pirfenidone.[106,107] Understanding the potential benefits of the antifibrotic agents, pirfenidone and nintedanib, post-lung-transplant requires further investigation.

IMMUNOSUPPRESSION MONITORING

Historically, immunosuppressant dosing has been primarily guided by trough levels, which provide limited insight into the individual intensity of immunosuppression. As we move toward an era of personalized immunosuppressive therapy, there is increasing interest in effect-related immune monitoring to minimize toxicity while maintaining efficacy.

Torque teno virus (TTV) is a latent, nonpathogenic, single-stranded, DNA anellovirus.[108] TTV DNA is detectable in the serum of up to 90% of healthy individuals[109] and evidence suggests that high or increasing TTV DNA levels precede infectious complications in solid organ transplant recipients, whereas low or decreasing viral loads are associated with the development of acute rejection.[110–112]

Viral replication is inversely correlated with the number and function of virus-specific T cells (VSTs) and containment of viral replication may be considered a marker of more general cellular immune defenses. The most well-recognized techniques used to quantify and characterize

VSTs are the enzyme-linked immunospot assay, enzyme-linked immunosorbent assay, intracellular cytokine staining followed by fluorescence-activated cell sorting analysis, and MHC multimer staining. Monitoring of VSTs (against cytomegalovirus (CMV), ADV, HSV, and other viruses) may provide an adjunct to trough-level monitoring to identify patients at risk of infection or rejection.[113,114]

Nonpathogen-specific immune monitoring involves the measurement of cell-mediated responses to antigenic stimuli. The commercially available Immunoknow and QuantiFERON Monitor have been evaluated as biomarkers of immunosuppression across solid organ transplant groups.[115-118]

Evidence from the liver transplant population suggests that adoption of immune response assays to guide therapy early posttransplant can result in CNI dose reduction, with a reduction in bacterial and fungal infections, and improved 1 year survival.[119] These findings have yet to be replicated in the lung transplant population, although randomized controlled trials are ongoing (NCT04198506).[120] For TTV monitoring and other immune response assays to be adopted into clinical practice, clarity is required regarding procedural methodology, standardization, quality control, and clinically relevant thresholds, along with robust definitions of sensitivity, specificity, and negative and positive predictive values.

TAILORING IMMUNOSUPPRESSION FOR RECIPIENT FACTORS

Mitigating the risks of immunosuppression requires consideration of recipient factors including age, hepatic and renal dysfunction, infection burden, genetic polymorphisms, drug–drug interactions, and total immunosuppression burden.

In highly sensitized patients, ATG induction may be preferred, whereas a less aggressive approach, avoiding induction immunosuppression, may be appropriate for recipients with CMV mismatch (donor positive, recipient negative) or colonized with highly resistant organisms. Notwithstanding their burden of infection, cystic fibrosis patients can still gain survival benefit with induction immunosuppression,[121,122] with suppression of chronic innate inflammation as the postulated mechanism.[122]

In older recipients, immunosenescence contributes to an increased risk of infection and posttransplant malignancy, but also a reduced risk of acute rejection, meaning that induction with an IL-2R antagonist may offer acceptable efficacy without the additional hazards associated with T-cell depleting therapies. In the maintenance phase, aging is associated with reduced CNI clearance, necessitating lower doses for similar trough levels compared with younger recipients.

Interpatient variability in CNI and mTORi pharmacokinetics has been reported with genotypic variants of cytochrome P-450 3A5 (CYP3A5) and ABCB1.[123-126] Polymorphisms that influence thiopurine S-methyl-transferase (TPMT) and NUDT15 activity are well recognized and can lead to inadequate metabolism of AZA and profound bone marrow suppression.[127,128] In patients with low TPMT activity, MMF is recommended in place of AZA.

Although thrombocytopenia, leukopenia, and anemia posttransplant are often multifactorial, their presence may prevent optimal maintenance immunosuppression. Patients with telomerase gene mutations have an increased risk of severe hematological complications, renal dysfunction, and susceptibility to infection following lung transplantation.[129,130] Avoidance of T-cell depleting induction may be beneficial in this cohort, along with dose modification or cessation of myelosuppressive medications for maintenance therapy.[129]

INFECTIOUS CONSIDERATIONS

Augmentation of immunosuppression for the treatment of rejection increases vulnerability to infection, and infection may drive alloimmune interactions that contribute to both acute rejection and CLAD.

Prophylaxis for common and opportunistic pathogens is routinely initiated, but there is a lack of consensus regarding strategy. Early posttransplant antibacterial prophylaxis typically includes a penicillin/cephalosporin and vancomycin and is tailored to culture results and clinical progress. Pneumocystis prophylaxis continues lifelong. Most centers favor universal CMV prophylaxis over monitoring at-risk patients and treating at predetermined thresholds. Options to mitigate invasive fungal infection include universal prophylaxis, targeted prophylaxis, and preemptive treatment, with no clear evidence for which of these is most effective.[131]

Infection risk is increased by recipient hypogammaglobulinaemia (HGG). A meta-analysis of 18 studies reported secondary HGG (immunoglobulin G [IgG] < 700 mg/dL) in 63% of lung transplant recipients at 1 year posttransplant, with severe HGG (IgG < 400 mg/dL) in 15%.[132] Replacement of IgG by intravenous or subcutaneous infusion is routine practice despite limited evidence of efficacy and may be best reserved for patients with severe HGG and recurrent infections.[133,134]

RENAL CONSIDERATIONS

Acute kidney injury (AKI) following lung transplantation is common, with up to 60% of patients experiencing an acute decline in renal function postoperatively[135–140] and may result in the need for renal replacement therapy in 5% to 10% of cases.[141–143] Even non-dialysis requiring AKI confers a poorer clinical outcome, with longer duration of mechanical ventilation, longer hospital stay, and increased early and late mortality.[135,139–141,143,144]

The development of progressive chronic kidney disease (CKD) after an AKI episode (even with biochemical recovery of renal function) is well-recognized[145] and at 1 year post-lung transplant, 4.8% of patients have severe CKD and 3.4% are dialysis-requiring.[27]

High and/or cumulative exposure to CNIs is an important factor in the development of both AKI and CKD post-solid organ transplantation due to nephrotoxicity.[146,147] One approach to facilitate minimization of CNI dose is induction treatment using the T-cell depleting agent alemtuzumab, which in a single-center retrospective analysis was associated with better renal function in the first 4 years post-lung transplant (compared with either no induction or ATG induction), without increasing infective episodes.[148]

Basiliximab induction has similarly been used to support the delayed introduction of CNIs in patients at risk of perioperative AKI, without increasing the risk of acute rejection.[149] Furthermore, there are case reports of basiliximab used to facilitate temporary "CNI holidays" in solid organ transplant recipients with AKI until restoration of renal function has been achieved.[150,151]

Another strategy has been the addition of an mTORi to standard triple therapy to facilitate lower trough CNI levels. The 4EVERLUNG prospective, multicenter, randomized trial assigned 130 lung transplant recipients (from 3 months posttransplant) to quadruple (everolimus) low CNI immunosuppression or standard triple CNI immunosuppression and demonstrated significantly superior renal function (eGFR 64.5 mL/min vs 54.6 mL/min) in the quadruple low CNI group at 12 months.[152] The NOCTET study randomized 282 patients from 1 year after heart or lung transplantation to continue conventional CNI therapy or to start everolimus with reduced-exposure CNI. Although an early renal benefit in lung transplant recipients was lost, long-term immunosuppressive efficacy was maintained albeit at the expense of a three-fold higher risk of pneumonia.[153] These trial data have led to a currently recruiting study using alemtuzumab induction for lung transplant recipients followed by either low-dose tacrolimus with low-dose everolimus or standard triple immunosuppression.[154]

Finally, there is retrospective data that replacing CNIs with the co-stimulation blocker, belatacept, in severe renal disease post-lung transplant may have a role in stabilizing kidney function without lung compromise.[155]

FUTURE FRONTIERS IN LUNG TRANSPLANT IMMUNOSUPPRESSION

Higher pretransplant DSA titers are associated with an increased risk of AMR and therein CLAD. A reduction in DSA levels pretransplant may reduce the risk of DSA-mediated allograft injury at the time of transplant and reperfusion. Imlifidase, a cysteine protease derived from the IgG-degrading enzyme of *Streptococcus pyogenes*, has been conditionally approved in Europe for desensitization of highly sensitized crossmatch-positive renal transplant patients. It acts to rapidly degrade DSA and create a 7 to 14-day window during which antibody levels remain sufficiently low to enable transplantation with an HLA-incompatible donor organ.[156,157] Outcomes and safety with Imlifidase-enabled renal allografts are comparable to those of other highly sensitized patients undergoing HLA-incompatible transplantation at 3 years,[158] but the treatment has yet to be trialed in lung transplant recipients.

New therapeutic strategies for AMR may be approved for use within the next decade. Phase II and III studies are ongoing to evaluate IL-6 antagonism, CD38-targeting antibodies, and selective inhibitors of complement.[159] The IL-6 inhibitor, tocilizumab, has come to prominence as a treatment to mitigate cytokine-release syndrome in solid organ transplant recipients with COVID-19, but may also be effective in suppressing DSA responses.[160,161]

The pivotal role of the CD28/CD80/CD86/CTLA-4 receptor–ligand system in the initiation and control of effector and Treg cell responses makes it an attractive target for immunosuppression.[162] Belatacept is a selective co-stimulation blocker that binds CD80 and CD86 to block CD28-mediated T-cell activation. It is administered intravenously once a month and requires no therapeutic drug monitoring. The safety and efficacy of belatacept, as an alternative to CNIs, has been demonstrated in renal transplant recipients.[163,164] Although it lacks many of the cardiovascular, metabolic, and renal adverse of effects of the CNIs,[165] there is an increased risk of posttransplant lymphoproliferative disease, especially in Epstein-Barr virus seronegative recipients.[163] This agent has been used more commonly as a calcineurin-sparing agent in patients with worsening renal function post-lung transplantation, in particular if patients' renal function failed to improve or have poor tolerance to mTOR inhibitors.

The field of engineered Tregs is early in development, and antigen-specific Tregs are a promising tool for immunosuppression. In rodent models, donor MHC-specific Tregs are more potent than polyclonal Tregs in preventing acute and chronic rejection.[166,167] The infusion of Tregs engineered with a chimeric antigen receptor (CAR) targeting donor-derived HLA may help facilitate allograft tolerance.[168] A pilot study demonstrated successful withdrawal of immunosuppression in 7 out of 10 adult liver transplant recipients given an ex vivo-generated autologous Treg-enriched cell product early posttransplant,[169] and the first clinical trial using CAR-Tregs to induce and maintain immunologic tolerance in HLA-mismatched kidney transplant recipients is ongoing (NCT04817774).

Based on success in murine and primate models, there has been some support for chimerism protocols in which depletion of the recipient immune system is followed by concomitant hematopoietic stem cell transplant and solid organ transplant from the same donor to achieve allograft tolerance.[170–172] These protocols have been successful in achieving tolerance in small numbers of human renal transplant recipients, but there have been concerns regarding morbidity and mortality from infection and GVHD.[173]

In the future, early alloimmune responses may be mitigated by donor organ modification before transplantation. Ex vivo lung perfusion (EVLP) promotes anti-inflammatory processes and offers the opportunity for depletion or transfer of cell populations and delivery of therapeutic agents including immunosuppressive elements.[174] In a rat model, the administration of cyclosporin A via EVLP has been associated with improved lung graft preservation.[175] Depletion of donor antigens may mitigate against posttransplant antibody-mediated injury and proof of concept was recently demonstrated via enzymatic depletion of A-antigen to convert blood group A lungs to blood group O lungs.[176]

SUMMARY

CNI-based immunosuppression regimens have remained the foundation of solid organ transplant immunosuppression for the past four decades. As we more clearly define allograft tolerance and rejection at a cellular and molecular level, there is scope to develop innovative and better targeted immunomodulatory therapies. Personalized therapy will demand greater understanding of the effects of each immunosuppressive agent or combination of agents on each individual lung transplant recipient via monitoring strategies that extend beyond measuring trough levels.

CLINICS CARE POINTS

- High intensity immunosuppression is initiated immediately post-transplant, when the risk of allograft rejection is greatest.
- To maximise preventive and therapeutic effects with the minimum toxicity, two or more immunosuppressive agents are used in combination and continued for the life of the recipient.
- Drug-drug interactions with immunosuppressive agents must be considered when prescribing additional medication.
- Antimicrobial prophylaxis is initiated after transplant to prevent opportunistic infection with pathogens such as Cytomegalovirus, Pneumocystis jirovecii and Aspergillus fumigatus.
- In the context of long-term immunosuppression, clinicians should be vigilant for increased cardiovascular risk, nephrotoxicity, osteoporosis and malignancy.

DISCLOSURE

C.M. Patterson and H. Lyster were involved in the conception of the article. All authors (C.M. Patterson, E.C. Jolly, F. Burrows, N.J. Ronan, and H. Lyster) were involved in the structuring the template of the article, undertaking literature review, drafting the article and providing critical revision of the article. All authors (C.M. Patterson, E.C. Jolly, F. Burrows, N.J. Ronan, and H. Lyster) have provided final approval of the version to be published.

CONFLICT OF INTEREST STATEMENT

All authors hereby certify that all affiliations with or financial involvement in, within the past 5 years and foreseeable future, any organization or entity with a financial interest in or financial conflict with the subject matter or materials discussed in the article are completely disclosed. None of the authors (C.M. Patterson, E.C. Jolly, F. Burrows, N.J. Ronan, and H. Lyster) have any financial interests related to the material in the article. None of the other authors (C.M. Patterson, E.C. Jolly, F. Burrows, N.J. Ronan, and H. Lyster) have any potential conflicts of interest related to the material in the article. The article has not been published previously and that it is not under consideration for publication elsewhere. All authors agree with the content of the article.

ACKNOWLEDGMENT

All authors hereby certify that all affiliations with or financial involvement in, within the past 5 years and foreseeable future, any organization or entity with a financial interest in or financial conflict with the subject matter or materials discussed in the manuscript are completely disclosed.

None of the authors have any financial interests related to the material in the manuscript.

None of the other authors have any potential conflicts of interest related to the material in the manuscript.

REFERENCES

1. Murphy JB. Heteroplastic tissue grafting effected through roentgen-ray lymphoid destruction. JAMA 1914;LXII(19):1459.
2. Silverstein AM. The lymphocyte in immunology: from James B. Murphy to James L. Gowans. Nat Immunol 2001;2(7):569–71.
3. Calne RY. The rejection of renal homografts. Inhibition in dogs by 6-mercaptopurine. Lancet 1960; 1(7121):417–8.
4. Schwartz R, Dameshek W. The effects of 6-mercaptopurine on homograft reactions. J Clin Invest 1960;39(6):952–8.
5. Murray JE, Merrill JP, Harrison JH, et al. Prolonged survival of human-kidney homografts by immunosuppressive drug therapy. N Engl J Med 1963; 268:1315–23.
6. Starzl TE, Marchioro TL, Waddell WR. The reversal of rejection in human renal homografts with subsequent development of homograft tolerance. Surg Gynecol Obstet 1963;117:385–95.
7. Borel JF, Feurer C, Gubler HU, et al. Biological effects of cyclosporine A: a new antilymphocytic agent. Agents Actions 1976;6(4):468–75.
8. Calne RY, Rolles K, White DJ, et al. Cyclosporine A initially as the only immunosuppressant in 34 recipients of cadaveric organs: 32 kidneys, 2 pancreases, and 2 livers. Lancet 1979;2(8151): 1033–6.
9. Calne RY, White DJ, Evans DB, et al. Cyclosporine A in cadaveric organ transplantation. Br Med J (Clin Res Ed 1981;282(6268):934–6.
10. Starzl TE, Weil R 3rd, Iwatsuki S, et al. The use of cyclosporine A and prednisone in cadaver kidney transplantation. Surg Gynecol Obstet 1980; 151(1):17–26.
11. Starzl TE, Klintmalm GB, Porter KA, et al. Liver transplantation with use of cyclosporine A and prednisone. N Engl J Med 1981;305(5):266–9.
12. Starzl TE, Todo S, Fung J, et al. FK 506 for liver, kidney, and pancreas transplantation. Lancet 1989; 2(8670):1000–4.
13. Reitz BA, Wallwork J, Hunt SA, et al. Heart lung transplantation: successful therapy for patients with pulmonary vascular disease. N Engl J Med 1982;306:557.
14. Cooper JD, Pearson FG, Patterson GA, et al. Technique of successful lung transplantation in humans. J Thorac Cardiovasc Surg 1987;93:173.
15. Witt CA, Puri V, Gelman AE, et al. Lung transplant immunosuppression - time for a new approach? Expert Rev Clin Immunol 2014;10(11):1419–21.
16. Shepherd HM, Gauthier JM, Kreisel D. Tolerance, immunosuppression, and immune modulation: impacts on lung allograft survival. Curr Opin Organ Transpl 2021;26(3):328–32.
17. Ingulli E. Mechanism of cellular rejection in transplantation. Pediatr Nephrol 2010;25(1):61–74.
18. Ng CY, Madsen JC, Rosengard BR, et al. Immunosuppression for lung transplantation. Front Biosci (Landmark Ed 2009;14(5):1627–41.
19. Ohm B, Jungraithmayr W. B cell immunity in lung transplant rejection - effector mechanisms and therapeutic implications. Front Immunol 2022;13: 845867.
20. Conlon TM, Saeb-Parsy K, Cole JL, et al. Germinal center Alloantibody responses are mediated exclusively by indirect-pathway CD4 T follicular helper cells. J Immunol 2012;188:2643–52.
21. Walters GD, Vinuesa CG. T follicular helper cells in transplantation. Transplantation 2016;100(8): 1650–5.
22. Wood KJ, Bushell A, Hester J. Regulatory immune cells in transplantation. Nat Rev Immunol 2012; 12(6):417–30.
23. Siu JHY, Surendrakumar V, Richards JA, et al. T cell allorecognition pathways in solid organ transplantation. Front Immunol 2018;9:2548.
24. Halloran PF, Venner JM, Madill-Thomsen KS, et al. Review: the transcripts associated with organ allograft rejection. Am J Transpl 2018;18(4): 785–95.
25. Shi T, Roskin K, Baker BM, et al. Advanced genomics-based approaches for defining allograft rejection with single cell resolution. Front Immunol 2021;12:750754.
26. Benazzo A, Bozzini S, Auner S, et al. Differential expression of circulating miRNAs after alemtuzumab induction therapy in lung transplantation. Sci Rep 2022;12(1):7072.
27. Chambers DC, Cherikh WS, Harhay MO, et al. The international thoracic organ transplant registry of the international society for heart and lung

transplantation: thirty-sixth adult lung and heart-lung transplantation report-2019; focus theme: donor and recipient size match. J Heart Lung Transpl 2019;38(10):1042–55.

28. Chambers DC, Cherikh WS, Goldfarb SB, et al. The international thoracic organ transplant registry of the international society for heart and lung transplantation: thirty-fifth adult lung and heart-lung transplant report-2018; focus theme: multiorgan transplantation. J Heart Lung Transpl 2018;37:1169–83.

29. Magliocca JF, Knechtle SJ. The evolving role of alemtuzumab (Campath-1H) for immunosuppressive therapy in organ transplantation. Transpl Int 2006;19(9):705–14.

30. Ippoliti G, Lucioni M, Leonardi G, et al. Immunomodulation with rabbit anti-thymocyte globulin in solid organ transplantation. World J Transpl 2015;5(4):261–6.

31. Hachem RR, Edwards LB, Yusen RD, et al. The impact of induction on survival after lung transplantation: an analysis of the International Society for Heart and Lung Transplantation Registry. Clin Transpl 2008;22(5):603–8.

32. Furuya Y, Jayarajan SN, Taghavi S, et al. The impact of Alemtuzumab and Basliliximab Induction on patient survival and time to bronchitis obliterates syndrome in double lung transplantation recipients. Am J Transpl 2016;16:2334–41.

33. Jaksch P, Ankersmit J, Scheed A, et al. Alemtuzumab in lung transplantation: an open-label, randomized, prospective single center study. Am J Transpl 2014;14:1839–45.

34. Shyu S, Dew MA, Pilewski JM, et al. Five-year outcomes with alemtuzumab induction after lung transplantation. J Heart Lung Transpl 2011;30:743–54.

35. Morris PJ, Russell NK. Alemtuzumab (Campath-1H): a systematic review in organ transplantation. Transplantation 2006;81(10):1361–7.

36. Peleg AY, Husain S, Kwak EJ, et al. Opportunistic infections in 547 organ transplant recipients receiving alemtuzumab, a humanized monoclonal CD-52 antibody. Clin Infect Dis 2007;44(2):204–12.

37. Penninga L, Møller CH, Penninga EI, et al. Antibody induction therapy for lung transplant recipients. Cochrane Database Syst Rev 2013;2013(11):CD008927.

38. Snell GI, Westall GP, Levvey BJ, et al. A randomized, double-blind, placebo-controlled, multicenter study of rabbit ATG in the prophylaxis of acute rejection in lung transplantation. Am J Transpl 2014;14(5):1191–8.

39. Fan Y, Xiao YB, Weng YG. Tacrolimus versus cyclosporine for adult lung transplant recipients: a meta-analysis. Transpl Proc 2009;41(5):1821–4.

40. Treede H, Glanville AR, Klepetko W, et al. Tacrolimus and cyclosporinee have differential effects on the risk of development of bronchiolitis obliterans syndrome: results of a prospective, randomized international trial in lung transplantation. J Heart Lung Transpl 2012;31(8):797–804.

41. Collin C, Boussaud V, Lefeuvre S, et al. Sublingual tacrolimus as an alternative to intravenous route in patients with thoracic transplant: a retrospective study. Transpl Proc 2010;42(10):4331–7.

42. Beckebaum S, Iacob S, Sweid D, et al. Efficacy, safety, and immunosuppressant adherence in stable liver transplant patients converted from a twice-daily tacrolimus-based regimen to once-daily tacrolimus extended-release formulation. Transpl Int 2011;24(7):666–75.

43. Doesch AO, Mueller S, Akyol C, et al. Increased adherence eight months after switch from twice daily calcineurin inhibitor based treatment to once daily modified released tacrolimus in heart transplantation. Drug Des Devel Ther 2013;7:1253–8.

44. Kolonko A, Chudek J, Wiecek A. Improved kidney graft function after conversion from twice daily tacrolimus to a once daily prolonged-release formulation. Transpl Proc 2011;43(8):2950–3.

45. Wagner M, Earley AK, Webster AC, et al. Mycophenolic acid versus azathioprine as primary immunosuppression for kidney transplant recipients. Cochrane Database Syst Rev 2015;3(12):CD007746.

46. Palmer SM, Baz MA, Sanders L, et al. Results of a randomized, prospective, multicenter trial of mycophenolate mofetil versus azathioprine in the prevention of acute lung allograft rejection. Transplantation 2001;71(12):1772–6.

47. McNeil K, Glanville AR, Wahlers T, et al. Comparison of mycophenolate mofetil and azathioprine for prevention of bronchiolitis obliterans syndrome in de novo lung transplant recipients. Transplantation 2006;81(7):998–1003.

48. Vos M, Plasmeijer EI, van Bemmel BC, et al. Azathioprine to mycophenolate mofetil transition and risk of squamous cell carcinoma after lung transplantation. J Heart Lung Transpl 2018;37(7):853–9.

49. Sabbatini M, Capone D, Gallo R, et al. EC-MPS permits lower gastrointestinal symptom burden despite higher MPA exposure in patients with severe MMF-related gastrointestinal side-effects. Fundam Clin Pharmacol 2009;23(5):617–24.

50. Barnes PJ. How corticosteroids control inflammation: quintiles prize lecture 2005. Br J Pharmacol 2006;148(3):245–54.

51. Bergmann TK, Barraclough KA, Lee KJ, et al. Clinical pharmacokinetics and pharmacodynamics of prednisolone and prednisone in solid organ transplantation. Clin Pharmacokinet 2012;51(11):711–41.

52. Sehgal SN. Rapamune (RAPA, rapamycin, siroli-mus): mechanism of action immunosuppressive effect results from blockade of signal transduction and inhibition of cell cycle progression. Clin Biochem 1998;31:335–40.

53. Bhorade S, Ahya VN, Baz MA, et al. Comparison of sirolimus with azathioprine in a tacrolimus-based immunosuppressive regimen in lung transplantation. Am J Respir Crit Care Med 2011;183(3): 379–87.

54. Snell GI, Valentine VG, Vitulo P, et al. Everolimus versus azathioprine in maintenance lung transplant recipients: an international, randomized, double-blind clinical trial. Am J Transpl 2006;6: 169–77.

55. Strueber M, Warnecke G, Fuge J, et al. Everolimus versus mycophenolate mofetil de novo after lung transplantation: a prospective, randomized, open-label trial. Am J Transpl 2016;16(11):3171–80.

56. Wijesinha M, Hirshon JM, Terrin M, et al. Survival associated with sirolimus plus tacrolimus maintenance without induction therapy compared with standard immunosuppression after lung transplant. JAMA Netw Open 2019;2(8):e1910297.

57. Knoll GA, Kokolo MB, Mallick R, et al. Effect of sirolimus on malignancy and survival after kidney transplantation: systematic review and meta-analysis of individual patient data. BMJ 2014;349: g6679.

58. Cullis B, D'Souza R, McCullagh P, et al. Sirolimus-induced remission of posttransplantation lymphoproliferative disorder. Am J Kidney Dis 2006; 47(5):e67–72.

59. Groetzner J, Kur F, Spelsberg F, et al. Airway anastomosis complications in de novo lung transplantation with sirolimus-based immunosuppression. J Heart Lung Transpl 2004;23(5):632–8.

60. King-Biggs MB, Dunitz JM, Park SJ, et al. Airway anastomotic dehiscence associated with use of sirolimus immediately after lung transplantation. Transplantation 2003;75(9):1437–43.

61. Lopez P, Kohler S, Dimri S. Interstitial lung disease associated with mTOR inhibitors in solid organ transplant recipients: results from a large phase III clinical trial program of everolimus and review of the literature. J Transpl 2014;2014:305931.

62. Sánchez-Fructuoso AI, Ruiz JC, Pérez-Flores I, et al. Comparative analysis of adverse events requiring suspension of mTOR inhibitors: everolimus versus sirolimus. Transpl Proc 2010;42(8): 3050–2.

63. de Pablo A, Santos F, Solé A, et al. Recommendations on the use of everolimus in lung transplantation. Transpl Rev (Orlando) 2013;27:9–16.

64. Meyer KC, Raghu G, Verleden GM, et al. An international ISHLT/ATS/ERS clinical practice guideline:

diagnosis and management of bronchiolitis obliterans syndrome. Eur Respir J 2014;44(6):1479–503.

65. Benden C, Haughton M, Leonard S, et al. Therapy options for chronic lung allograft dysfunction-bronchiolitis obliterans syndrome following first-line immunosuppressive strategies: a systematic review. J Heart Lung Transpl 2017;36(9):921–33.

66. Vos R, Vanaudenaerde BM, Verleden SE, et al. Anti-inflammatory and immunomodulatory properties of azithromycin involved in treatment and prevention of chronic lung allograft rejection. Transplantation 2012;94(2):101–9.

67. Verleden GM, Dupont LJ. Azithromycin therapy for patients with bronchiolitis obliterans syndrome after lung transplantation. Transplantation 2004;77: 1465–7.

68. Verleden GM, Vanaudenaerde BM, Dupont LJ, et al. Azithromycin reduces airway neutrophilia and interleukin-8 in patients with bronchiolitis obliterans syndrome. Am J Respir Crit Care Med 2006; 174:566–70.

69. Gottlieb J, Szangolies J, Koehnlein T. Long-term azithromycin for bronchiolitis obliterans syndrome after lung transplantation. Transplantation 2008; 85(1):36–41.

70. Vos R, Vanaudenaerde BM, Ottevaere A, et al. Long-term azithromycin therapy for bronchiolitis obliterans syndrome: divide and conquer? J Heart Lung Transpl 2010;29:1358–68.

71. Kingah PL, Muma G, Soubani A. Azithromycin improves lung function in patients with post-lung transplant bronchiolitis obliterans syndrome: a meta-analysis. Clin Transpl 2014;28(8):906–10.

72. Jain R, Hachem RR, Morrell MR, et al. Azithromycin is associated with increased survival in lung transplant recipients with bronchiolitis obliterans syndrome. J Heart Lung Transpl 2010;29(5):531–7.

73. Vos R, Vanaudenaerde BM, Verleden SE, et al. A randomised controlled trial of azithromycin to prevent chronic rejection after lung transplantation. Eur Respir J 2011;37(1):164–72.

74. Meloni F, Cascina A, Miserere S, et al. Peripheral CD4(+)CD25(+) TREG cell counts and the response to extracorporeal photopheresis in lung transplant recipients. Transpl Proc 2007;39(1): 213–7.

75. George J, Gooden C, Guo W, et al. Role for CD4 CD25 T cells in inhibition of graft rejection by extracorporeal photopheresis. J Heart Lung Transpl 2008;27:616–22.

76. Gatza E, Rogers CE, Clouthier SG, et al. Extracorporeal photopheresis reverses experimental graft-versus-host disease through regulatory T cells. Blood 2008;112(4):1515–21.

77. Hachem R, Corris P. Extracorporeal photopheresis for bronchiolitis obliterans syndrome after lung

transplantation. Transplantation 2018;102(7): 1059–65.

78. Benden C, Speich R, Hofbauer GF, et al. Extracorporeal photopheresis after lung transplantation: a 10-year single-center experience. Transplantation 2008;86:1625–1627.41.

79. Morrell MR, Despotis GJ, Lublin DM, et al. The efficacy of photopheresis for bronchiolitis obliterans syndrome after lung transplantation. J Heart Lung Transpl 2010;29:424–31.

80. Jaksch P, Scheed A, Keplinger M, et al. A prospective interventional study on the use of extracorporeal photopheresis in patients with bronchiolitis obliterans syndrome after lung transplantation. J Heart Lung Transpl 2012;31:950–7.

81. Del Fante C, Scudeller L, Oggionni T, et al. Long-term off-line extracorporeal photochemotherapy in patients with chronic lung allograft rejection not responsive to conventional treatment: a 10-year single-centre analysis. Respiration 2015;90: 118–28.

82. Pecoraro Y, Carillo C, Diso D, et al. Efficacy of extracorporeal photopheresis in patients with bronchiolitis obliterans syndrome after lung transplantation. Transpl Proc 2017;49(4):695–8.

83. Greer M, Dierich M, De Wall C, et al. Phenotyping established chronic lung allograft dysfunction predicts extracorporeal photopheresis response in lung transplant patients. Am J Transpl 2013;13(4): 911–8.

84. Halperin EC. Total lymphoid irradiation as an immunosuppressive agent for transplantation and the treatment of 'autoimmune' disease: a review. Clin Radiol 1985;36(2):125–30.

85. Diamond DA, Michalski JM, Lynch JP, et al. Efficacy of total lymphoid irradiation for chronic allograft rejection following bilateral lung transplantation. Int J Radiat Oncol Biol Phys 1998;41:795.

86. Fisher AJ, Rutherford RM, Bozzino J, et al. The safety and efficacy of total lymphoid irradiation in progressive bronchiolitis obliterans syndrome after lung transplantation. Am J Transpl 2005;5: 537–43.

87. Verleden GM, Lievens Y, Dupont LJ, et al. Efficacy of total lymphoid irradiation in azithromycin nonresponsive chronic allograft rejection after lung transplantation. Transpl Proc 2009;41(5):1816–20.

88. Miller R, Hartog B, Frewet J, et al. Total lymphoid irradiation (TLI) for the management of bronchiolitis obliterans syndrome (BOS) post lung transplant: a single centre experience [abstract]. J Heart Lung Transpl 2016;35(S4):70.

89. Lebeer M, Kaes J, Lambrech M, et al. Total lymphoid irradiation in progressive bronchiolitis obliterans syndrome after lung transplantation: a single-center experience and review of literature. Transpl Int 2020;33(2):216–28.

90. Ruttens D, Verleden SE, Demeyer H, et al. Montelukast for bronchiolitis obliterans syndrome after lung transplantation: a randomized controlled trial. PLoS One 2018;13:e0193564.

91. Vos R, Eynde RV, Ruttens D, et al. Montelukast in chronic lung allograft dysfunction after lung transplantation. J Heart Lung Transpl 2019;38(5): 516–27.

92. Iacono AT, Keenan RJ, Duncan SR, et al. Aerosolized cyclosporine in lung recipients with refractory chronic rejection. Am J Respir Crit Care Med 1996; 153:1451–5.

93. Iacono AT, Corcoran TE, Griffith BP, et al. Aerosol cyclosporine therapy in lung transplant recipients with bronchiolitis obliterans. Eur Respir J 2004;23: 384–90.

94. Iacono AT, Johnson BA, Grgurich WF, et al. A randomized trial of inhaled cyclosporine in lung-transplant recipients. N Engl J Med 2006; 354(2):141–50.

95. Neurohr C, Kneidinger N, Ghiani A, et al. A randomized controlled trial of liposomal cyclosporine A for inhalation in the prevention of bronchiolitis obliterans syndrome following lung transplantation. Am J Transpl 2022;22(1):222–9.

96. Iacono A, Wijesinha M, Rajagopal K, et al. A randomised single-centre trial of inhaled liposomal cyclosporine for bronchiolitis obliterans syndrome post-lung transplantation. ERJ Open Res 2019;5:00167.

97. Deuse T, Blankenberg F, Haddad M, et al. Mechanisms behind local immunosuppression using inhaled tacrolimus in preclinical models of lung transplantation. Am J Respir Cell Mol Biol 2010; 43(4):403–12.

98. Sahakijpijarn S, Beg M, Levine SM, et al. A safety and tolerability study of thin film freeze-dried tacrolimus for local pulmonary drug delivery in human subjects. Pharmaceutics 2021;13(5):717.

99. Hayes D, Zwischenberger JB, Mansour HM. Aerosolized tacrolimus: a case report in a lung transplant recipient. Transpl Proc 2010;42(9): 3876–9.

100. Li Y, Gottlieb J, Ma D, et al. Graft-protective effects of the HMG-CoA reductase inhibitor pravastatin after lung transplantation–a propensity score analysis with 23 years of follow-up. Transplantation 2011;92(4):486–92.

101. Szczepanik A, Hulbert A, Lee HJ, et al. Effect of HMG CoA reductase inhibitors on the development of chronic lung allograft dysfunction. Clin Transpl 2018;32(1). https://doi.org/10.1111/ctr.13156.

102. Veit T, Leuschner G, Sisic A, et al. Pirfenidone exerts beneficial effects in patients with IPF

undergoing single lung transplantation. Am J Transpl 2019;19(8):2358–65.

103. Ihle F, von Wulffen W, Neurohr C. Pirfenidone: a potential therapy for progressive lung allograft dysfunction? J Heart Lung Transpl 2013;32(5):574–5.

104. Vos R, Verleden SE, Ruttens D, et al. Pirfenidone: a potential new therapy for restrictive allograft syndrome? Am J Transpl 2013;13(11):3035–40.

105. Vos R, Wuyts WA, Gheysens O, et al. Pirfenidone in restrictive allograft syndrome after lung transplantation: a case series. Am J Transpl 2018;18(12):3045–59.

106. Focosi D, Antonelli G, Pistello M, et al. Torquetenovirus: the human virome from bench to bedside. Clin Microbiol Infect 2016;22(7):589–93.

107. Hino S, Miyata H. Torque teno virus (TTV): current status. Rev Med Virol 2007;17(1):45–57.

108. De Vlaminck I, Khush KK, Strehl C, et al. Temporal response of the human virome to immunosuppression and antiviral therapy. Cell 2013;155(5):1178–87.

109. Jaksch P, Kundi M, Görzer I, et al. Torque teno virus as a novel biomarker targeting the efficacy of immunosuppression after lung transplantation. J Infect Dis 2018;218(12):1922–8.

110. Redondo N, Navarro D, Aguado JM, et al. Viruses, friends, and foes: the case of Torque Teno Virus and the net state of immunosuppression. Transpl Infect Dis 2022;24(2):e13778.

111. Ahlenstiel-Grunow T, Koch A, Grosshennig A, et al. A multicenter, randomized, open-labeled study to steer immunosuppressive and antiviral therapy by measurement of virus (CMV, ADV, HSV)-specific T cells in addition to determination of trough levels of immunosuppressants in pediatric kidney allograft recipients (IVIST01-trial): study protocol for a randomized controlled trial. Trials 2014;15:324.

112. Sester M, Leboeuf C, Schmidt T, et al. The "ABC" of virus-specific T cell immunity in solid organ transplantation. Am J Transpl 2016;16(6):1697–706.

113. Shino MY, Weigt SS, Saggar R, et al. Usefulness of immune monitoring in lung transplantation using adenosine triphosphate production in activated lymphocytes. J Heart Lung Transpl 2012;31(9):996–1002.

114. Piloni D, Magni S, Oggionni T, et al. Clinical utility of CD4+ function assessment (ViraCor-IBT ImmuKnow test) in lung recipients. Transpl Immunol 2016;37:35–9.

115. Gardiner BJ, Lee SJ, Cristiano Y, et al. Evaluation of Quantiferon®-Monitor as a biomarker of immunosuppression and predictor of infection in lung transplant recipients. Transpl Infect Dis 2021;23(3):e13550.

116. Mian M, Natori Y, Ferreira V, et al. Evaluation of a novel global immunity assay to predict infection in organ transplant recipients. Clin Infect Dis 2018;66(9):1392–7.

117. Ravaioli M, Neri F, Lazzarotto T, et al. Immunosuppression modifications based on an immune response assay: results of a randomized, controlled trial. Transplantation 2015;99(8):1625–32.

118. Gottlieb J, Reuss A, Mayer K, et al. Viral load-guided immunosuppression after lung transplantation (VIGILung)-study protocol for a randomized controlled trial. Trials 2021;22(1):48.

119. Jaksch P, Wiedemann D, Augustin V, et al. Antithymocyte globulin induction therapy improves survival in lung transplantation for cystic fibrosis. Transpl Int 2013;26(1):34–41.

120. Kirkby S, Whitson BA, Wehr AM, et al. Survival benefit of induction immunosuppression in cystic fibrosis lung transplant recipients. J Cyst Fibros 2015;14(1):104–10.

121. Wang J, Zeevi A, McCurry K, et al. Impact of ABCB1 (MDR1) haplotypes on tacrolimus dosing in adult lung transplant patients who are CYP3A5 *3/*3 non-expressors. Transpl Immunol 2006;15(3):235–40.

122. Staatz CE, Goodman LK, Tett SE. Effect of CYP3A and ABCB1 single nucleotide polymorphisms on the pharmacokinetics and pharmacodynamics of calcineurin inhibitors: Part I. Clin Pharmacokinet 2010;49(3):141–75.

123. Li Y, Yan L, Shi Y, et al. CYP3A5 and ABCB1 genotype influence tacrolimus and sirolimus pharmacokinetics in renal transplant recipients. Springerplus 2015;4:637.

124. Brazeau DA, Attwood K, Meaney CJ, et al. Beyond single nucleotide polymorphisms: CYP3A5*3*6*7 composite and ABCB1 haplotype Associations to tacrolimus pharmacokinetics in black and white renal transplant recipients. Front Genet 2020;11:889.

125. Krynetski EY, Evans WE. Genetic polymorphism of thiopurine S-methyltransferase: molecular mechanisms and clinical importance. Pharmacology 2000;61(3):136–46.

126. Daniel LL, Dickson AL, Zanussi JT, et al. Predicted expression of genes involved in the thiopurine metabolic pathway and azathioprine discontinuation due to myelotoxicity. Clin Transl Sci 2022;15(4):859–65.

127. Silhan LL, Shah PD, Chambers DC, et al. Lung transplantation in telomerase mutation carriers with pulmonary fibrosis. Eur Respir J 2014;44(1):178–87.

128. Borie R, Kannengiesser C, Hirschi S, et al. Severe hematologic complications after lung transplantation in patients with telomerase complex mutations. J Heart Lung Transpl 2015;34(4):538–46.

129. Bitterman R, Marinelli T, Husain S. Strategies for the prevention of invasive fungal infections after lung transplant. J Fungi (Basel) 2021;7(2):122.

130. Florescu DF, Kalil AC, Qiu F, et al. What is the impact of hypogammaglobulinemia on the rate of infections and survival in solid organ transplantation? A meta-analysis. Am J Transpl 2013;13(10): 2601–10.

131. Petrov AA, Traister RS, Crespo MM, et al. A prospective observational study of hypogammaglobulinemia in the first year after lung transplantation. Transpl Direct 2018;4(8):e372.

132. Lederer DJ, Philip N, Rybak D, et al. Intravenous immunoglobulin for hypogammaglobulinemia after lung transplantation: a randomized crossover trial. PLoS One 2014;9(8):e103908.

133. Rocha PN, Rocha AT, Palmer SM, et al. Acute renal failure after lung transplantation: incidence, predictors and impact on perioperative morbidity and mortality. Am J Transpl 2005;5(6):1469–76.

134. Arnaoutakis GJ, George TJ, Robinson CW, et al. Severe acute kidney injury according to the RIFLE (risk, injury, failure, loss, end stage) criteria affects mortality in lung transplantation. J Heart Lung Transpl 2011;30(10):1161–8.

135. Jacques F, El-Hamamsy I, Fortier A, et al. Acute renal failure following lung transplantation: risk factors, mortality, and long-term consequences. Eur J Cardiothorac Surg 2012;41(1):193–9.

136. Wehbe E, Brock R, Budev M, et al. Short-term and long-term outcomes of acute kidney injury after lung transplantation. J Heart Lung Transpl 2012; 31(3):244–51.

137. Fidalgo P, Ahmed M, Meyer SR, et al. Incidence and outcomes of acute kidney injury following orthotopic lung transplantation: a population-based cohort study. Nephrol Dial Transpl 2014;29(9):1702–9.

138. Doricic J, Greite R, Vijayan V, et al. Kidney injury after lung transplantation: long-term mortality predicted by post-operative day-7 serum creatinine and few clinical factors. PLoS One 2022;17(3): e0265002.

139. George TJ, Arnaoutakis GJ, Beaty CA, et al. Acute kidney injury increases mortality after lung transplantation. Ann Thorac Surg 2012;94(1):185–92.

140. Mason DP, Solovera-Rozas M, Feng J, et al. Dialysis after lung transplantation: prevalence, risk factors and outcome. J Heart Lung Transpl 2007; 26(11):1155–62.

141. Ojo AO. Renal disease in recipients of nonrenal solid organ transplantation. Semin Nephrol 2007; 27(4):498–507.

142. Wehbe E, Duncan AE, Dar G, et al. Recovery from AKI and short- and long-term outcomes after lung transplantation. Clin J Am Soc Nephrol 2013;8(1): 19–25.

143. Sawhney S, Marks A, Fluck N, et al. Post-discharge kidney function is associated with subsequent ten-year renal progression risk among survivors of acute kidney injury. Kidney Int 2017; 92(2):440–52.

144. Bentata Y. Tacrolimus: 20 years of use in adult kidney transplantation. What we should know about its nephrotoxicity. Artif Organs 2020;44(2):140–52.

145. Nankivell BJ, P'Ng CH, O'Connell PJ, et al. Calcineurin inhibitor nephrotoxicity through the lens of longitudinal histology: comparison of cyclosporine and tacrolimus eras. Transplantation 2016;100(8): 1723–31.

146. Benazzo A, Schwarz S, Muckenhuber M, et al. Alemtuzumab induction combined with reduced maintenance immunosuppression is associated with improved outcomes after lung transplantation: a single centre experience. PLoS One 2019;14(1): e0210443.

147. Kim HE, Paik HC, Jeong SJ, et al. Basiliximab induction with delayed calcineurin inhibitors for high-risk lung transplant candidates. Yonsei Med J 2021;62(2):164–71.

148. Cantarovich M, Metrakos P, Giannetti N, et al. Anti-CD25 monoclonal antibody coverage allows for calcineurin inhibitor "holiday" in solid organ transplant patients with acute renal dysfunction. Transplantation 2002;73(7):1169–72.

149. Alonso P, Sanchez-Lazaro I, Almenar L, et al. Use of a "CNI holidays" strategy in acute renal dysfunction late after heart transplant. Report of two cases. Heart Int 2014;9(2):74–7.

150. Gottlieb J, Neurohr C, Müller-Quernheim J, et al. A randomized trial of everolimus-based quadruple therapy vs standard triple therapy early after lung transplantation. Am J Transpl 2019;19(6):1759–69.

151. Gullestad L, Eiskjaer H, Gustafsson F, et al. Long-term outcomes of thoracic transplant recipients following conversion to everolimus with reduced calcineurin inhibitor in a multicenter, open-label, randomized trial. Transpl Int 2016;29(7):819–29.

152. Benazzo A, Cho A, Nechay A, et al. Combined low-dose everolimus and low-dose tacrolimus after Alemtuzumab induction therapy: a randomized prospective trial in lung transplantation. Trials 2021;22(1):6.

153. Timofte I, Terrin M, Barr E, et al. Belatacept for renal rescue in lung transplant patients. Transpl Int 2016; 29(4):453–63.

154. Jordan SC, Lorant T, Choi J, et al. IgG endopeptidase in highly sensitized patients undergoing transplantation. N Engl J Med 2017;377(5):442–53.

155. Jordan SC, Legendre C, Desai NM, et al. Imlifidase desensitization in crossmatch-positive, highly sensitized kidney transplant recipients: results of an international phase 2 trial (highdes). Transplantation 2021;105(8):1808–17.

156. Kjellman C, Maldonado AQ, Sjöholm K, et al. Outcomes at 3 years posttransplant in imlifidase-desensitized kidney transplant patients. Am J Transpl 2021;21(12):3907–18.

157. Mayer KA, Budde K, Jilma B, et al. Emerging drugs for antibody-mediated rejection after kidney transplantation: a focus on phase II & III trials. Expert Opin Emerg Drugs 2022;27(2):151–67.

158. Pearl M, Weng PL, Chen L, et al. Long term tolerability and clinical outcomes associated with tocilizumab in the treatment of refractory antibody mediated rejection (AMR) in pediatric renal transplant recipients. Clin Transpl 2022;36(8):e14734.

159. Jordan SC, Choi J, Kim I, et al. Interleukin-6, A cytokine critical to mediation of inflammation, autoimmunity and allograft rejection: therapeutic implications of IL-6 receptor blockade. Transplantation 2017;101(1):32–44.

160. Beyersdorf N, Kerkau T, Hünig T. CD28 co-stimulation in T-cell homeostasis: a recent perspective. Immunotargets Ther 2015;4:111–22.

161. Vincenti F, Charpentier B, Vanrenterghem Y, et al. A phase III study of belatacept-based immunosuppression regimens versus cyclosporine in renal transplant recipients (BENEFIT study). Am J Transpl 2010;10(3):535–46.

162. Vincenti F, Rostaing L, Grinyo J, et al. Belatacept and long-term outcomes in kidney transplantation. N Engl J Med 2016;374(4):333–43.

163. Masson P, Henderson L, Chapman JR, et al. Belatacept for kidney transplant recipients. Cochrane Database Syst Rev 2014;2014(11):CD010699.

164. Joffre O, Santolaria T, Calise D, et al. Prevention of acute and chronic allograft rejection with CD4+CD25+Foxp3+ regulatory T lymphocytes. Nat Med 2008;14(1):88–92.

165. Bézie S, Charreau B, Vimond N et al. Human CD8+ Tregs expressing a MHC-specific CAR display enhanced suppression of human skin rejection and GVHD in NSG mice. Blood Adv 2019;3(22):3522–38.

166. Muller YD, Ferreira LMR, Ronin E, et al. Precision engineering of an anti-HLA-A2 chimeric antigen receptor in regulatory T cells for transplant immune tolerance. Front Immunol 2021;12:686439.

167. Todo S, Yamashita K, Goto R, et al. A pilot study of operational tolerance with a regulatory T-cell-based cell therapy in living donor liver transplantation. Hepatology 2016;64(2):632–43.

168. Sasaki H, Oura T, Spitzer TR, et al. Preclinical and clinical studies for transplant tolerance via the mixed chimerism approach. Hum Immunol 2018;79(5):258–65.

169. Lee KW, Park JB, Park H, et al. Inducing transient mixed chimerism for allograft survival without maintenance immunosuppression with combined kidney and bone marrow transplantation: protocol optimization. Transplantation 2020;104(7):1472–82.

170. Szabolcs P, Buckley RH, Davis RD, et al. Tolerance and immunity after sequential lung and bone marrow transplantation from an unrelated cadaveric donor. J Allergy Clin Immunol 2015;135(2):567–70.

171. Issa F, Strober S, Leventhal JR, et al. The fourth international workshop on clinical transplant tolerance. Am J Transpl 2021;21(1):21–31.

172. Iske J, Hinze CA, Salman J, et al. The potential of ex vivo lung perfusion on improving organ quality and ameliorating ischemia reperfusion injury. Am J Transpl 2021;21(12):3831–9.

173. Haam S, Noda K, Philips BJ, et al. Cyclosporin A administration during ex vivo lung perfusion preserves lung grafts in rat transplant model. Transplantation 2020;104(9):e252–9.

174. Wang A, Ribeiro RVP, Ali A, et al. Ex vivo enzymatic treatment converts blood type A donor lungs into universal blood type lungs. Sci Transl Med 2022;14(632):eabm7190.

175. Haam S, Noda K, Philips BJ, et al. Cyclosporin A Administration During Ex Vivo Lung Perfusion Preserves Lung Grafts in Rat Transplant Model. Transplantation 2020;104(9):e252–9.

176. Wang A, Ribeiro RVP, Ali A, et al. Ex vivo enzymatic treatment converts blood type A donor lungs into universal blood type lungs. Sci Transl Med 2022;14(632):eabm7190.

Acute Rejection and Chronic Lung Allograft Dysfunction
Obstructive and Restrictive Allograft Dysfunction

Hanne Beeckmans, MD[a,1], Saskia Bos, MD[b,c,1], Robin Vos, MD, PhD[a,b,*,2], Allan R. Glanville, MD[d,2]

KEYWORDS

- Acute cellular rejection • Bronchiolitis obliterans syndrome • Chronic lung allograft dysfunction
- Lung transplantation • Restrictive allograft syndrome • T-cell-mediated rejection

KEY POINTS

- Multifactorial injuries to the secondary pulmonary lobule precipitate post-transplant immune-driven airway/vascular remodeling, resulting in a pathophysiological decline in lung allograft function over time after transplantation.
- Better diagnostic methods are needed to identify subclinical rejection and allograft health status.
- Targeting treatable traits after lung transplantation can help to mitigate CLAD onset and progression.
- Efforts should be made to improve therapeutic management, aiming at preventing acute and chronic rejection after lung transplantation.

INTRODUCTION

Lung transplantation is an established therapeutic procedure for well-selected patients with end-stage respiratory diseases Appendix. However, the lung is characterized by the highest rates of acute rejection and chronic allograft dysfunction among transplanted solid organs, and long-term outcomes, therefore, remain inferior to other solid organ transplants.[1,2] Ongoing alloimmune (non-self) recognition and ensuing immune activation, together with the initial ischemic-reperfusion insult to the small airways, constant environmental exposure, and increased susceptibility of the lung to endogenous or exogenous injuries, resulting in local innate immune activation, likely contribute to these high rates of allograft dysfunction.[3] Multifactorial injuries to the bronchovascular axis of the secondary pulmonary lobule may indeed precipitate the post-transplant immune-driven airway/vascular remodeling, resulting in a pathophysiological decline of the lungs over time after transplantation, which may become evident either functionally and/or structurally. As neither alloimmune recognition nor non-alloimmune stimulation can be avoided, most lung transplant recipients will at some point in time develop structural and/or functional abnormalities of their graft,

[a] Department of Chronic Diseases and Metabolism, KU Leuven, Laboratory of Respiratory Diseases and Thoracic Surgery (BREATHE), Leuven, Belgium; [b] Department of Respiratory Diseases, University Hospitals Leuven, Leuven, Belgium; [c] Newcastle University, Translational and Clinical Research Institute, Newcastle upon Tyne, UK; [d] Lung Transplant Unit, St. Vincent's Hospital, Sydney, Australia
[1] Contributed equally as first author.
[2] Contributed equally as senior author.
* Corresponding author. Department of Respiratory Diseases, University Hospitals Leuven, 49 Herestraat, Leuven B-3000, Belgium.
E-mail address: robin.vos@uzleuven.be

Clin Chest Med 44 (2023) 137–157
https://doi.org/10.1016/j.ccm.2022.10.011
0272-5231/23/© 2022 Elsevier Inc. All rights reserved.

depending on the efficacy of their immunosuppressive regimen to suppress immune alloimmune responses and the number/severity of injuries encountered by the lung allograft. This review focuses on current knowledge and concepts, barriers, and gaps in acute cellular rejection (ACR), the most significant risk factor for chronic lung allograft dysfunction (CLAD)—the greatest impediment to the long-term survival of lung transplant recipients. Antibody-mediated rejection (AMR) will be discussed in another article in this issue; yet AMR is indisputably related to both ACR and CLAD development, through direct and indirect cellular interactions within the graft.

ACUTE CELLULAR REJECTION

Despite the availability of improved immunosuppressive agents, acute lung allograft rejection remains a relevant problem, especially in the first-year post-transplant. Its incidence varies depending on different data sources, up to 30% to 50% during the first-year post-transplant. Moreover, ACR accounts for 3.8% and 1.8% of deaths within the first month and between 1 month and 1 year after transplantation, respectively.[1,3,4] More importantly, ACR is one of the strongest risk factors for the subsequent development of CLAD.[5,6]

Mechanism

ACR is an alloimmune 'host-versus-graft' response, primarily driven by T lymphocytes recognizing circulating or tissue–resident donor major histocompatibility complexes, also called human leukocyte antigens (HLA), or other (non-HLA) antigens.[7] Major histocompatibility complexes are presented by antigen-presenting cells and regulate the immune response by presenting antigenic peptides to T cells.[3] This allorecognition is the central mechanism of ACR, although increasingly greater emphasis is given to the role of B-cells and natural killer cells.[7,8] Following allorecognition, T cells undergo clonal expansion and differentiation into alloreactive cytotoxic T cells.[3] Unlike other solid organ transplants, the lung allograft is continuously exposed to the external environment and has a more intense local innate immunity primed to respond to environmental or microbiological challenges. Therefore, the process of allorecognition is typically enhanced by local innate immune activation in the lung allograft.[3]

Acute Cellular Rejection as a Risk Factor for Chronic Lung Allograft Dysfunction

Although the etiology of CLAD is multifactorial, ACR has been consistently reported as a substantial risk factor. Thus, acute rejection is not only an important cause of acute allograft dysfunction and/or failure, but both perivascular (A-grade) and peribronchiolar (B-grade) rejection also predispose patients to subsequent development of CLAD.[5,6] Studies examining the impact of A-grade ACR noted a strong association between high-grade ACR ($\geq$A2), recurrent episodes of ACR, a cumulative burden of ACR, and episodes of late ACR with the long-term development of CLAD, although even single episodes can increase the risk for later CLAD.[7,9–12] Likewise, B-grade ACR (lymphocytic bronchiolitis, LB) is a precursor of obliterative bronchiolitis (OB) and its severity is linked to the development of bronchiolitis obliterans syndrome (BOS), and possibly also restrictive allograft syndrome (RAS).[5,6,13]

So, although histopathologic signs of ACR often resolve with treatment, the alloimmune responses that occur can generate a profibrotic environment contributing to CLAD.

Classic Histopathology

The clinical presentation of ACR is variable, ranging from asymptomatic to symptoms that overlap with other complications frequently seen in this patient population (ie, respiratory infection) to acute graft failure.[7] A decrease in forced expiratory volume in 1 s (FEV1) is often the main finding, which can be accompanied by non-specific signs and symptoms including dyspnea, cough, hypoxia, fever; and radiographic abnormalities (eg, ground glass opacities, septal thickening, and pleural effusion).[3,4] As clinical findings lack specificity, tissue diagnosis is necessary to support a diagnosis of ACR. Histopathologic analysis of transbronchial biopsies (TBB) therefore remains the gold standard.[4,7] ACR may affect the vasculature and/or small airways of the lung allograft, and the diagnosis relies on the presence of perivascular and/or peribronchiolar mononuclear cell infiltration. Episodes of ACR are often clinically silent, hence, many transplant centers have implemented surveillance bronchoscopies, as will be discussed later.[7,14,15]

The latest International Society for Heart and Lung Transplantation (ISHLT) update of the Working formulation for the standardization of nomenclature in the diagnosis of lung rejection dates from 2007 and these recommendations have become widely adopted by transplant centers worldwide.[14,15]

The severity of A-grade rejection depends on the degree of perivascular mononuclear infiltrates, cellular invasion into the interstitial and alveolar spaces, and the presence or absence of accompanying acute lung injury, with grades ranging from A0 (none) to A4 (severe)[7,14] (**Table 1**). Accurate grading is important as treatment and follow-up are often adjusted accordingly.[4,7]

B-grade rejection (LB) is characterized by peribronchiolar mononuclear inflammation and its presence is more common in higher grades of A-grade rejection (≥A2). Owing to poor reproducibility, quantification of its severity has been simplified over time and is rated as low (B1R) or high (B2R) grade.[7,14] However, many TBB contain no or minimal airway tissue, making accurate evaluation and grading difficult. In addition, airway biopsies are susceptible to tangential cutting and other artifacts. Therefore, further investigation of the correlation between TBB and endobronchial biopsies of larger airways and the clinical use of the latter in interpreting bronchial/bronchiolar inflammation would be interesting. Lastly, airway inflammation is also commonly seen in respiratory infections—a common complication in lung transplant recipients, and viral infections, in particular, can cause mononuclear inflammation. Therefore, ascribing and grading the histomorphologic findings to an alloimmune reaction are generally

recommended after the exclusion of acute infection.[3,4,7]

The ISHLT recommends at least five pieces of well-expanded alveolated lung tissue for adequate morphologic evaluation and sensitivity, either from a target lobe based on radiological findings or the (better-perfused) lower lobe.[14–16] Different rejection grades can be seen in different lung lobes, but the grade is often worse in the lower lobes, which relates to better perfusion at the base of the lungs, promoting local cellular migration across the blood vessel walls into the surrounding tissue.[16,17]

TBB should be thoroughly reviewed and higher-power analysis should be used as abnormalities can be very focal, especially in low-grade rejection.[7] The issue of intra- and inter-reader variability has been recognized and may be further challenged by the fact that histologic features of ACR can be mimicked by other conditions, such as infection, drug toxicity, aspiration, or ischemia-reperfusion injury.[3,7] Finally, it is important to note that the finding of "no rejection" does not completely rule out the absence of ACR, due to the patchy nature of the disease. Similarly, the

Table 1
Grading of acute cellular rejection

Category	Grade	Severity	Findings
A: perivascular	0	None	Normal lung parenchyma
	1	Minimal	Scattered, infrequent, small mononuclear perivascular cellular infiltrates
	2	Mild	More frequent perivascular mononuclear cellular infiltrates, eosinophils may be present
	3	Moderate	Dense perivascular mononuclear cellular infiltrates, extension into interstitial space, can involve endothelialitis, eosinophils and neutrophils may be present
	4	Severe	Diffuse perivascular, interstitial, and air-space infiltrates of mononuclear cells, endothelialitis, neutrophils may be present
	X	Ungradable	No or scarce alveolar tissue present
B: small airway inflammation – lymphocytic bronchiolitis	0	None	No evidence of bronchiolar inflammation
	1R	Low grade	Infrequent, scattered or single layer mononuclear cells in bronchiolar submucosa
	2R	High grade	Larger infiltrates of larger and activated lymphocytes in bronchiolar submucosa, can involve eosinophils and plasmacytoid cells, epithelial damage with necrosis, metaplasia, and intra-epithelial lymphocytic infiltration
	X	Ungradable	No or scarce bronchiolar tissue present

Acute cellular rejection grading based on the ISHLT lung rejection working group.
Data from Stewart S, Fishbein MC, Snell GI, et al. Revision of the 1996 working formulation for the standardization of nomenclature in the diagnosis of lung rejection. J Heart Lung Transplant. 2007;26(12):1229-1242.

finding of A1 rejection does not preclude (unsampled) areas of $\geq$ A2 elsewhere in the lung. These and other relevant issues regarding grading and analyzing ACR are further discussed below and in the Appendix.

Interobserver and Intraobserver Variability

The reported incidence of ACR varies widely, and a high degree of intra- and interobserver variability exists in the pathologic interpretation of ACR, even if scored by experienced pathologists.[9,18,19] Particularly, the quantification of more subtle forms of perivascular infiltration carries considerable variation, with interobserver agreement concordance rates varying between 50% and 80%.[18–20] There may also be variation in the way in which centers interpret perivascular infiltrates in the presence of infection.[21] Generally, A grades are more reliable, whereas B grades only have fair reliability.[11,19,20] Importantly, inaccurate grading could potentially impact treatment and outcome, especially the detrimental effects of undertreatment as reported.[15]

Surveillance Bronchoscopy for Subclinical Acute Cellular Rejection

The arguments for clinically indicated bronchoscopy and TBB are strong. However, less certainty remains on the merits of surveillance bronchoscopy with well-established arguments both for and against surveillance biopsies.[15] A significant number of ACR cases, particularly low-grade forms, are clinically silent ("subclinical") and are only diagnosed at the time of surveillance TBB in an otherwise clinically stable and asymptomatic patient.[9,11] The yield of detection of subclinical ACR varies between 15% to 40% with relatively high percentages of grade A2 and higher acute rejection.[22] Given the relatively high detection rates of subclinical ACR $\geq$ A2, there is a rationale for surveillance biopsies because of the risk of recurrent or persistent ACR, the association of LB, and subsequent development of CLAD. Other arguments in favor are the lack of adequate surrogate markers at this time, the relatively low risks of the procedure, and the intent of treating before there is any impact on allograft function.[3,11,12] Therefore, many transplant centers screen for subclinical ACR through scheduled surveillance bronchoscopy, however, the optimal duration of such screening is unclear.[22]

On the other hand, the impact of surveillance bronchoscopy and the relevance of these findings on long-term outcomes, and the necessity of treatment in asymptomatic patients remain questioned, and its practice is not universal.[15,22]

Within the first year, subclinical ACR is the most prevalent in the first 3 to 6 months post-transplant, but the yield is also still relevant after those first months, although a preponderance of A1 lesions was seen later post-transplant.[22] In addition to the duration of surveillance bronchoscopy (ie, beyond the first year), the yield might also be affected by the number of biopsies taken and the areas of the lung sampled, differences in clinical thresholds for performing bronchoscopy (ie, low threshold) and different treatment protocols, making it difficult to truly validate the role of surveillance bronchoscopy.[22] Soon, not only biopsies, but likely a combination evaluation of circulating donor-derived cell-free DNA, gene expression profile analysis of activated/inhibited genes, and/or intrapulmonary microbiome signatures could perhaps better determine the presence of T-cell-mediated rejection (TCMR), ABMR, and infection in the lung graft. For this, however, results of ongoing trials are awaited.

Minimal Acute Cellular Rejection

ACR has been identified as the primary risk factor for CLAD, but the true impact of minimal grade A1 ACR, especially a solitary episode, remains unclear.[9] There is consensus in most centers to treat clinically manifest and/or higher grade ($\geq$A2) ACR with increased immunosuppression.[7,9] However, there is still debate as to whether subclinical A1 and isolated LB should be treated because of controversy regarding clinical significance and long-term outcome implications.[7,9,23] The main reason why treatment of minimal ACR in asymptomatic patients is questioned is the increased susceptibility to infections and other side effects associated with augmented immunosuppression, the mainstay of ACR treatment.[9,11] Consequently, treatment remains controversial and different practices have been implemented throughout lung transplant centers.[7,9]

Several studies have demonstrated the importance of subclinical minimal ACR in lung transplant recipients and its impact on the risk of subsequent CLAD, in which grade A1 rejection (even without recurrence or subsequent progression to a higher grade) and isolated LB were both risk factors for CLAD.[3,10,24] The risk to evolve to BOS was higher in the case of multiple episodes of minimal rejection or a higher grade of LB.[23,25] As such, the treatment seems appropriate. However, these studies often had a mixed population of clinically stable and unstable patients.[9]

On the other hand, other studies failed to substantiate this increased CLAD risk, and in a recent large study, Levy and colleagues showed that an episode of untreated subclinical A1 in the first year post-transplant did not significantly increase the risk of CLAD, implying that a watchful-waiting approach might be acceptable in clinically stable patients.[9] However, other factors that may impact the risk for later CLAD development were not included in this study.

From a theoretic perspective, every A1 rejection needs to be seen as an early sign of (increased) alloreactivity with the risk of persistent smoldering alloreactivity, progression to higher ACR grades, and/or association of LB in the absence of increased immunosuppression.[23] Careful consideration, clinical assessment, and follow-up are strongly recommended to guide treatment, especially in patients with multiple A1 lesions in the absence of high-grade rejection, or a history of A1 episodes.[23]

Late-Onset Acute Cellular Rejection

The incidence of ACR is highest within the first year post-transplant, but acute rejection can also be seen thereafter, and late ACR is strongly associated with subsequent CLAD development.[21,22] Burton and colleagues even reported that around 20% to 25% of patients developed ACR $\geq$ A2 1 to 2 years after transplantation, with a 44% incidence of $\geq$ A1 at 2-year surveillance bronchoscopy.[21] This could mean that the up to 12-month surveillance schedule currently used by most centers is too short, implying some value in performing late surveillance bronchoscopy (beyond the first year), especially in those patients with a history of $\geq$ A2 who are at risk for subsequent episodes of ACR requiring treatment.[21]

Acute Cellular Rejection: Time to Rename?

It has been acknowledged that acute graft rejection can be either cell-mediated (ACR), antibody-mediated (AMR), or mixed (ACR + AMR).[4] However, it is well-known that "acute" cellular rejection can be detected at later times post-transplant, and also AMR can occur at later stages after transplantation (ie, > 1 year post-transplant).[21,26] Indeed, the name "acute" cellular rejection implicitly suggests an acute onset, whereas the process of ACR might in fact have been going on for some time before detection, and thus, may be more subacute or chronic in nature. However, the duration or chronicity of the underlying cellular process cannot be determined on TBB, which only gives a limited snapshot view of a highly dynamic immunologic process affecting the lung allograft.

This makes us wonder whether TCMR would be a more appropriate name comparable to the terminology of TCMR and AMR used in the kidney transplant population.[27] Indeed, ACR is mainly mediated by T lymphocytes recognizing donor HLA and other donor-mediated antigens, although this name might sound as if no other mechanisms (eg, natural killer cells and B-cells) are involved though T cells remain the main culprit and cause of TCMR.[4] Renaming ACR would dispel any notion that cell-mediated rejection (in the form of A- and B-grade rejection) can only occur *early* after transplantation, or with an *acute* clinical onset, and could make the treating physicians more aware of its probabilistic causation, *independent* of time post-transplant. It is also important to note that, although poorly described, TCMR and AMR can coexist at the same time in the lung allograft (mixed rejection).[26] This is better described in kidney transplants, where mixed TCMR-AMR was found more frequently than commonly assumed, and was shown to be associated with poorer outcomes and higher rates of graft loss compared with pure TCMR.[28,29] Notably, a major shortcoming at the moment is the lack of a Banff Lung Report on TCMR.

T-Cell-Mediated Rejection and Its Effect on Lung Allograft Function

By separately describing the underlying process (TCMR, AMR, or mixed rejection) and the impact on allograft function, the histopathological processes and clinical presentation may perhaps be better distinguished (**Table 2**). As such, we can describe the impact of TCMR on lung allograft function as follows:

- *Subclinical* TCMR in which there is no deterioration of allograft function and the diagnosis was made on surveillance biopsies.
- TCMR with *acute* deterioration of allograft function.
- TCMR with *chronic* deterioration of allograft function (eg, persistent or recurrent TCMR despite treatment).
- TCMR with *acute on chronic* deterioration of allograft function (eg, detection of TCMR on indication biopsy in a patient with established CLAD).

Analogous to current terminology describing the syndromes of AMR or CLAD, which incorporates both histologic, functional, and/or radiologic features, once could speak of 'minimal clinical TCMR' in case of A1 TCMR with clinical symptoms, chest imaging abnormalities, and/or pulmonary function decline, for example, or of 'severe subclinical TCMR' in case of A2 TCMR in a stable patient without clinical symptoms, chest imaging

Table 2
Impact of acute rejection on lung allograft function

Mechanisms of Rejection	Time After Transplant	Impact on Lung Allograft Function
TCMR AMR Mixed rejection	Early (≤1 y post-transplant) Late onset (>1 y post-transplant)	No deterioration of lung allograft function (subclinical) Acute deterioration of lung allograft function Chronic deterioration of lung allograft function Acute on chronic deterioration of lung allograft function

Abbreviations: AMR, antibody-mediated rejection; TCMR, T-cell mediated rejection.

abnormalities, and/or pulmonary function (eg, with A2 detected on surveillance biopsy).

ACR in CLAD Progression and/or CLAD Phenotype Transition.

Little is known about the incidence of TCMR and AMR in patients with established CLAD and their role in CLAD progression. The incidence of TCMR decreases beyond the first-year post-transplant, and the likelihood during CLAD is possibly low, although data are scarce. AMR episodes have been described in CLAD patients and this again raises the question of whether an AMR episode can accelerate the process of CLAD.[26,30] Similarly, in some patients who transitioned from one CLAD phenotype to another (mostly BOS to RAS), an episode of AMR occurred, possibly triggering this transition via a mixed CLAD phenotype.[30] Consequently, it is very plausible that subclinical TCMR and/or AMR processes, which are difficult to detect by imaging, spirometry, or TBB, are an important driving factor for the onset and progression of CLAD.

CHRONIC LUNG ALLOGRAFT DYSFUNCTION

CLAD is the major long-term complication after lung transplantation, characterized by progressive deterioration of pulmonary function.[5] Our understanding of the pathophysiology of CLAD has evolved over time with changing definitions of CLAD.

Definition

CLAD is a *syndromic* term that refers to persistent lung dysfunction after transplantation not explained by other conditions. As such, it is a *diagnosis by exclusion* as there are several possible causes of the chronic decline of allograft function.[31] These can be either allograft-related (eg, infection, TCMR, AMR, anastomotic strictures, and disease recurrence) or non-allograft-related

(eg, pleural disorders, diaphragmatic dysfunction, obesity, ascites, and chronic kidney failure), or a combination of both. These factors are not included in the current CLAD definition. CLAD is defined as (**Figs. 1** and **2**):[6]

- *Absolute* FEV1 decline (L) ≥ 20% from baseline
  - Baseline = average of the two best post-transplant values for FEV1 obtained ≥ 3 weeks apart
- In function of the *duration* of FEV1 decline with
  - '*Possible* CLAD': FEV1 decline for less than 3 weeks
  - '*Probable* CLAD': FEV1 decline for ≥ 3 weeks
  - '*Definite* CLAD': FEV1 decline for ≥ 3 months
- In function of the *severity* of FEV1 decline, with stages 1 to 4
- '*Potential* CLAD' is defined as FEV1 decline ≥ 10% from baseline

Potential CLAD should always trigger an in-depth investigation of possible causes for the observed pulmonary function decline that could respond to therapy (ie, infection, TCMR, and AMR), including full pulmonary function test (PFT) (with measurement of total lung capacity [TLC] and residual volume, in addition to spirometry), chest imaging, preferably by high-resolution computed tomography (HRCT) with inspiratory and expiratory phase imaging, blood sampling (anti-HLA-antibodies, infection parameters), bronchoscopy with bronchoalveolar lavage for total and differential cell count and TBB. If a specific cause is found, it should be treated appropriately. If patients are not already on macrolide therapy, a prolonged course (at least 8 weeks) of macrolide therapy (usually azithromycin) should be completed (see **Fig. 1**), which may cause some patients to respond with a substantial FEV1 increase so-called azithromycin responsive allograft dysfunction.

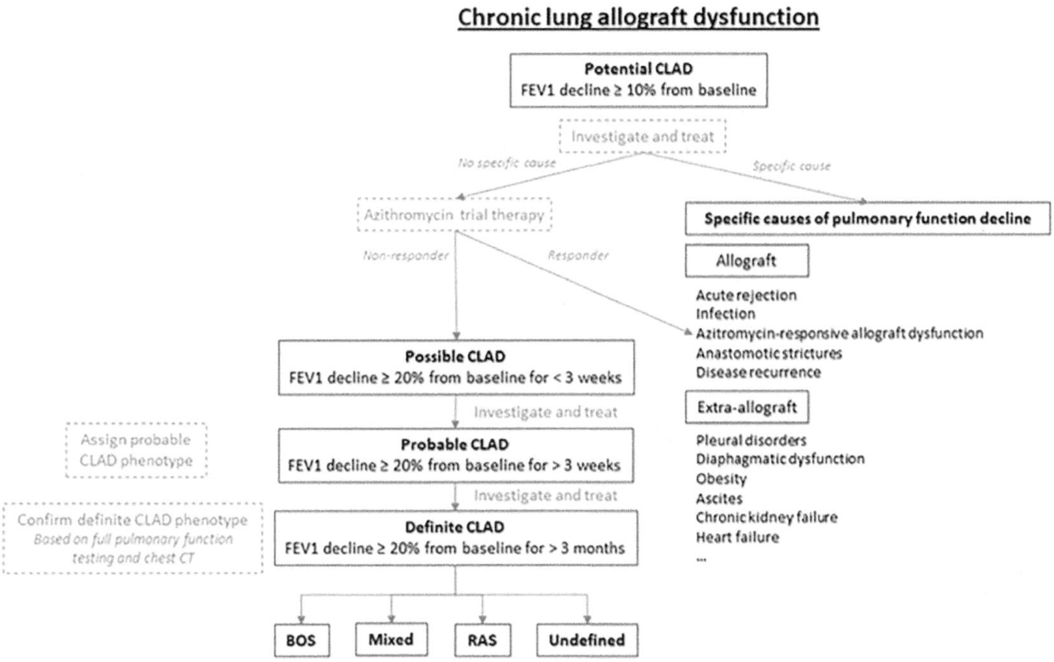

Chronic lung allograft dysfunction

Fig. 1. CLAD flowchart.

Chronic Lung Allograft Dysfunction Phenotypes

The most common manifestation of CLAD is BOS, characterized by often progressive obstructive airflow limitation, defined as a FEV1 decline of $\geq$ 20% with an obstructive PFT pattern, and without persistent radiologic opacities or TLC decline. RAS is a less frequent manifestation of CLAD and is defined as a FEV1 decline of $\geq$ 20% accompanied by a restrictive PFT pattern (TLC decline of $\geq$ 10% compared with baseline) and persistent opacities on chest radiograph or computed tomography (CT). In a mixed phenotype, an obstructive-restrictive PFT and persistent opacities are present. Importantly, CLAD subtypes are not permanent and may change over time because of various reasons described below.

Radiological Findings

Chest CT is not a sensitive diagnostic tool for BOS; however, it should always be performed to assess the presence of opacities, which would exclude the patient from the BOS phenotype or may suggest infection, TCMR, or AMR. Typical CT features of BOS include air trapping and mosaicism as a consequence of small airway disease and hypoxic vasoconstriction, bronchial wall thickening, and bronchiectasis (see **Fig. 2**).[32,33] To adequately assess air trapping, CT scans should be performed both at full inspiration and at end-tidal expiration.

Pleuroparenchymal abnormalities on CT are a key diagnostic feature of RAS and can refer to ground glass opacities, parenchymal consolidations, septal and pleural thickening, and architectural distortion (**Fig. 3**).[32,33] In the early stages of RAS, ground glass opacities seem to be the most prominent feature on CT whereas consolidations are more observed in later stages.[5]

Risk Factors

Several risk factors for the development of CLAD have been identified (see **Fig. 2**). However, earlier studies did not recognize RAS as a separate phenotype and pooled different phenotypes of CLAD together making it difficult to distinguish individual risk factors for each phenotype. Moreover, several risk factors seem to be similar for BOS and RAS (see **Fig. 2**).[34–48]

New Insights

Pathogenesis of chronic lung allograft dysfunction—"multiple hits" theory

The exact pathophysiology of CLAD remains unclear but is likely multifactorial. The similarity in risk factors could indicate that the underlying molecular mechanisms of the two main clinical phenotypes (BOS and RAS) also bear similarities. The driving factor of CLAD is (innate and adaptive) immune activation, provoked by alloimmune triggers (because of non-self-recognition by the recipient's immune system of donor HLA and non-HLA

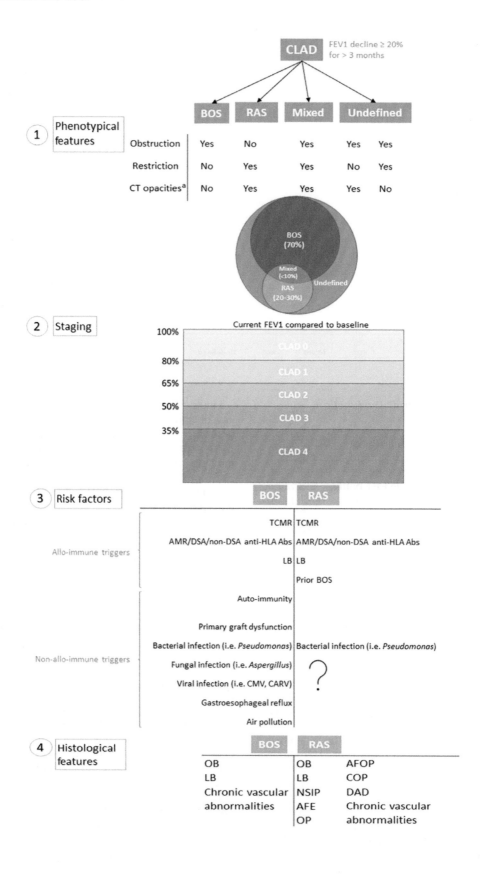

antigens) and non-alloimmune triggers (ie, sterile inflammation in ischemia-reperfusion injury, infection, gastroesophageal reflux, and air pollutants). In this way, CLAD is an inevitable consequence of lung transplantation. Pending on the efficacy of the used immunosuppressive regimen to adequately suppress immune activation, and the number and severity of post-transplant hits, CLAD may develop sooner or later after lung transplantation. As neither ongoing alloimmune recognition nor non-alloimmune stimulation can be fully avoidable, most lung transplant recipients will, therefore, at some point in time, develop structural and/or functional abnormalities of their graft due to the underlying post-transplant immune-driven airway/vascular remodeling, which may be exaggerated by subsequent injuries (hits) to the bronchovascular axis of the secondary pulmonary lobule.

Different injury processes induced by allo- and auto-immune responses and external stimuli can indeed result in inflammation of the bronchovascular axis leading to small airway remodeling and fibrosis resulting in clinical small airway disease, the hallmark of BOS.[49] Histologically, this is represented by different findings, such as LB, OB, and vascular sclerosis.[49,50] The initial bronchovascular inflammation can further augment tissue injury (with exposure of allo- or auto-antigens, vascular damage, and epithelial damage), resulting in a vicious cycle of injury and remodeling. Although in BOS the bronchovascular axis is predominantly affected, other parts of the lung (alveoli, pleura) can be affected to a greater or lesser degree as described below (**Fig. 4**).[50]

In RAS, similar injuries can induce inflammation of the bronchovascular axis, but may also affect other regions of the secondary pulmonary lobule, specifically the alveoli, pleura, interlobular septa, and interstitial space.[49] The resulting remodeling and fibrosis are evidenced by a variety of histologic findings, such as non-specific interstitial pneumonia, alveolar fibroelastosis, diffuse alveolar damage, (acute fibrinous) organizing pneumonia, and vascular sclerosis, resulting in gross parenchymal fibrosis and pleural/septal thickening, typical for the RAS phenotype.[5,51] In addition, small airway inflammation and remodeling with findings of LB and OB can also be seen in RAS.

Although some external stimuli may affect several compartments of the secondary pulmonary lobule (eg, infectious diseases affecting the alveolar spaces), others may be more airway-specific (eg, aspiration and gastroesophageal reflux), thus, resulting in an airway-predominant disease pattern. Some endogenous factors such as TCMR, AMR/anti-HLA antibodies, or auto-antibodies may be directed against the vascular compartment (endothelial cells) of the lung, whereas some auto-antibodies may be directed against antigens present in the airways (epithelial cells) and parenchyma.[49,52]

CLAD should thus be regarded as a common end point due to multifactorial injuries, which helps to explain the different phenotypes with the predominant anatomic localization of the injury determining the dominant phenotype and transition from one CLAD phenotype to another. For example, in a BOS patient, most injuries occur in the airways, and in a mixed or RAS phenotype, several injuries may have occurred spread over the different anatomic compartments. In conclusion, this theory shifts our understanding of CLAD as an umbrella term with distinct entities toward CLAD as a common endpoint of several mechanisms of tissue damage affecting the secondary pulmonary lobule as a whole.

Treatment of Chronic Lung Allograft Dysfunction—Treatable Traits

The concept of 'treatable traits' (TT) has increasingly been used in the management of obstructive pulmonary diseases.[53] Translating this model to lung transplantation, identification of TT (eg, ischemia-reperfusion injury, therapeutic malcompliance, *Pseudomonas aeruginosa* or *Aspergillus* colonization/infection, gastroesophageal reflux, exposure to pollutants, and de novo anti-HLA antibodies) could direct us toward a more personalized and precise management of CLAD. As is depicted in **Fig. 5**, lung injury may occur long before it is detectable by PFT (subclinical injury). Actively searching for TT during post-transplant

Fig. 2. Overview of CLAD phenotyping, staging, risk factors, and histology. [a]CT opacities refer to parenchymal opacities and/or increasing pleural thickening. Ab, antibody; AFE, alveolar fibroelastosis; AFOP, acute fibrinous and organizing pneumonia; AMR, antibody-mediated rejection; BOS, bronchiolitis obliterans syndrome; CARV, community-acquired respiratory viruses; CLAD, chronic lung allograft dysfunction; CMV, cytomegalovirus; CT, computed tomography; DAD, diffuse alveolar damage; DSA, donor-specific antibodies; FEV1, forced expiratory volume in 1 s; HLA, human leukocyte antigen; LB, lymphocytic bronchiolitis; NSIP, non-specific interstitial pneumonia; OB, obliterative bronchiolitis; OP, organizing pneumonia; RAS, restrictive allograft syndrome; TCMR, T-cell-mediated rejection.

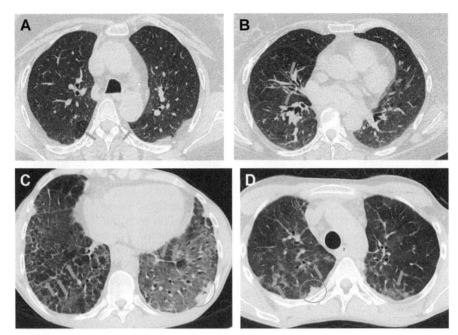

Fig. 3. Chest CT in CLAD. Chest CT of patient with BOS, with air trapping (*left, arrow*) (*A*) and bronchial dilatation (*right, arrow*) (*B*) Chest CT of patient with RAS, with septal thickening (*left, big arrow*), peripheral consolidation (*left, circle*) (*C*), ground glass opacities (*right, big arrow*) and (traction) bronchiectasis (*left, small arrow*) (*D*).

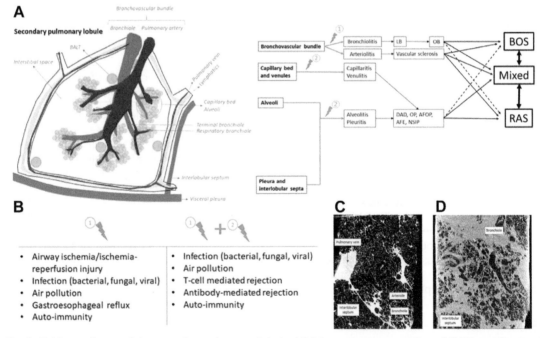

Fig. 4. CLAD as a disease of the secondary pulmonary lobule. (*A*) Schematic representation of CLAD as a disease of the secondary pulmonary lobule. (*B*) Possible distribution of injuries. Micro-CT of lung tissue of an explanted BOS lung (*left*) (*C*) showing perivascular/peribronchiolar fibrosis. Lung tissue of the explanted RAS lung (*right*) (*D*) demonstrating seriously distorted anatomy by fibrosis, showing the thickened interlobular septum, diffuse interstitial fibrosis, and a distorted bronchiole. AFE, alveolar fibroelastosis; AFOP, acute fibrinous and organizing pneumonia; BALT, bronchus associated lymphoid tissue; BOS, bronchiolitis obliterans syndrome; DAD, diffuse alveolar damage; NSIP, non-specific interstitial pneumonia; OP, organizing pneumonia; RAS, restrictive allograft syndrome.

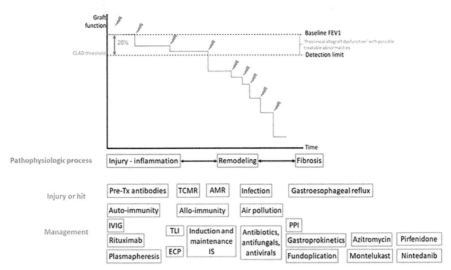

Fig. 5. Multiple injuries and treatable traits in CLAD. AMR, antibody-mediated rejection; ECP, extracorporeal photopheresis; FEV1, forced expiratory volume in one second; IS, immunosuppression; IVIG, intravenous immunoglobulin; PPI, proton pump inhibitor; TCMR, T-cell-mediated rejection; TLI, total lymphoid irradiation; Tx, transplant.

follow-up and specifically targeting TT before and after CLAD onset could mitigate the decline of allograft function after lung transplantation. This is even more important as effective prevention and treatment of CLAD remain a significant unmet medical need. A schematic overview of the current therapeutic approaches is summarized in **Fig. 6**.

Current Controversies and Future Considerations Mixed and Undefined Chronic Lung Allograft Dysfunction

A particular CLAD phenotype diagnosed in a patient may change over time as some patients initially display a typical FEV1 decline compatible with BOS but may subsequently develop CT

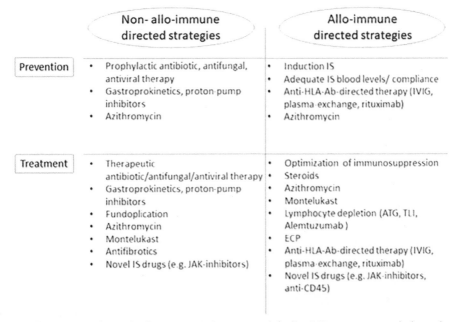

Fig. 6. Approach to CLAD. Ab, antibody; ATG, anti-thymocyte globulin; ECP, extracorporeal photopheresis; HLA, human leukocyte antigen; IS, immunosuppressive/immunosuppression; IVIG, intravenous immunoglobulins; JAK, janus kinase; RTx, rituximab; TLI, total lymphoid irradiation.

opacities and a restrictive PFT pattern compatible with RAS progressing through a mixed phenotype. The undefined phenotype indicates patients who do not fit the current definitions of BOS, RAS, or mixed phenotypes.[6]

Thinking about CLAD as a disease of the secondary pulmonary lobule (see **Fig. 4**) might help explain the undefined and mixed phenotype. If the location of the injury determines the phenotype, the development of parenchymal infiltrates in the BOS phenotype might be the result of injuries to the alveoli, pleura, and/or interlobular septa that are not (yet) detected by PFT, resulting in a patient with obstruction, CT opacities but no restriction. Following this hypothesis, some patients with the classic BOS phenotype might have subclinical injuries to the alveoli, pleura, and/or interlobular septa that are yet to be detected by CT and PFT. Indeed, the presence of parenchymal and interstitial fibrotic changes on histopathology has recently been described in up to 54% of end-stage BOS patients suggesting that BOS and RAS might represent different ends of the same disease continuum (**Fig. 7**).[50]

Preclinical Chronic Lung Allograft Dysfunction

As per the current ISHLT consensus, a patient is only diagnosed with CLAD if FEV1 declines $\geq$ 20% from baseline. However, as previously mentioned, allograft injury (especially of the small airways) may occur long before it is detectable by FEV1 (which is not a sensitive measure for small airways dysfunction) and we will give some examples of such patients with 'preclinical CLAD'.

Example 1: Small airway disease with 80%< FEV1 $\leq$100% of baseline.

Patients might display (often heterogenous, multi-lobar) air trapping on expiratory chest CT and a significant decline in forced expiratory flow at 25% to 75% of forced vital capacity (FEF$_{25-75}$) but without a significant FEV1 or forced vital capacity (FVC) decline. FEF$_{25-75}$, a sensitive marker

of airflow in small airways, may decline before subsequent CLAD onset in these patients (**Fig. 8**, patient A–B), indicating preclinical BOS, which may evolve to true BOS (per current ISHLT-definition) with longer follow-up in case of ongoing airway remodeling.

Example 2: Persistent CT changes with 80%< FEV1 $\leq$ 100% of baseline and 90%< TLC $\leq$100% of baseline.

Patients may demonstrate clear, chronic interstitial changes on subsequent CTs (ie, reticulations and subpleural parenchymal opacities) without significant FEV1 or TLC decline, thus, not qualifying for RAS as per the current definition (see **Fig. 8**, patient C–D). There are no clear guidelines on the management of this subgroup of patients with documented structural abnormalities of the lung allograft, yet they may evolve to true RAS with longer follow-up in case of ongoing remodeling of the alveoli/pleura/interstitial space.

Incorporating FEF$_{25-75}$ and routine CT imaging during follow-up to the current guidelines could, therefore, help to better detect allograft dysfunction at an earlier stage, allowing for timely intervention in the hope of stabilizing preclinical CLAD progression before patients further deteriorate and develop more advanced, irreversible structural lung disease presenting as CLAD.

Need for Redefining Chronic Lung Allograft Dysfunction by Incorporating Other Pulmonary Function Test Parameters?

The need for a more sensitive marker to detect BOS has long been clear as FEV1 is insufficiently sensitive to detect (early) small airway disease. FEF$_{25-75}$, on the other hand, measures airflow in the small airways, where primary airflow obstruction originates in BOS and is increasingly used in other obstructive pulmonary diseases.[54] Multiple lung transplant groups demonstrated that FEF$_{25-75}$ declines before FEV1 drops. Of note, FEF$_{25-75}$ was indeed also included in previous BOS

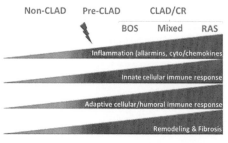

Fig. 7. CLAD: from separate phenotypes to a disease continuum of the allograft. Schematic representation of the different pathophysiologic mechanisms involved in CLAD. AMR, antibody-mediated rejection; BOS, bronchiolitis obliterans syndrome; CARV, community-acquired respiratory virus; CLAD, chronic lung allograft dysfunction; CR, chronic rejection; CMV, cytomegalovirus; PM10, particulate matter of 10 microns in diameter or smaller; RAS, restrictive allograft syndrome; TCMR, T-cell mediated rejection.

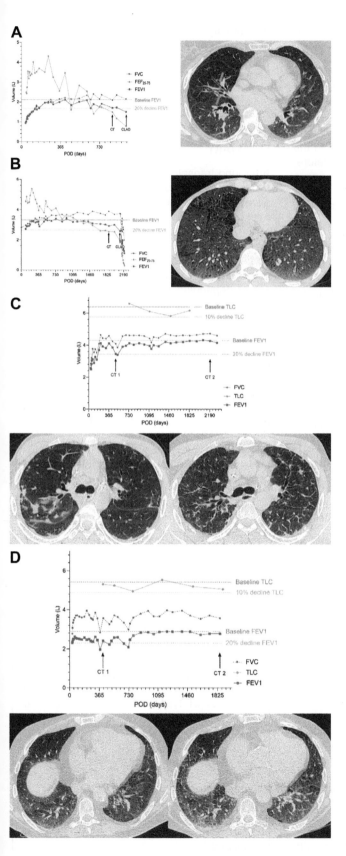

Fig. 8. Case studies of subclinical CLAD. (*A*) This patient underwent a bilateral lung transplantation for emphysema in 2007. Her FEF$_{25-75}$ declined gradually from a baseline of 4.16 to 2.83 L (32% from baseline) on POD 540, 1.77 L (57% from baseline) on POD 730 and 1.17 L (72% from baseline) on POD 892. Expiratory chest CT on POD 852 (*arrow*) showed signs of air trapping. Diagnosis of CLAD phenotype BOS was not made until POD 982 (*arrow*), when FEV1 declined from a baseline of 2.11 to 1.5 L. (*B*) This patient underwent a bilateral lung transplantation for bronchiectasis in 2015. His FEF$_{25-75}$ declined gradually from a baseline of 5.25 to 3.95 L (25% from baseline) on POD 641, 3.28 L (37% from baseline) on POD 1193 and 2.6 L (50% from baseline) on POD 1684. Expiratory chest CT on POD 1866 (*narrow arrow*) showed signs of air trapping. CLAD BOS phenotype did not occur until POD 2111 (*arrow*), when FEV1 declined from a baseline of 2.11 to 1.5 L after refractory AMR. (*C*) This patient underwent a bilateral lung transplantation for cystic fibrosis in 2015. His FEV1 and TLC remained stable through follow-up, but the patient developed ground glass opacities and consolidations without air trapping on expiratory chest CT on POD 494 (upper CT). Abnormalities persisted and aggravated through follow-up regardless of exclusion and treatment of other causes, evolving to thickened interlobular septa, opacities and bronchiectasis without air trapping on expiratory chest CT on POD 2195 (lower CT). (*D*) This patient underwent a bilateral lung transplantation for emphysema in 2016. His FEV1 and TLC remained stable through follow-up, but the patient developed ground glass opacities on expiratory chest CT POD 409 (upper CT), worsening throughout follow-up (lower CT POD 1890).

guidelines: BOS stage 0p was defined as a persistent decrease in FEV1 of 10% to 19% and/or FEF_{25-75} of $\geq 25\%$ compared with baseline.[55] As a poor specificity of FEF_{25-75} decline for CLAD was reported, FEF_{25-75} was no longer included in the current ISHLT consensus for CLAD.[6] Likely, this poor specificity for CLAD is in part because of the inclusion of non-obstructive phenotype (RAS) and single-lung transplant recipients in the former studies regarding FEF_{25-75}. Therefore, better-designed studies regarding FEF_{25-75} as a tool for the detection of obstructive CLAD phenotypes (BOS, mixed, undefined) are needed stratified by transplant modality.

Another parameter to assess the function of the secondary pulmonary lobule is diffusion capacity for carbon monoxide (DLCO), which measures the alveolar and vascular compartment of the lung allograft. DLCO has been reported as an important prognostic factor in outcomes after lung transplantation.[56] Also, it was demonstrated that DLCO may be a more sensitive tool compared with FEV1 and lung volumes in interstitial lung disease suggesting it could also be useful in the early detection of RAS.[57] However, further studies are needed to evaluate its utility for early RAS diagnosis. DLCO is a marker for the vascular compartment and recent in-dept histopathologic research of end-stage BOS lungs has revealed chronic vascular abnormalities in up to 42% of patients; therefore, DLCO might also be useful to detect early BOS or for follow-up of vascular changes in established BOS.[50,58]

Next to DLCO, lung clearance index (LCI), derived from multiple breath washout testing, is a global measure of ventilation heterogeneity which has previously been shown to be a more sensitive measure of obstructive small airway diseases than spirometry.[59] In double-lung transplant recipients, LCI was shown to increase with increasing BOS severity.[60,61] Of note, a significant proportion of adult and pediatric lung transplant recipients demonstrated to have an abnormal LCI with preserved FEV1, suggesting early subclinical small airway dysfunction. LCI, however, is less useful after single lung transplantation as the native lung may significantly affect pulmonary gas clearance.

Finally, impulse oscillometry could be another technique to detect small airway dysfunction in double-lung transplant recipients.[62] Indeed, oscillometry may detect physiologic changes associated with ACR that were not discernible by spirometry and may detect BOS earlier than by conventional spirometry.[63,64] Again, the test is less useful after single lung transplantation, but the lack of a need for deep inspiration with oscillometry facilitates its use in children and the acute postoperative lung transplant period.

Importantly, many of the above-described issues are equally relevant for bone marrow transplant recipients suffering from BOS, which bears many similarities to post-lung transplant BOS, as summarized elsewhere.[65]

SUMMARY

After lung transplantation, almost all patients will suffer from a pathophysiological decline of their allograft because of multifactorial injuries on a background of an alloimmune-mediated remodeling process affecting the secondary pulmonary lobule. Such is the nature of organ transplantation. Allograft dysfunction probably occurs in all lung transplant recipients to a greater or lesser extent depending on the number and severity of injuries and the efficacy of how these can be prevented/treated by appropriate immunosuppressive and prophylactic management. Development of improved therapeutic (mainly preventive) options as well as more sensitive PFT or biomarkers to detect lung allograft dysfunction is paramount as a decline in FEV1 and FVC are late signals of lung allograft damage and often irreversible. HRCT follow-up may detect structural allograft remodeling even before this results in significant dysfunction. Yet it is currently unclear how this should be best managed.

CLINICS CARE POINTS

- Adequate surrogate biomarkers would be useful to identify patients at risk for TCMR, to support TCMR grading, and to distinguish patients with minimal TCMR who are at higher risk. Therefore, studies on donor-derived cell-free DNA, gene expression profile analysis, and/or intrapulmonary microbiome signatures are eagerly awaited as these could perhaps better determine the presence of TCMR, ABMR, and infection in the lung graft.

- Renaming ACR to TCMR, AMR or mixed rejection with a separate description of the impact on allograft function might better reflect the causative process and its repercussion on allograft function.

- Further research on the incidence and impact of (subclinical) TCMR and AMR on CLAD onset and during CLAD progression is needed.

- FEF_{25-75} and DLCO are useful PFT markers for early CLAD and would be informative if incorporated into routine follow-up. Also, LCI and oscillometry may provide additional information on small airway dysfunction after lung transplantation.
- Routine HRCT with inspiratory and expiratory images should be a part of follow-up after lung transplantation.
- Targeting TT after lung transplantation can help to delay/mitigate CLAD onset and progression.

FUNDING

- H. Beeckmans is supported by a pre-doctoral research grant from KU Leuven.
- S. Bos is supported by the Paul Corris International Clinical Research Training Scholarship.
- R. Vos is a Senior Clinical Research Fellow of the Research Foundation—Flanders (FWO) and is supported by a Research Grant from the FWO (G060322N).

DISCLOSURE

None of the authors of this article have any conflicts of interest to disclose concerning this article. The authors confirm that the work described has not been published previously, that it is not under consideration for publication elsewhere, that its publication is approved by all authors and tacitly or explicitly by the responsible authorities where the work was carried out, and that, if accepted, it will not be published elsewhere in the same form in English or any other language, without the written consent of the copyright holder.

The data that support the findings of this study are available on request from the corresponding author. The data are not publicly available because of privacy or ethical restrictions. All authors contributed importantly to the study design, data collection, and analysis, or writing of the article according to the guidelines of the International Committee of Medical Journal Editors. All authors have read and approved the article. All authors take responsibility for the article, and the submitting author has permission from all authors to submit the article on their behalf.

REFERENCES

1. Yusen RD, Edwards LB, Kucheryavaya AY, et al. The Registry of the international Society for heart and lung transplantation: Thirty-second Official adult lung and heart-lung transplantation report–2015; Focus theme: early graft failure. J Heart Lung Transpl 2015;34(10):1264–77. https://doi.org/10.1016/j.healun.2015.08.014.
2. Chambers DC, Cherikh WS, Harhay MO, et al. The international Thoracic organ transplant Registry of the international Society for heart and lung transplantation: Thirty-sixth adult lung and heart-lung transplantation report-2019; Focus theme: donor and recipient size match. J Heart Lung Transpl 2019;38(10):1042–55. https://doi.org/10.1016/j.healun.2019.08.001.
3. Martinu T, Chen DF, Palmer SM. Acute rejection and humoral sensitization in lung transplant recipients. Proc Am Thorac Soc 2009;6(1):54–65. https://doi.org/10.1513/pats.200808-080GO.
4. Werlein C, Seidel A, Warnecke G, et al. Lung transplant pathology: an overview on current entities and procedures. Surg Pathol Clin 2020;13(1):119–40. https://doi.org/10.1016/j.path.2019.11.003.
5. Glanville AR, Verleden GM, Todd JL, et al. Chronic lung allograft dysfunction: definition and update of restrictive allograft syndrome-A consensus report from the Pulmonary Council of the ISHLT. J Heart Lung Transpl 2019;38(5):483–92. https://doi.org/10.1016/j.healun.2019.03.008.
6. Verleden GM, Glanville AR, Lease ED, et al. Chronic lung allograft dysfunction: definition, diagnostic criteria and approaches to treatment. A consensus report from the pulmonary Council of the ISHLT. ISHLT 2019;38(5):493–503.
7. Roden AC, Aisner DL, Allen TC, et al. Diagnosis of acute cellular rejection and antibody-mediated rejection on lung transplant biopsies: a perspective from Members of the pulmonary pathology Society. Arch Pathol Lab Med 2017;141(3):437–44. https://doi.org/10.5858/arpa.2016-0459-SA.
8. Bergantini L, d'Alessandro M, De Vita E, et al. Regulatory and effector cell Disequilibrium in patients with acute cellular rejection and chronic lung allograft dysfunction after lung transplantation: comparison of Peripheral and alveolar distribution. Cells 2021;10(4):780. https://doi.org/10.3390/cells10040780.
9. Levy L, Huszti E, Tikkanen J, et al. The impact of first untreated subclinical minimal acute rejection on risk for chronic lung allograft dysfunction or death after lung transplantation. Am J Transpl 2020;20(1):241–9. https://doi.org/10.1111/ajt.15561.
10. Hachem RR, Khalifah AP, Chakinala MM, et al. The significance of a single episode of minimal acute rejection after lung transplantation. Transplantation 2005;80(10):1406–13.
11. Yousem SA. Significance of clinically silent untreated mild acute cellular rejection in lung allograft recipients. Hum Pathol 1996;27(3):269–73. https://doi.org/10.1016/S0046-8177(96)90068-4.
12. Kim DW, Dacic S, Iacono A, et al. Significance of a solitary perivascular mononuclear infiltrate in lung

allograft recipients with mild acute cellular rejection. J Heart Lung Transpl 2005;24(2):152–5. https://doi.org/10.1016/j.healun.2003.10.024.

13. Glanville AR, Aboyoun CL, Havryk A, et al. Severity of lymphocytic bronchiolitis predicts long-term outcome after lung transplantation. Am J Respir Crit Care Med 2008;177(9):1033–40. https://doi.org/10.1164/rccm.200706-951OC.

14. Stewart S, Fishbein MC, Snell GI, et al. Revision of the 1996 working formulation for the standardization of nomenclature in the diagnosis of lung rejection. J Heart Lung Transpl 2007;26(12):1229–42. https://doi.org/10.1016/j.healun.2007.10.017.

15. Greer M, Werlein C, Jonigk D. Surveillance for acute cellular rejection after lung transplantation. Ann Transl Med 2020;8(6):410. https://doi.org/10.21037/atm.2020.02.127.

16. Hasegawa T, Iacono AT, Yousem SA. The anatomic distribution of acute cellular rejection in the allograft lung. Ann Thorac Surg 2000;69(5):1529–31. https://doi.org/10.1016/s0003-4975(00)01226-1.

17. Jaksch P, Scheed A, Geleff S, et al. Transbronchial lung biopsy after lung transplantation: different A and B scores in different lobes. Eur Respir J 2011;38(Suppl 55). Available at: https://erj.ersjournals.com/content/38/Suppl_55/p3075. Accessed February 24, 2022.

18. Arcasoy SM, Berry G, Marboe CC, et al. Pathologic interpretation of transbronchial biopsy for acute rejection of lung allograft is highly variable. Am J Transpl 2011;11(2):320–8. https://doi.org/10.1111/j.1600-6143.2010.03382.x.

19. Chakinala MM, Ritter J, Gage BF, et al. Reliability for grading acute rejection and airway inflammation after lung transplantation. J Heart Lung Transpl 2005;24(6):652–7. https://doi.org/10.1016/j.healun.2004.04.002.

20. Stephenson A, Flint J, English J, et al. Interpretation of transbronchial lung biopsies from lung transplant recipients: inter- and intraobserver agreement. Can Respir J 2005;12(2):75–7. https://doi.org/10.1155/2005/483172.

21. Burton CM, Iversen M, Scheike T, et al. Minimal acute cellular rejection remains prevalent up to 2 years after lung transplantation: a retrospective analysis of 2697 transbronchial biopsies. Transplantation 2008;85(4):547–53. https://doi.org/10.1097/TP.0b013e3181641df9.

22. Chakinala MM, Ritter J, Gage BF, et al. Yield of surveillance bronchoscopy for acute rejection and lymphocytic bronchitis/bronchiolitis after lung transplantation. J Heart Lung Transpl 2004;23(12):1396–404. https://doi.org/10.1016/j.healun.2003.09.018.

23. Hopkins PM, Aboyoun CL, Chhajed PN, et al. Association of minimal rejection in lung transplant recipients with obliterative bronchiolitis. Am J Respir Crit Care Med 2004;170(9):1022–6. https://doi.org/10.1164/rccm.200302-165OC.

24. Khalifah AP, Hachem RR, Chakinala MM, et al. Minimal acute rejection after lung transplantation: a risk for bronchiolitis obliterans syndrome. Am J Transpl 2005;5(8):2022–30. https://doi.org/10.1111/j.1600-6143.2005.00953.x.

25. Burton CM, Iversen M, Scheike T, et al. Is lymphocytic bronchiolitis a marker of acute rejection? An analysis of 2,697 transbronchial biopsies after lung transplantation. J Heart Lung Transpl 2008;27(10):1128–34. https://doi.org/10.1016/j.healun.2008.06.014.

26. Levine DJ, Glanville AR, Aboyoun C, et al. Antibody-mediated rejection of the lung: a consensus report of the international Society for heart and lung transplantation. J Heart Lung Transpl 2016;35(4):397–406. https://doi.org/10.1016/j.healun.2016.01.1223.

27. Loupy A, Haas M, Roufosse C, et al. The Banff 2019 Kidney Meeting Report (I): Updates on and clarification of criteria for T cell- and antibody-mediated rejection. Am J Transpl 2020;20(9):2318–31. https://doi.org/10.1111/ajt.15898.

28. Matignon M, Muthukumar T, Seshan SV, et al. Concurrent acute cellular rejection is an independent risk factor for renal allograft failure in patients with C4d-positive antibody-mediated rejection. Transplantation 2012;94(6):603–11. https://doi.org/10.1097/TP.0b013e31825def05.

29. Willicombe M, Roufosse C, Brookes P, et al. Acute cellular rejection: impact of donor-specific antibodies and C4d. Transplantation 2014;97(4):433–9. https://doi.org/10.1097/01.TP.0000437431.97108.8f.

30. Verleden SE, Von Der Thüsen J, Van Herck A, et al. Identification and characterization of chronic lung allograft dysfunction patients with mixed phenotype: a single-center study. Clin Transpl 2020;34(2):e13781. https://doi.org/10.1111/ctr.13781.

31. Verleden GM, Raghu G, Meyer KC, et al. A new classification system for chronic lung allograft dysfunction. J Heart Lung Transpl 2014;33(2):127–33. https://doi.org/10.1016/j.healun.2013.10.022.

32. Byrne D, Nador RG, English JC, et al. Chronic lung allograft dysfunction: review of CT and pathologic findings. Radiol Cardiothorac Imaging 2021;3(1):e200314. https://doi.org/10.1148/ryct.2021200314.

33. Brun AL, Chabi ML, Picard C, et al. Lung transplantation: CT assessment of chronic lung allograft dysfunction (CLAD). Diagnostics (Basel) 2021;11(5):817. https://doi.org/10.3390/diagnostics11050817.

34. Verleden SE, Ruttens D, Vandermeulen E, et al. Bronchiolitis obliterans syndrome and restrictive allograft syndrome: do risk factors differ? Transplantation 2013;95(9):1167–72. https://doi.org/10.1097/TP.0b013e318286e076.

35. Davis WA, Finlen Copeland CA, Todd JL, et al. Spirometrically significant acute rejection increases the risk for BOS and death after lung transplantation. Am J Transpl 2012;12(3):745–52. https://doi.org/10.1111/j.1600-6143.2011.03849.x.

36. Snyder LD, Wang Z, Chen DF, et al. Implications for human leukocyte antigen antibodies after lung transplantation: a 10-year experience in 441 patients. Chest 2013;144(1):226–33. https://doi.org/10.1378/chest.12-0587.

37. Verleden SE, Vanaudenaerde BM, Emonds MP, et al. Donor-specific and -nonspecific HLA antibodies and outcome post lung transplantation. Eur Respir J 2017;50(5). https://doi.org/10.1183/13993003.01248-2017.

38. Muynck BD, Herck AV, Sacreas A, et al. Successful Pseudomonas aeruginosa eradication improves outcomes after lung transplantation: a retrospective cohort analysis. Eur Respir J 2020. https://doi.org/10.1183/13993003.01720-2020.

39. Weigt SS, Copeland CAF, Derhovanessian A, et al. Colonization with small Conidia Aspergillus Species is associated with bronchiolitis obliterans syndrome: a two-center validation study. Am J Transplant 2013; 13(4):919–27. https://doi.org/10.1111/ajt.12131.

40. Moore CA, Pilewski JM, Venkataramanan R, et al. Effect of aerosolized antipseudomonals on Pseudomonas positivity and bronchiolitis obliterans syndrome after lung transplantation. Transpl Infect Dis 2017;19(3). https://doi.org/10.1111/tid.12688.

41. Le Pavec J, Pradère P, Gigandon A, et al. Risk of lung allograft dysfunction associated with Aspergillus infection. Transpl Direct 2021;7(3):e675. https://doi.org/10.1097/TXD.0000000000001128.

42. Allyn PR, Duffy EL, Humphries RM, et al. Graft loss and CLAD-onset is Hastened by viral pneumonia after lung transplantation. Transplantation 2016; 100(11):2424–31. https://doi.org/10.1097/TP.0000000000001346.

43. Hartwig MG, Anderson DJ, Onaitis MW, et al. Fundoplication after lung transplantation prevents the allograft dysfunction associated with reflux. Ann Thorac Surg 2011;92(2):462–8. https://doi.org/10.1016/j.athoracsur.2011.04.035. discussion; 468-469.

44. Ruttens D, Verleden SE, Bijnens EM, et al. An association of particulate air pollution and traffic exposure with mortality after lung transplantation in Europe. Eur Respir J 2017;49(1):1600484. https://doi.org/10.1183/13993003.00484-2016.

45. Huang HJ, Yusen RD, Meyers BF, et al. Late primary graft dysfunction after lung transplantation and bronchiolitis obliterans syndrome. Am J Transpl 2008;8(11):2454–62. https://doi.org/10.1111/j.1600-6143.2008.02389.x.

46. Sarma NJ, Tiriveedhi V, Angaswamy N, et al. Role of antibodies to self-antigens in chronic allograft rejection: potential mechanism and therapeutic implications. Hum Immunol 2012;73(12):1275–81. https://doi.org/10.1016/j.humimm.2012.06.014.

47. Koutsokera A, Royer PJ, Antonietti JP, et al. Development of a Multivariate Prediction model for early-onset bronchiolitis obliterans syndrome and

48. Paraskeva M, Bailey M, Levvey BJ, et al. Cytomegalovirus Replication within the lung allograft is associated with bronchiolitis obliterans syndrome. Am J Transplant 2011;11(10):2190–6. https://doi.org/10.1111/j.1600-6143.2011.03663.x.

49. Sato M. Bronchiolitis obliterans syndrome and restrictive allograft syndrome after lung transplantation: why are there two distinct forms of chronic lung allograft dysfunction? Ann Transl Med 2020;8(6):418. https://doi.org/10.21037/atm.2020.02.159.

50. Vanstapel A, Verleden SE, Verbeken EK, et al. Beyond bronchiolitis obliterans: in-depth histopathologic characterization of bronchiolitis obliterans syndrome after lung transplantation. J Clin Med 2021; 11(1):111. https://doi.org/10.3390/jcm11010111.

51. Verleden SE, Von der Thüsen J, Roux A, et al. When tissue is the issue: a histological review of chronic lung allograft dysfunction. Am J Transpl 2020; 20(10):2644–51. https://doi.org/10.1111/ajt.15864.

52. Meyer KC, Raghu G, Verleden GM, et al. An international ISHLT/ATS/ERS clinical practice guideline: diagnosis and management of bronchiolitis obliterans syndrome. Eur Respir J 2014;44(6):1479–503. https://doi.org/10.1183/09031936.00107514.

53. Agusti A, Barnes N, Cruz AA, et al. Moving towards a Treatable Traits model of care for the management of obstructive airways diseases. Respir Med 2021; 187:106572. https://doi.org/10.1016/j.rmed.2021.106572.

54. Qin R, An J, Xie J, et al. FEF25-75% is a more sensitive measure reflecting airway dysfunction in patients with Asthma: a comparison study using FEF25-75% and FEV1. J Allergy Clin Immunol Pract 2021;9(10):3649–59. https://doi.org/10.1016/j.jaip.2021.06.027. e6.

55. Estenne M, Maurer JR, Boehler A, et al. Bronchiolitis obliterans syndrome 2001: an update of the diagnostic criteria. J Heart Lung Transplant 2002;21(3):297–310. https://doi.org/10.1016/S1053-2498(02)00398-4.

56. Darley DR, Ma J, Huszti E, et al. Diffusing capacity for carbon monoxide (DLCO): association with long-term outcomes after lung transplantation in a 20-year longitudinal study. Eur Respir J 2021;25:2003639. https://doi.org/10.1183/13993003.03639-2020.

57. Hildebrandt J, Rahn A, Kessler A, et al. Lung clearance index and diffusion capacity for CO to detect early functional pulmonary impairment in children with rheumatic diseases. Pediatr Rheumatol Online J 2021;19(1):23. https://doi.org/10.1186/s12969-021-00509-1.

58. Winkler A, Kahnert K, Behr J, et al. Combined diffusing capacity for nitric oxide and carbon monoxide as predictor of bronchiolitis obliterans syndrome

following lung transplantation. Respir Res 2018;19: 171. https://doi.org/10.1186/s12931-018-0881-1.

59. Stanojevic S, Bowerman C, Robinson P. Multiple breath washout: measuring early manifestations of lung pathology. Breathe 2021;17(3):210016. https://doi.org/10.1183/20734735.0016-2021.

60. Driskel M, Horsley A, Fretwell L, et al. Lung clearance index in detection of post-transplant bronchiolitis obliterans syndrome. ERJ Open Res 2019;5(4):00164–2019. https://doi.org/10.1183/23120541.00164-2019.

61. Nyilas S, Carlens J, Price T, et al. Multiple breath washout in pediatric patients after lung transplantation. Am J Transpl 2018;18(1):145–53. https://doi.org/10.1111/ajt.14432.

62. Kaminsky DA, Simpson SJ, Berger KI, et al. Clinical significance and applications of oscillometry. Eur Respir Rev 2022;31(163):210208. https://doi.org/10.1183/16000617.0208-2021.

63. Cho E, Wu JKY, Birriel DC, et al. Airway oscillometry detects Spirometric-silent episodes of acute cellular rejection. Am J Respir Crit Care Med 2020;201(12):1536–44. https://doi.org/10.1164/rccm.201908-1539OC.

64. Ochman M, Wojarski J, Wiórek A, et al. Usefulness of the impulse oscillometry system in graft function Monitoring in lung transplant recipients. Transpl Proc 2018;50(7):2070–4. https://doi.org/10.1016/j.transproceed.2017.12.060.

65. Bos S, Beeckmans H, Vanstapel A, et al. Pulmonary graft-versus-host disease and chronic lung allograft dysfunction: two sides of the same coin? Lancet Respir Med 2022;10(8):796–810. https://doi.org/10.1016/S2213-2600(22)00001-7.

APPENDIX: GRADING AND ANALYZING ACR: TOWARD A NEW PARADIGM

Analysis
  Fallacy of Ordinal Analysis
    Ordinal analysis of ACR grades makes the untested and ultimately unverifiable assumption that there is an orderly and mathematical progression from grade to grade. In a Cox proportional hazards model, it assumes that an A2 or B2 for that matter carries twice the impact as an A1 or B1. Similarly, an A3 carries three times the impact of an A1.

    This flawed logic underpins many analyses that have been published in reputable journals and has not seriously been challenged (until now). It has direct implications for how we interpret the burden of rejection, and hence, the propensity for critical downstream events such as chronic lung allograft dysfunction, let alone the decision to treat or not to treat a particular grade.

Advantages of categorical determination and analysis
  Conversely, utilizing a categorical analysis of ACR grade has several advantages. First, it cohorts so that a more precise determination of risk and management can be performed. Second, it facilitates a more robust description of the burden of disease, providing always that histopathological assessment is at once informed and experienced but most importantly constant over time. Changes in grading criteria need to be based on hard data, consensus, and have the wide agreement of the global community otherwise they will not be used.

How does this change how we view prior literature?
  Clearly, the prior literature largely uses an ordinal system, in part, for ease of analysis but predominantly out of ignorance of the potential for introducing a flawed analysis. Most would agree an A4 ACR is life and graft-threatening. How many times worse than an A1 is it? The question is rather moot. We do not know, and in truth should not think this way, rather consider the gravitas of an A4 as a stand-alone phenomenon, with severe sequelae, if the patient survives.

Burden of disease and risk
  Sum of Scores
    The value of using a sum of scores is that it allows at best a semi-quantitative assessment of ACR burden over a period, but it is also seriously flawed. It adds apples and oranges so to speak as explained above. Bias is introduced by the duration of time of observation, and importantly, the frequency and adequacy of sampling. In this regard, the performance of transbronchial biopsies requires adequate supervision to ensure the number and quality of biopsies meet the ISHLT criteria as it is a critical investigation that determines major care decisions. That is not to say that teaching is not important, but rather that oversight is part of that process to ensure quality. Quality and the number of pieces weigh on the benefit side to justify the known risks of the procedure. In all programs, some bronchoscopies will yield Ax and/or Bx biopsies for various reasons. If the decision to re-biopsy is indicated, the possible associated risks must be weighed carefully against the putative

benefits to resolve a diagnostic dilemma, and thereby, guide the best possible treatment of a given patient.

Average score

Similarly, computing an average score assumes an evenly time-weighted biopsy schedule and also compares apples with oranges as above, and does not truly allow a between-patient comparison unless a rigid schedule is adhered to, and even then, bias is introduced by the duration of time of observation as well as the frequency and adequacy of sampling, such that any comparisons between units will be subject to criticism.

Consider two hypothetical cases, albeit drawn from real-life experience.

Patient 1: An 18-year-old man with cystic fibrosis who undertakes a long vacation trip with friends on the first anniversary of his bilateral lung transplant. A vast quantity of alcohol is consumed, in celebration, and he misplaces his immunosuppressive medications. After he recovers from the effects of inebriation, he realizes his predicament but, advised by his friends, he delays returning from his journey. When he reports to the transplant unit a week or so later, he is mildly short of breath, has a 20% fall in his FEV1, and subtle diffuse infiltrates on chest radiography. Blood examination reveals significant eosinophilia and relative thrombocytosis but otherwise is unremarkable. Urgent bronchoscopy with transbronchial lung biopsy is performed with respiratory support as his resting SaO2 has fallen to 91%. A comprehensive examination for bacterial, viral, and fungal agents is all negative. Transbronchial biopsy pieces (×12) are taken from the right lower and middle lobes. The pieces are all 2-4 mm in diameter and float in formalin. While awaiting formal results from histopathology, he receives a dose of intravenous methylprednisolone at 15 mg/kg body weight with empiric antibacterial cover. However, he deteriorates further and that evening needs invasive ventilation in the ICU. Pathology returns a result of A4B3 with evidence of early diffuse alveolar damage (DAD) but without clear evidence suggestive of antibody-mediated rejection indicates severe T-cell-mediated rejection. Urgent Luminex screen finds no donor-specific antibodies.

Review of prior biopsies performed at 3 weeks, 6 weeks, 3 months, and 6 months show A0B0 for each. Assuming a low risk of acute cellular rejection, he has been weaned off prednisolone at 9 months and was maintained on tacrolimus (target range 8–10 ng/mL) and azathioprine at 50 mg/day, as he was intolerant of mycophenolate and higher doses of azathioprine caused leukopenia while on cytomegalovirus prophylaxis with valganciclovir. After a 2-week period of ventilation and further methylprednisolone, under viral and fungal prophylaxis, a slow wean is successful and he is liberated from the ICU. Three months later, he has established CLAD Stage 3, remained oxygen dependent, and preparations to evaluate him for retransplantation are underway.

Sum of A scores: 4 (using ordinal analysis)
Average A score: 0.8 (using ordinal analysis)
Worst A score: 4 (categorical analysis)

Patient 2: A 25-year-old woman with cystic fibrosis, now 1 year post-bilateral lung transplant, who needed early post-transplant inpatient management for distal intestinal obstruction syndrome, managed conservatively with close therapeutic drug monitoring. By 1 year, she was asymptomatic from a respiratory perspective, otherwise well, and had normal renal function and normal graft function, CLAD Stage 0. Surveillance transbronchial lung biopsies taken at 3 weeks, 6 weeks, 3 months, 6 months, and 12 months showed A1B1, A1B0, A1B0, A1B0, and A0B0, respectively. In view of the low-level ACR, prednisolone had been maintained at 0.1 mg/kg body weight. The tacrolimus target level was 8 to 10 ng/mL. After 3 months, mycophenolate was reduced to maintenance levels in part because of gastrointestinal symptoms.

Sum of A scores: 4 (using ordinal analysis)
Average A score: 0.8 (using ordinal analysis)
Worst A score: 1 (categorical analysis)

The outcome analysis demonstrates a stark difference between these two patients, emphasizing the importance of considering the implications of analyzing ACR scores as ordinal. When this type of discrepancy is multiplied many times within a large series, a biased conclusion may be drawn. One area in which this may be relevant is in the assessment of whether there is a change in the frequency and/or severity of ACR in different eras, perhaps reflecting changes in immune-suppressive protocols, differing indications, and differing ages plus increasing team experience.

Worst Score

The value of the analysis of categorical variables, in this case, the worst score, is highlighted above. Some studies have taken this approach and by using the worst ACR score as a time-dependent variable, the true risk of downstream events, such as CLAD and death, to name two key outcomes, may be assessed without breaching the dictates of proportional hazards modeling. Unfortunately, many reputable studies have not utilized such robust methodologies for which reason further analysis is appropriate and future studies should aim, a priori , to incorporate this strategy. Evidence to support the clear division of outcomes based on categorical analysis both of A and B grades has been demonstrated in prior studies.[1–4]

Duration of ACR

There are several seemingly unanswered questions regarding the implications of the duration of ACR in an individual patient. A close review of the literature, in fact, does provide some insights, but as so commonly occurs, raises additional questions. Early studies suggested that certain grades of ACR were apt to resolve spontaneously, that is, without augmented immune suppression.[5] The problem with interpreting such studies is the lack of granularity of the data. We do not know whether subtle changes to ambient immune suppression were made, such as ensuring target levels were achieved or a slightly higher target range was used. Nor do we know the quality of the sampling. Sampling error is frequent when taking TBBx. The ISHLT criteria recommend analyzing at least five pieces of alveolated lung tissue, each with ~100 alveoli to have reasonable confidence that ACR can be excluded. The study by Scott and colleagues from the Harefield group computes that 18 TBBx should be analyzed to provide a 95% confidence that ACR is not present.[6] It is likely, therefore, that at least some cases of "spontaneous" resolution reflect sampling error. To compound this potential error, open lung biopsy samples have demonstrated that different manifestations of ACR may coexist within one lung at the same time. Convention decrees that for grading purposes, the highest grade is reported. Finally, we do not know the within-observer kappa scores for grading ACR as no study has ever reported them. We do know the between observers' kappa scores are low for A grades and even lower for B grades. This potential source of error can be mitigated when a single pathologist grades all of the biopsies.

There is evidence in the literature, however, that persistent ACR, as judged by a positive follow-up biopsy, is at risk for CLAD and mortality, even for so-called low-grade ACR, Grade A1 or B1. Herein lies a further confounding variable to the analysis of ACR outcomes. Large series should delineate surveillance biopsies (asymptomatic patient) from clinically mandated biopsies (symptomatic and or follow-up of a prior positive biopsy managed with or without augmented immune suppression). Some do, but often, the time interval between biopsies is not specified. Real-world experience does suggest that persistent higher grade ACR, in particular, which is refractory to usual therapies, portends a poor prognosis.

This discussion is, of course, predicated on the premise that TBBx biopsies are performed as the arbiter of the presence of ACR. However, some studies refer to "clinical ACR" as an entity defined usually in a symptomatic patient often with chest X-Ray opacities and a fall in lung function both of which respond to augmented immune suppression usually with pulse dose methylprednisolone. The number of treated who did not, in effect, have ACR in these studies, as judged by treatment failure or an alternative diagnosis, is usually not provided, but is clearly of great importance. Nor is the risk of augmented immune suppression usually evaluated. It is, after all, a risk–benefit equation both in the short and long term. Further, several studies pool so-called "clinical ACR" with "biopsy-proven ACR", thereby, creating data pollution which is impossible to properly evaluate. This is akin to equating apples and oranges with watermelons!

REFERENCES (APPENDIX)

1. Burton CM, Iversen M, Scheike T, et al. Is lympho-cytic bronchiolitis a marker of acute rejection? An analysis of 2,697 transbronchial biopsies after lung transplantation. J Heart Lung Transplant 2008; 27(10):1128–34.
2. Glanville AR, Aboyoun CL, Havryk A, et al. Severity of lymphocytic bronchiolitis predicts long-term outcome after lung transplantation. Am J Respir Crit Care Med 2008;177(9):1033–40. https://doi.org/10.1164/rccm.200706-951OC.
3. Burton CM, Iversen M, Scheike T, et al. Minimal acute cellular rejection remains prevalent up to 2 years after lung transplantation: a retrospective analysis of 2697 transbronchial biopsies. Transplantation 2008; 85(4):547–53. https://doi.org/10.1097/TP.0b013e318 1641df9.
4. Hachem RR, Khalifah AP, Chakinala MM, et al. The significance of a single episode of minimal acute rejection after lung transplantation. Transplantation 2005;80(10):1406–13. https://doi.org/10.1097/01.tp. 0000181161.60638.fa.
5. Sibley RK, Berry GJ, Tazelaar HD, et al. The role of transbronchial biopsies in the management of lung transplant recipients. J Heart Lung Transplant 1993; 12(2):308–24. doi: not available.
6. Scott JP, Fradet G, Smyth RL, et al. Prospective study of transbronchial biopsies in the management of heart-lung and single lung transplant patients. J Heart Lung Transplant 1991;10(5 Pt 1):626–36 [dis-cussion: 636-7].

Opportunistic Infections Post-Lung Transplantation: Viral, Fungal, and Mycobacterial

Gabriela Magda, MD

KEYWORDS

- Lung transplant • Opportunistic infection • Immunocompromised hosts

KEY POINTS

- Comprehensive donor and recipient screening for infection risk pre-transplant can reduce infection incidence post-transplant and guide prophylaxis.
- Certain infections (eg, cytomegalovirus, *Aspergillus*, community-acquired respiratory viruses affecting the lower respiratory tract) are more strongly associated with the development of chronic lung allograft dysfunction; prevention, early diagnosis, and aggressive treatment are critical to preserving long-term allograft function.
- Antifungal prophylaxis strategies are variable across transplant centers; there are supportive data for universal prophylaxis, but available evidence has not proven it to be a clearly superior strategy to preemptive approaches.

INTRODUCTION

Lung transplant recipient (LTR) outcomes have improved significantly but remain inferior to other solid organ transplant (SOT) outcomes despite advances in surgical techniques and immunosuppressive strategies, partly because of infection-related complications.[1] Between the first 30 days and 1-year post-transplant, infections are the leading cause of LTR mortality. Certain infections are associated with the development of acute rejection and chronic lung allograft dysfunction (CLAD).[2] Gram-negative bacterial infections are most common, but viruses, fungi, and mycobacteria are also important contributors to LTR outcomes. Risk factors for infection include continuous exposure of the lung allograft to the external environment, high immunosuppression levels, disruptions to allograft bronchial blood supply, lymphatic drainage, and vagal nerve paths causing impaired mucociliary clearance from airway epithelium changes and decreased cough reflex, and impact of the native lung microbiome in single LTRs.[3,4] Infection risk is mitigated through careful pre-transplant screening of recipients and donors, implementation of antimicrobial prophylaxis strategies, and routine post-transplant surveillance.[5] This review describes common viral, fungal, and mycobacterial infectious after lung transplant and provides prevention and treatment recommendations.

INFECTION SCREENING AND PREVENTION

LTR infections can be derived from the donor, reactivated latent infections in the recipient, or newly acquired (**Fig. 1**). Donors and recipients should undergo thorough pre-transplant evaluation of infection risk. Prior infectious exposures can be ascertained through taking comprehensive medical, social, travel, and immunization histories. Serostatus, sputum, and nucleic acid tests should

Columbia University Lung Transplant Program, Division of Pulmonary, Allergy, and Critical Care Medicine, Columbia University Irving Medical Center, Columbia University Vagelos College of Physicians and Surgeons, 622 West 168th Street PH-14, New York, NY 10032, USA
E-mail address: gm2339@cumc.columbia.edu

Clin Chest Med 44 (2023) 159–177
https://doi.org/10.1016/j.ccm.2022.10.012
0272-5231/23/© 2022 Elsevier Inc. All rights reserved.

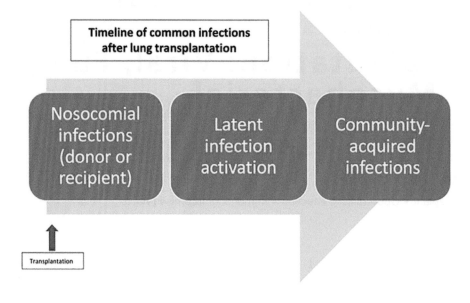

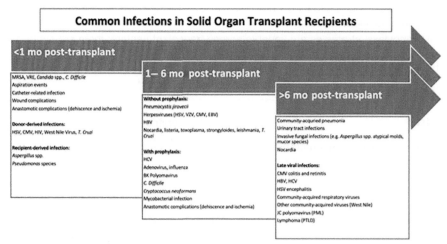

Fig. 1. Types and timing of infections after lung transplantation. (*Modified from* Fishman JA. Infection in solid-organ transplant recipients. N Engl J Med. 2007;357(25):2606.)

be confirmed pre-transplant to risk stratify donor to recipient transmission and guide post-transplant infectious prophylaxis (**Table 1**). LTRs with suppurative underlying lung diseases, who have been frequently hospitalized, or who have received broad-spectrum antimicrobials may be colonized with fungi or bacteria. Antimicrobial susceptibilities of colonizing organisms should be known pre-transplant for appropriate perioperative and postoperative antimicrobial selection.[6,7]

Effort should be made to vaccinate potential LTRs when absence of immunity to specific pathogens is identified (**Table 2**). Vaccination timing may be impacted by degree of immunosuppression pre-transplant and post-transplant and transplant urgency. Vaccination may be deferred until

immunosuppression levels are significantly reduced post-transplant to better ensure protective immune response. Live attenuated vaccines are contraindicated after SOT.[8–10] Household members and close contacts of LTRs also should adhere to routine immunization schedules.

Infection risk depends on time since transplant surgery. In the first month post-transplant, infections are generally due to donor allograft transmission, reactivation of recipient infections, or acquired from the hospitalization or surgical procedures. Infection risk may be increased in LTRs with comorbid immunodeficiencies or who received immunosuppression pre-transplant. Bacterial infections are most common. Pleural effusions within the first 3 months posttransplant

Table 1
Infection risk screening of lung transplant donors and recipients

Pathogen	Donor and Recipient Screening Test	Special Considerations
Cytomegalovirus (CMV)	CMV Immunoglobulin G (IgG)	
Epstein–Barr virus (EBV)	EBV nuclear antigen, viral capsid IgG	
Varicella-Zoster virus (VZV)	VZV IgG	
Herpes simplex 1 and 2 (HSV-1/HSV-2)	HSV-1 IgG HSV-2 IgG	
Hepatitis B virus (HBV)	HBV nucleic acid test (NAT), anti-HBc antibody, HBsAG	
Hepatitis C virus (HCV)	HCV NAT anti-HCV antibody	Perform testing in LTR immediately before transplant and 4–6 wk post-transplant
HIV	NAT and anti-HIV antibody	Repeat testing in LTR 4–6 wk post-transplant
SARS-CoV-2	Nasopharyngeal PCR	BAL can be considered in donor lung
Measles, mumps, rubella	Measles IgG, mumps IgG, rubella IgG	
Tuberculosis	Tuberculin skin testing (TST) or interferon gamma release assay (IGRA)	TST and IGRA are not validated in donors BAL and sputum can be obtained from donor for AFB smear, culture, and molecular testing Repeat testing in LTR 4–6 wk post-transplant
Treponema pallidum (syphilis)	Venereal Disease Research Laboratory or Rapid Plasma Reagin	
Toxoplasma gondii	Toxoplasma IgG	Toxoplasma IgG
Strongyloides stercoralis	Strongyloides IgG	Can limit screening to endemic areas
Region Specific Screening		
Pathogen	Endemic Regions	Special Considerations
Schistosoma spp	Africa, South America, Caribbean, Middle East, southern China, southeast Asia	Cystoscopy may be indicated in renal transplant patients
Trypanosoma cruzi (Chagas disease)	Mexico, Central America, South America	
Leishmania spp	Africa, Asia, Middle East, southern Europe, Mexico, Central America, South America	May cross-react with *T Cruzi*
Coccidioides spp	Southeastern United States, California Central Valley, Mexico, part of Central and South America	
Histoplasma spp	Central and Eastern North America, Central America, South America, Africa, Asia, Australia	
Blastomyces spp.	Midwestern/South-Central/Southeastern United States, Eastern Canada, Africa, South Asia	

(continued on next page)

Table 1
(continued)

Region Specific Screening		
Pathogen	**Endemic Regions**	**Special Considerations**
HTLV1 and HTLV2	Southern Japan, South America, Caribbean, Middle East, Sub-Saharan Africa, Central Australia, Papua New Guinea	Screening tests may be suboptimal in low prevalence areas
Hepatitis A	Areas with contaminated food and water supply, inadequate sanitation	Consider consultation with infectious diseases experts to determine if testing is indicated

should not be presumed to benign without infection evaluation.[11] Up to 6 months post-transplant, opportunistic infections predominate, though donor-derived infections may still occur. After the first 6 months, infections from broader range bacteria become more common.[12,13]

VIRUSES

Viral infections in LTRs can be grouped into pathogens primarily affecting extrapulmonary tissues (eg, the herpesviruses) and pathogens primarily affecting the respiratory tract (eg, the community-acquired respiratory viruses [CARVs]).

Cytomegalovirus

Cytomegalovirus (CMV) is a ubiquitous herpesvirus that can reactivate from latent infection in SOT recipients; transmission also occurs through allografts or blood product transfusions from CMV-infected donors or close contact with CMV-infected people. Over half of United States adults have serologic evidence of prior CMV infection.[14,15] Owing to relatively increased immunosuppression levels in LTRs and higher viral load transmission from seropositive lung allografts, CMV infection occurs more frequently in LTRs than other SOTs.[16,17] Immunomodulatory effects of CMV increase risks of infection from other opportunistic pathogens, Epstein–Barr virus (EBV)-related post-transplant lymphoproliferative disease, and allograft dysfunction.[18–20] CMV infection is variably associated with acute rejection and CLAD.[21–23] Without antiviral prophylaxis, 54% to 92% of LTRs develop CMV infection or disease.[24,25] Negative serostatus recipients with positive serostatus donors (CMV D+/R-) are at highest risk. CMV D+/R+ recipients have higher rate of infection than CMV D-/R+ recipients (69% and 58%, respectively) due to potential for CMV reactivation or infection with new strains.[26–29] CMV prophylaxis significantly decreases rates of CLAD.[30,31]

CMV disease requires evidence of viral replication in the presence of attributable symptoms or tissue invasion, whereas CMV infection is defined by viral replication regardless of symptom presence.[32] CMV disease most frequently occurs in the early post-transplant period and times of augmented immunosuppression. CMV pneumonitis is the most common presentation in LTRs; characteristics include fever, dyspnea, dry cough, lung function decline on spirometry, and radiographic findings such as ground-glass opacities and patchy consolidations.[33] Some tissue-invasive disease (CMV enteritis) presents with negative serum viral loads. Tissue biopsy with histopathologic findings of CMV inclusion bodies and/or viral antigens confirms diagnosis. Viral shedding in bronchoalveolar lavage (BAL) or bronchial washings cannot be distinguished from tissue-invasive disease and must be interpreted in clinical context.[34–39]

Although no trials have compared the approaches, universal antiviral prophylaxis in the first 6 to 12 months post-transplant with either oral valganciclovir or intravenous ganciclovir is recommended over preemptive serial monitoring of CMV viral loads with initiation of antivirals on viral replication detection.[31,40–42] A recently developed CMV T-Cell immunity panel, measuring CMV-specific CD4+ and CD8+ T-cell immunity by flow cytometry and intracellular cytokine staining has potential to personalize prophylaxis choice and duration and to predict clinically significant CMV events or inability to clear viremia. A measure of 0.2% of CMV reactive CD4+ and CD8+ T cells indicates existing immunity to CMV in a healthy population. The utilization of this test in combination with CMV polymerase chain reaction (PCR) testing is currently being studied in LTRs and could guide treating physicians in deciding continuation of CMV prophylaxis beyond 3 months post-transplant.[43–46]

Table 2
Vaccination recommendations for lung transplant recipients

Pathogen Target	Vaccine Type	Current Recommendation	Special Considerations
Influenza	Nonlive	Before and after transplant	Only inactivated, nonlive vaccine should be administered Annual administration to account for changing seasonal strains
Hepatitis B	Nonlive	Before and after transplant if not previously immunized of inadequate immunity	Monitor serostatus to confirm immunity
Hepatitis A	Nonlive	Before and after transplant	
Streptococcus pneumoniae	Nonlive	Before and after transplant if not previously immunized	
Neisseria meningitidis	Nonlive	Before and after transplant for high-risk patients not previously immunized	Risk factors include impaired splenic function and treatment with eculizumab
Haemophilus influenzae	Nonlive	Before and after transplant for high-risk patients not previously immunized	Risk factors include impaired splenic function
Human papillomavirus	Nonlive	Before and after transplant	
Tetanus, diphtheria, pertussis (Tdap)	Nonlive	Before and after transplant	
SARS-CoV-2	Nonlive	Before and after transplant	Boosters should be administered at recommended intervals
Zoster	Nonlive (recombinant zoster vaccine)	Before and after transplant in LTRs > 19 year old	
Zoster	Live, attenuated zoster vaccine	Before transplant in candidates > 50 year old; *contraindicated posttransplant and in immunosuppressed patients*	
Varicella	Live, attenuated	Before transplant; *contraindicated posttransplant and in immunosuppressed patients*	
Measles, mumps, rubella	Live, attenuated	Before transplant; *contraindicated posttransplant and in immunosuppressed patients*	
Rotavirus	Live, attenuated	Before transplant; *contraindicated posttransplant and in immunosuppressed patients*	

Ongoing prophylaxis may be considered in CMV D+/R+ or CMV D-/R+ recipients receiving augmented immunosuppression with high-dose glucocorticoids or antilymphocyte antibodies. Myelosuppression is a common treatment toxicity. Oral letermovir lacks the myelosuppressive effects of valganciclovir and has been approved for CMV prophylaxis in hematopoietic stem cell transplant recipients.[47] Successful letermovir use in LTRs has been described in small studies, but there reports of breakthrough viremia and letermovir resistance exist.[48–50]

CMV treatment consists of valganciclovir or ganciclovir and concomitant immunosuppression reduction (particularly in moderate to severe disease). Treatment of asymptomatic viremia to prevent the development of invasive disease is advised. Valganciclovir is equivalent to ganciclovir for mild to moderate disease.[51,52] Ganciclovir is recommended for CMV pneumonitis, with transition to oral medication on clinical and virologic resolution. Treatment duration depends on clinical response and virologic clearance. Antiviral drug dosing should not be reduced if leukopenia emerges because of risk of drug resistance. Treatment with CMV immune globulin (CytoGam) might be considered in severe disease, though data are limited. If no virologic or clinical improvement is observed after 2 weeks of therapy, genotypic resistance testing should be performed.[53–56] The most common mutation conferring resistance is UL97 phosphotransferase. Resistant CMV treatment includes immunosuppression reduction and changing antivirals to foscarnet or cidofovir.[26] Oral maribavir is an alternative salvage treatment of resistant CMV disease approved for use in SOTs, with limited data in LTRs.[56–58] Letermovir can also be considered.

Non-Cytomegalovirus Herpesviruses

Herpes simplex 1 (HSV-1) and HSV-2 disease in LTRs is usually due to reactivation of latent virus in the dorsal root ganglia when herpesvirus prophylaxis is not used.[59] Acyclovir, valacyclovir, or famciclovir should be used in patients not receiving CMV prophylaxis.[60] Patients with limited mucocutaneous infection should be treated with oral medications until lesions are fully healed.[61] LTRs with severe or disseminated infection should be treated with intravenous acyclovir.

Varicella-zoster virus (VZV) infection occurs by airborne acquisition or reactivation from primary infection and presents as herpes zoster in up to 20% of LTRs in the first 5 years post-transplant.[62,63] Prophylaxis is similar in HSV; treatment is with valacyclovir or famciclovir. If lesions progress or new lesions develop despite therapy, treatment should be changed to intravenous acyclovir. Intravenous acyclovir is recommended for primary VZV infection, disseminated disease, or VZV affecting the trigeminal nerve.

Community-Acquired Respiratory Viruses

CARVs are associated with significant morbidity and mortality in LTRs.[64–66] Infection incidence in LTRs may be underestimated because historically studies have been retrospective and only of inpatient populations, whereas severity may be over-estimated because studies used culture-based diagnostics in patients with severe respiratory symptoms.[66–68] Seasonal and geographic patterns of CARV infection in LTRs and immunocompetent individuals are similar.[69] Infection prevention strategies generally focus on contact avoidance and isolation and vaccination when available.

Immunosuppression can mute systemic inflammatory responses to CARV infection, and lung function declines from baseline on spirometry might be the sole infection indicators. Radiographic parenchymal abnormalities include ground-glass opacities, tree-in-bud opacities, nodules, and/or airspace consolidations.[70] Progression to lower respiratory tract disease or severe illness increases in LTRs who have had early post-transplant infections and who are receiving augmented immunosuppression or rejection treatment.[64,71]

Definitive diagnosis is achieved through testing respiratory tract samples. Initial testing should be through nasopharyngeal swab or washing and include a wide range of viruses to account for high likelihood of coinfection. Available tests and techniques vary by institution. Washings are more sensitive than swabs.[72] Molecular diagnostic tests are more sensitive than viral culture, direct fluorescent antibody, or rapid antigen detection in symptomatic and asymptomatic immunocompromised patients in outpatient and inpatient settings.[73–78] If initial testing is negative but clinical suspicion remains high, repeat confirmatory testing is advised, particularly if effective antiviral therapeutics are available. BAL may be indicated. When prolonged viral shedding is detected, serial quantitative molecular testing can guide treatment responsiveness.[79]

CARV infection stimulates cytokine and chemokine production that attracts damaging inflammatory cells, thereby changing mucosal epithelium integrity and composition.[80–83] Risk of secondary infection with locally invading bacterial or fungal airway colonizers is increased. Local alloantigen production can incite immune-mediated injury leading to episodes of acute rejection and CLAD development.[84,85] High BAL chemokine concentration prognosticates significant forced expiratory volume in the first second (FEV1) decline 6 months after initial infection.[86] CARV infections (particularly in the lower respiratory tract) are independent risk factors for CLAD, but contemporary studies have failed to demonstrate a strong relationship to acute rejection, possibly because most studies are retrospective single center analyses with variable definitions of acute rejection.[87–96] As expected host response to viral infection is perivascular lymphocytic infiltrate, the presence of lymphocytes on allograft biopsy can signify appropriate response to infection or rejection.

Influenza

LTRs have the highest incidence of influenza among SOTs. Unlike in immunocompetent patients, antiviral therapies are advised for all LTRs with suspected or confirmed influenza infection, regardless of illness severity or interval between symptom onset and diagnosis, due to secondary infections and rejection risks.[79,97] Confirmatory testing to guide antiviral therapy should be obtained when drug resistance is a concern. Neuraminidase inhibitors (oseltamivir, zanamivir, peramivir) are typical first-line treatments; M2 inhibitors (amantadine, rimantadine) are no longer recommended because of resistance and inactivity.[74,98] Therapy should continue until viral shedding is undetectable. Resistance testing should be performed in patients with prolonged symptom duration or clinical deterioration with ongoing viral shedding; empiric treatment with alternative antivirals should be considered while awaiting testing results. Antiviral prophylaxis is generally avoided to minimize development of resistance, except in LTRs likely to have inadequate immunity due to augmented immunosuppression or recent transplantation.[79]

Adenovirus

Adenovirus infection can be acquired throughout the year or reactivate from latent childhood infection to cause pneumonia or disseminated disease.[99] Mild disease is generally managed through immunosuppression reduction. Disseminated disease carries 50% mortality. Cidofovir is recommended for severe pneumonia or disseminated disease. Treatment can cause nephrotoxicity, neutropenia, and Fanconi-type anemia. Weekly quantitative serum viral load is recommended in addition to serial monitoring of renal function, serum electrolytes, and urine protein content.[100]

Respiratory syncytial virus

Respiratory syncytial virus (RSV) is a common cause of childhood bronchiolitis that carries 10% to 20% mortality in LTRs. Infection ranges from mild upper respiratory to severe lower respiratory tract disease associated with allograft dysfunction.[101,102] Prophylaxis with palivizumab can be considered. Ribavirin has in vitro activity against RSV; limited data in LTRs suggest ribavirin, with or without concomitant glucocorticoids or intravenous immunoglobulin (IVIG), successfully prevents progression to lower respiratory infection.[103,104]

Human metapneumovirus

Human metapneumovirus has similar presentation to RSV infection in LTRs and has been associated with allograft dysfunction. The main therapy is supportive care; ribavirin with or without IVIG has been used in few severe cases with successful outcome.[102,105]

Parainfluenza

Parainfluenza infects up to 10% of LTRs, with peak seasonal distribution in spring and summer. Infection is usually mild but can progress to severe lower respiratory tract illness and be associated with CLAD.[106,107] Ribavirin has been used in few reported cases with successful outcome.[108] Antivirals, adjunctive steroids, and IVIG generally have not proven beneficial.[71]

FUNGAL INFECTIONS

Invasive fungal infections (IFIs) have an 8% to 10% yearly cumulative incidence in LTRs. Aspergillus and Candida spp are the most common causative organisms; other culprits include the geographically endemic mycoses (Histoplasma, Blastomyces, and Coccidioides spp), Pneumocystis, Cryptococcus spp, mucormycosis agents, and non-Aspergillus molds (Scedosporium and Fusarium spp).[109] Incidence and type of IFI are influenced by immunosuppression intensity, pretransplant airway colonization and ischemia, microbiome alterations from antimicrobial usage, timing since transplant, and antifungal prophylaxis. Invasive Candida spp (IC) infections typically occur in the early post-transplant period as complications associated with surgery, hospitalization, and ICU length of stay. Most non-Candida IFIs are acquired through inhalation or develop from recipient airway colonization. Aspergillus infections occur most frequently within the first 6 to 12 months posttransplant.[109] Non-Aspergillus mold infections occur later post-transplant and are associated with significantly higher mortality than Aspergillus (60.5% vs 39.5%, respectively).[110] IFIs are notably associated with allograft

Table 3
Diagnosis and treatment of invasive fungal infections in lung transplant recipients

Pathogen	Diagnostic Tests	Treatment	Special Considerations
Aspergillus sp	• Cultures • Histopathology • Serum galactomannan • BAL galactomannan • Serum PCR: single negative test rules out IA; two positive tests help rule in IA • BAL PCR: Identifies the presence of mold but cannot distinguish infection from colonization without appropriate clinical context • 1,3-beta-D-glucan variably helpful	First-line for IA: voriconazole Alternative agents: • Azoles: posaconazole, isavuconazole • Echinocandins: caspofungin, anidulafungin • Combination therapy can be considered Tracheobronchitis: inhaled amphotericin B in combination with systemic therapy	Treatment considerations: • Azoles: monitoring of hepatic function and calcineurin/mTOR inhibitor levels is advised • Liposomal amphotericin: monitoring of electrolytes, renal and hepatic function is advised • Caspofungin and micafungin: monitoring of hepatic function is advised • Anidulafungin and caspofungin: role as single agent therapy is controversial • Trimethoprim-sulfamethoxazole (TMP-SMX): correct for renal function and maintain adequate hydration • Pentamidine side effects include pancreatitis, hypo- and hyperglycemia, myelosuppression, renal failure, electrolyte disturbances • Avoid primaquine and dapsone in G6PD deficiency
Candida spp.	• Cultures • Histopathology • 1,3-beta-D-glucan can be helpful in clinical context T2 Candida assay (detects whole blood Candida cells of the 5 most common species with high sensitivity and specificity) • PCR testing not clinically available	IC and candidemia: • Echinocandins (micafungin, anidulafungin) are initial empiric therapy • Fluconazole as empiric therapy when azole resistance is not a concern • Liposomal amphotericin B Mild oropharyngeal disease: • Clotrimazole, fluconazole • Nystatin Endovascular infection/implantable Device infection: • Liposomal amphotericin B as initial therapy • High-dose echinocandin as alternative therapy	
Mucormycosis	• Mucorales PCR is not clinically available • Cultures grow within 24–48 h • Cultures might be negative despite positive tissue staining • Galactomannan notably not useful	Invasive mucormycosis: • Induction therapy with high dose liposomal amphotericin B • Combination of liposomal amphotericin B with echinocandin or posaconazole can be considered for refractory cases but data are weak • Posaconazole or isavuconazole can be used in patients not tolerating amphotericin but data are weak	

(*continued on next page*)

Table 3
(continued)

Pathogen	Diagnostic Tests	Treatment	Special Considerations
Cryptococcus	• Cryptococcus antigen testing of CSF and serum • CSF culture and stain • BAL culture and stain • Biopsy whenever possible	• Surgical excision and debridement for all extrapulmonary manifestations CNS disease: • Induction with liposomal amphotericin B and flucytosine for 2–4 wk • Consolidation with high-dose fluconazole for 8 wk • Maintenance with lower dose fluconazole for a year • Lumbar puncture as needed to relieve elevated intracranial pressure Pulmonary disease: • Asymptomatic or mild to moderate disease: Fluconazole for 6–12 mo • Severe pulmonary disease: same as CNS treatment	
Fusarium	• Cultures • Histopathology	Invasive fusariosis: • No treatment is clearly superior; voriconazole is typically first line • Amphotericin B in combination with voriconazole for resistant cases • Posaconazole as alternative • Surgical excision and debridement where indicated	
Scedosporium	• Cultures • Histopathology	Invasive scedosporiosis • Voriconazole is first line • Amphotericin B, voriconazole, posaconazole, isavuconazole are all options and can be considered in combination • Surgical excision and debridement	
Pneumocystis jirovecii	• BAL or tissue biopsy • Immunofluroscent assays are the most sensitive diagnostics	*Pneumocystis* Pneumonia: • Trimethoprim–sulfamethoxazole is first-line treatment	

(continued on next page)

Table 3
(continued)

Pathogen	Diagnostic Tests	Treatment	Special Considerations
	• Nucleic acid testing in BAL cannot distinguish colonization from disease without clinical context • Silver stain on BAL excludes *Pneumocystis* pneumonia (PCP) if negative • LDH is nonspecific • 1,3-beta-D-glucan can be a helpful adjunct but is not specific for PCP	• Alternatives: inhaled pentamidine: dapsone and trimethoprim • For mild to moderate disease only: atovaquone; combination primaquine and clindamycin • Combination echinocandins and TMP-SMX have shown benefit in animal models but clinical benefit is unknown • Adjunctive steroids are not clearly beneficial in non-HIV populations	

dysfunction. *Aspergillus* colonization is an independent risk factor for CLAD.[111] IFI testing and treatment is summarized in **Table 3**.

For all suspected IFIs, early bronchoscopy is recommended to evaluate anastomotic integrity, inspect airways for tracheobronchial abnormalities (pseudomembranes, erythema, ulcerations, or necrosis), and obtain BAL. Anastomotic dehiscence can be confirmed by chest imaging. Cavitary and nodular lesions are characteristic radiographic features. Cultures and fungal stains are positive in 50% to 70% of cases.[112] *Aspergillus* BAL PCR sensitivity is over 90% but testing cannot distinguish between infection and colonization.[113] Definitive IFI diagnosis necessitates tissue biopsy for visualization of fungal presence or tissue invasion at the suspected infection site.

Galactomannan antigen and 1,3-beta-D-glucan serum assays have variable utility in diagnosing IFIs in LTRs. Galactomannan is a cell wall component of *Aspergillus* sp released during fungal replication that can be detected in serum using enzyme immunoassay (EIA).[114] Serum galactomannan sensitivity is greatest in severely neutropenic patients because preserved immune systems consume circulating galactomannan; sensitivity in LTRs is 30%, versus over 70% in hematopoietic stem cell transplants.[115,116] In BALs of nonneutropenic SOT recipients, sensitivity increases to 88%.[114] Serum and BAL specificity are over 90% in all patients.[115,117,118] Galactomannan EIA cross-reactivity can occur with non-*Aspergillus* molds (*Fusarium* and *Penicillium*) and penicillin antibiotics (less so recently due to improved antibiotic purification).[109] The 1,3-beta-D-glucan is present in most fungal cell walls and particularly abundant

in *Candida* spp; 1,3-beta-D-glucan sensitivity and specificity for IC is 80% and 60%, respectively. Patients with *Pneumocystis* pneumonia also have characteristically high levels; 1,3-beta-D-glucan is notably absent in cell walls of *Blastomyces*, *Cryptococcus*, and *Mucorales*. Falsely elevated levels of 1,3-beta-D-glucan can occur in patients on hemodialysis or who have received blood transfusions and intravenous immunoglobulin.[119,120] There is paucity of evidence on 1,3-beta-D-glucan testing in LTRs, and it is best used as a diagnostic adjunct in clinical context.

Prophylaxis strategies targeting both *Candida* spp and molds vary among transplant centers.[116] Questions remain regarding universal versus preemptive prophylaxis, choice of drug, need for monotherapy versus combination therapy, and prophylaxis duration. Studies of IFI prophylaxis have been limited by retrospective, single-center, and nonrandomized designs.[121] Some transplant centers begin universal antifungal prophylaxis immediately post-transplant, whereas others limit prophylaxis to recipients with high risk for IFIs (underlying cystic fibrosis or bronchiectatic lung diseases, evidence of airway colonization, primary graft dysfunction, and history of CMV infection).[122–126] Data on superiority of either strategy are mixed.[127–129] Most centers use monotherapy with aerosolized amphotericin B, or systemic voriconazole or itraconazole; the remainder use combination therapy with inhaled and systemic antifungals. Isavuconazole has been demonstrated to be a safe and effective alternative agent.[130] Duration of prophylaxis varies from 3 to over 12 months post-transplant. In one large retrospective study, incidences of IC and mold IFI were greater than previously reported despite micafungin and amphotericin B prophylaxis, suggesting breakthrough infection because of inadequate tissue penetration of echinocandins, reduced systemic drug concentration in the presence of ECMO circuits, and resistance to inhaled amphotericin B. A recent meta-analysis of 12 antifungal prophylactic strategies among 13 studies did not establish a strong recommendation for a particular regimen.[131,132]

Aspergillus

Aspergillus spp is the most common cause of IFIs after lung transplantation. Owing to higher immunosuppression levels, invasive aspergillosis (IA) occurs more frequently in LTRs than other SOTs. Other risk factors include airway ischemia and prior airway colonization. Aspergillus fumigatus most commonly causes IA; other causative species include Aspergillus terreus (notable for in vitro resistance to amphotericin B), Aspergillus flavus, and Aspergillus niger. Aspergillus infection can present as tracheobronchitis, anastomotic dehiscence, pneumonia, aspergilloma, and disseminated disease to the sinuses, central nervous system (CNS), spine, pleural or pericardial spaces, or skin. Tracheobronchial aspergillosis typically occurs within 3 months posttransplant with fever, cough, wheezing, hemoptysis, or can be asymptomatic. Pulmonary aspergillosis generally presents 6 months post-transplant.[133,134] Single LTRs are at an increased risk of developing IA posttransplant and consequently experience higher mortality than bilateral or combined heart-LTRs. Among bilateral LTRs cystic fibrosis patients are at higher risk of aspergillosis.[133,135,136]

Voriconazole is the preferred initial treatment for IA; alternative agents include caspofungin and isavuconazole.[137] Azoles increase levels of tacrolimus, cyclosporine, and sirolimus; therefore, immunosuppression reduction and close serum drug concentration monitoring is required during treatment. Nebulized amphotericin B can be an adjunct therapy at the devascularized anastomotic site in tracheobronchial aspergillosis. Anastomotic debridement of necrotic tissue or debris is necessary when there is a threat of airway obstruction. Severe pulmonary and disseminated aspergillosis is typically treated in combination with echinocandins. Treatment duration is not well established but at least 3 months is advised with therapy extension if there is no clinical improvement.

Candida

Candida spp is the second most common cause of IFIs in LTRs. Infections typically occur within the first 3 months post-transplant and are associated with prolonged hospital exposure or critical illness, indwelling catheters, prolonged antibacterial therapy, and neutropenia.[138] Presentation ranges from candidemia to deep tissue infection in the pleural space and at the incision or anastomoses. Although Candida is frequently isolated from sputum and BAL specimens, invasive pulmonary disease is rare. Species identification is crucial for guiding treatment because of variable antifungal therapy resistance (fluconazole resistance in C krusei; dose-dependent susceptibility to fluconazole and amphotericin, respectively C glabrata and C lusitaniae). Echinocandins (micafungin, caspofungin) are suggested initial empiric therapy; high-dose fluconazole can alternatively be used in mild to moderate IC with low risk for glabrata, pending organism identification. Prompt source control including removal of infected catheters improves outcomes.

Mucormycosis

Mucormycosis is the third most common IFI in LTRs in the first-year post-transplant (2% incidence) and carries high morbidity and mortality (76% in pneumonia, 95% in disseminated disease). Rhizopus, Mucor, and Rhizomucor are the most implicated organisms.[139] Disease can be pulmonary, rhinocerebral, gastrointestinal, cutaneous, anastomotic, or disseminated. Fungal cell wall biomarkers are classically negative, making diagnosis challenging. Successful treatment depends on early diagnosis and resection of involved tissue when there is evidence of vascular invasion and tissue necrosis.

Cryptococcus

Yearly cumulative incidence of Cryptococcus in LTRs is under 1%, but infection risk is higher than other SOTs. Disease onsets within the first 6 to 12 months posttransplant; presentation can be pulmonary or disseminated. Concomitant immunosuppression reduction at the initiation of antifungal therapy is associated with the development of immune reconstitution inflammatory syndrome (IRIS).[140,141]

Non-Aspergillus Molds

Fusarium spp are environmentally ubiquitous but uncommonly pathogenic in LTRs; when they cause IFIs, mortality is high (65% in disseminated disease). Infection occurs through inhalation or mucosal or cutaneous invasion with potential for hematogenous spread.[142] LTRs, especially those with underlying cystic fibrosis (CF), are at increased risk for focal or disseminated IFI with

Scedosporium. Treatment involves voriconazole, immunosuppression reduction, and surgical debridement.

Pneumocystis Jirovecii

Immunocompromised hosts with depleted T-cell immunity are at increased risk for *Pneumocystis* infection. LTRs are at higher risk than other SOTs. Before universal prophylaxis with trimethoprim–sulfamethoxazole, incidence of *Pneumocystis* pneumonia in LTRs ranged from 10% to 40%; lifelong prophylaxis reduces incidence to 5%.[143,144] Diagnostic testing sensitivity is decreased in LTRs because of reduced organismal burden in non-HIV patients with severe infection.[145]

Endemic Fungi

Infection with *Histoplasma*, *Coccidioides*, and *Blastomyces* may be reactivation of latent recipient infection, transmitted from donors from endemic areas, or acquired de novo from the environment. LTRs are more likely to present with severe pneumonia and disseminated disease.[146]

MYCOBACTERIAL INFECTIONS

Over 200 species of genus *Mycobacterium* exist with wide heterogeneity in prevalence, pathogenicity, and management. Mycobacteria are further divided into species complexes, the most notable being *Mycobacterium tuberculosis* complex which causes tuberculosis (TB). Active pulmonary TB affects more than 10 million people worldwide, and number of latent infections exceeds that. Nontuberculous mycobacteria (NTM) are ubiquitously found in soil and water and more frequently encountered in areas with low TB prevalence. Most NTM infections arise from environmental exposure, though nosocomial infections have also been described.[147,148]

Tuberculosis

Incidence of active TB in LTRs is less than 2% but mortality is highest among SOTs; mortality in all SOT is between 10% and 20%.[149,150] All donors and LTRs should be screened with tuberculin skin test (TST) or interferon gamma release assay (IGRA) and preferably treated for latent TB infection (LTBI) pre-transplant. Transplant urgency may preclude full treatment pre-transplant; if active TB is excluded, LTBI is not a contraindication for transplant and treatment should continue post-transplant.[151,152] Negative recipients should undergo repeat IGRA testing at an interval post-transplant to verify donor transmission (noting that IGRA sensitivity is decreased with immunosuppression). LTBI treatment options are isoniazid for 9 months, rifampin for 4 months, or combination therapy with isoniazid and rifapentine for 3 months; rifampin and rifapentine are generally avoided post-transplant because of immunosuppressant drug interactions.

Active TB is an absolute contraindication for transplant because of dissemination risk and poor outcomes post-transplant.[153,154] It is not clear when a patient who has been successfully treated for active TB can safely undergo transplant. Diagnosing active TB after SOT can be difficult because of muted immune response, atypical radiographic presentation, and difficulty isolating organisms in culture; late diagnosis increases disseminated disease risk. First-line treatment of susceptible active TB is combination therapy with isoniazid, rifampin, pyrazinamide, and ethambutol for 2 months followed by at least an additional 4 months of rifampin and isoniazid.[155] Prolonged treatment is challenging because of drug toxicities and immunosuppressant interactions.

Nontuberculous Mycobacteria

NTM infection incidence in LTRs may be underestimated due to asymptomatic colonization and lack of reporting to public health agencies. Difficulty in diagnosis and treatment leads to significant morbidity and mortality. There is no clear association between NTM infection and CLAD. LTRs colonized or infected with NTM pretransplant should receive multidrug treatment to reduce disease burden; delay of transplant to complete at least 6 months of therapy can be considered.[156] Infection generally occurs 12 months posttransplant.[157,158] *Mycobacterium avium* complex species are the most common causative organisms. *Mycobacterium abscessus*, *Mycobacterium chelonae*, and *Mycobacterium kansasii* are most frequently associated with disseminated infection.[159] *M abscessus* is a virulent, fast growing NTM notable for human-to-human transmission among CF patients and high mortality without significant allograft dysfunction.[160,161] CF patients are at higher risk for NTM infection; risk increases with chronic macrolide therapy or airway colonization with *Pseudomonas aeruginosa* or *Burkholderia cepacia*.[162–164] CF patients with pretransplant *M abscessus* colonization have higher rates of disseminated infection.[165]

Symptoms depend on organism and infection site. In all SOTs, pleuropulmonary disease is the most common presentation with features including chronic productive cough, occasional hemoptysis, and nodular, bronchiectatic, or cavitary parenchymal abnormalities on imaging.[166] Cutaneous, musculoskeletal, and disseminated infection can occur. Immunosuppression might mute expected constitutional symptoms. Treatment is based on distinguishing NTM colonization from disease. Positive BAL acid-fast bacilli (AFB) culture can represent infection or contaminant from the laboratory or environment.[164] Molecular testing is available for some NTM species. Suspicious dermatologic lesions should be evaluated by skin biopsy with AFB staining and culture. The presence of virulent NTM such as *M abscessus* is highly suspicious for infection.

There are limited data and no randomized trials on NTM treatment in LTRs. Initial management involves combination therapy with multiple antimycobacterial drugs and surgical resection for complicated skin or soft tissue involvement. Typical combination therapies can include macrolides, rifamycins, ethambutol, isoniazid, fluoroquinolones, linezolid, tetracyclines, or aminoglycosides for duration of months to years depending on infection site and severity. Treatment is generally longer in LTRs than immunocompetent patients to prevent relapse.[156,167] Bacteriophages are being investigated as potential therapeutic options for management of drug resistant NTM.[168] Immunosuppression reduction should be considered with caution because of risk of IRIS. A minimum 12 months of treatment following negative sputum cultures is recommended for pulmonary disease. At least 4 to 6 months of therapy is recommended for focal soft tissue or bone infections. The rifamycins, particularly rifampin, reduce serum concentration of tacrolimus, cyclosporine, sirolimus, and everolimus through cytochrome p450 induction. Careful immunosuppressive drug monitoring and adjustment must be made to prevent rejection. Macrolides such as clarithromycin can increase serum concentrations of calcineurin inhibitors and sirolimus through cytochrome p450 inhibition; azithromycin is less likely to cause this effect. Outcomes of treatment are not well established due to relatively low incidence of infection.

SUMMARY

LTR outcomes are compromised by the wide range of infections to which the allograft is exposed. Comprehensive pre-transplant screening and careful post-transplant prophylaxis can mitigate infection risk and prevent infectious complications including development of allograft dysfunction. Future research in infection prevention, diagnostics, and therapeutics can further reduce LTR morbidity and mortality from infection.

CLINICS CARE POINTS

- Risk factors for infection in lung transplant recipients (LTRs) include continuous exposure of the lung allograft to the external environment, high levels of immunosuppression, impaired mucociliary clearance from airway epithelium changes due to disruptions in allograft blood supply and lymphatic drainage, and impact of the native lung microbiome in single LTRs.

- In the first month post-transplant, infections are generally due to donor allograft transmission, reactivation of recipient infections, or acquired from the hospitalization or surgical procedures; bacterial infections are the most common.

- Up to 6 months post-transplant, opportunistic infections predominate, though donor-derived infections may still occur; after the first 6 months, infections from broader range bacteria become more common.

- Comprehensive donor and recipient screening for infection risk pre-transplant, and vaccination of potential LTRs when absence of immunity to specific pathogens is identified, can reduce infection incidence post-transplant and guide prophylaxis choice and duration.

- Cytomegalovirus, *Aspergillus*, and community-acquired respiratory viruses affecting the lower respiratory tract are among the infections more strongly associated with the development of chronic lung allograft dysfunction; prevention, early diagnosis, and aggressive treatment are critical to preserving long-term allograft function.

- There are supportive data for the use of universal antifungal prophylaxis in lung transplant recipients, but available evidence has not proven it to be a clearly superior strategy to preemptive approaches in preventing invasive fungal infections, and antifungal prophylaxis strategies are variable across transplant centers

DISCLOSURE

The author has nothing to disclose.

REFERENCES

1. Chambers DC, Perch M, Zuckerman A, et al. The international thoracic organ transplant Registry of the international Society for heart and lung transplantation: Thirty-eighth adult lung transplantation

report- 2021; focus on recipient characteristics. J Heart Lung Transpl 2021;40(10):1060–72.

2. Martin-Gandul C, Mueller NJ, Pascual M, et al. The impact of infection on chronic allograft dysfunction and allograft survival after solid organ transplantation. Am J Transpl 2015;15(12):3024–40.

3. Adegunsoye A, Strek ME, Garrity E, et al. Comprehensive care of the lung transplant patient. Chest 2017;152(1):150–64.

4. Bos S, Vos R, Van Raemdonck DR, et al. Survival in adult lung transplantation: where are we in 2020? Curr Opin Organ Transpl 2020;25(3):268–73.

5. Costa J, Benvenuto LJ, Sonett JR. Long-term outcomes and management of lung transplant recipients. Best Pract Res Clin Anaesthesiol 2017; 31(2):285–97.

6. Avery RK. Recipient screening prior to solid-organ transplantation. Clin Infect Dis 2002;35(12):1513–9.

7. Trachuk P, Bartash R, Abbasi M, et al. Infectious complications in lung transplant Recipients. Lung 2020;198(6):879–87.

8. Malinas M, Boucher HW. Screening of donor and candidate prior to solid organ transplantation-guidelines from the American Society of transplantation infectious diseases community of practice. Clin Transpl 2019;33(9):e13548.

9. Danziger-Isakov L, Kumar D. Vaccination of solid organ transplant candidates and recipients: guidelines from the American Society of transplantation infectious diseases community of practice. Clin Transpl 2019;33(9):e13563.

10. Wolfe CR, Ison MG. Donor-derived infections: guidelines from the American Society of transplantation infectious diseases community of practice. Clin Transpl 2019;33(9):e13547.

11. Fishman JA. Infection in organ transplantation. Am J Transpl 2017;17(4):856–79.

12. Wahidi MM, Willner DA, Snyder LD, et al. Diagnosis and outcome of early pleural space infection following lung transplantation. Chest 2009;135(2): 484–91.

13. Fishman JA. Infections in solid organ transplant recipients. N Engl J Med 2007;357(25):2606–14.

14. Munting A, Manuel O. Viral infections in lung transplantation. J Thorac Dis 2021;13(11):6673–94.

15. Bate SL, Dollard SC, Cannon MJ. Cytomegalovirus seroprevalence in the United States: the national health and nutrition examination surveys, 1988-2004. Clin Infect Dis 2010;50(11):1439–47.

16. Humar A, Snydman D. Cytomegalovirus in solid organ transplant recipients. Am J Transpl 2009; 9(Suppl 4):S78–86.

17. Zamora MR. Cytomegalovirus and lung transplantation. Am J Transpl 2004;4(8):1219–26.

18. Rubin RH. The indirect effects of cytomegalovirus infection on the outcome of organ transplantation. JAMA 1989;261:3607–9.

19. Hakimi Z, Aballea S, Ferchichi S, et al. Burden of cytomegalovirus disease in solid organ transplant recipients: a national matched cohort study in an inpatient setting. Transpl Infect Dis 2017;19(5): 1–11.

20. Reinke P, Prosch S, Kern F, et al. Mechanisms of human cytomegalovirus (HCMV) (re)activation and its impact on organ transplant pateints. Transpl Infect Dis 1999;1(3):157–64.

21. Snyder LD, Finlen-Copeland CA, Turbyfill WJ, et al. Cytomegalovirus pneumonitis is a risk for bronchiolitis obliterans syndrome in lung transplantation. Am J Respir Crit Care Med 2010; 181(12):1391–6.

22. Paraskeva M, Bailey M, Levvey NJ, et al. Cytomegalovirus replication within the lung allograft is associated with bronchiolitis obliterans syndrome. Am J Transpl 2011;11(10):2190–6.

23. Stern M, Hirsch H, Cusini A, et al. Cytomegalovirus serology and replication remain associated with solid organ graft rejection and graft loss in the era of prophylactic treatment. Transplantation 2014;98(9):1013–8.

24. Duncan AJ, Dummer JS, Paradis IL, et al. Cytomegalovirus infection and survival in lung transplant recipients. J Heart Lung Trnasplant 1991; 10(5 Pt 1):638.

25. Zamora MR, Davis RD, Leonard C, CMV Adviso4y Board Expert Committee. Management of cytomegalovirus infection in lung transplant recipients: evidence-based recommendations. Transplantation 2005;80(2):157.

26. Razonable RR, Humar A. Cytomegalovirus in solid organ transplant recipients-guidelines of the American Society of transplantation infectious diseases community of practice. Clin Transpl 2019;33:e13512.

27. Manuel O, Husain S, Kumar D, et al. Assessment of cytomegalovirus-specific cell-mediated immunity for the prediction of cytomegalovirus disease in high-risk solid organ transplant recipients: a multicenter cohort study. Clin Infec Dis 2013;56(6):817–24.

28. Hammond SP, Martin ST, Roberts K, et al. Cytomegalovirus disease in lung transplantation: impact of recipient seropositivity and duration of antiviral prophylaxis. Transpl Infect Dis 2013; 15(2):163–70.

29. Zamora MR. Controversies in lung transplantation: management of cytomegalovirus infections. J Heart Lung Transpl 2002;21(8):841.

30. Chmiel C, Speich R, Hofer M, et al. Ganciclovir/valganciclovir prophylaxis decreases cytomegalovirus-related events and bronchiolitis obliterans syndrome after lung transplantation. Clin Infect Dis 2008;46(6): 831–9.

31. Jaamei N, Koutsoker A, Pasquier J, et al. Clinical significance of post-prophylaxis cytomegalovirus

infection in lung transplant recipients. Transpl Infect Dis 2018;20(4):e12893.

32. Ljungman P, Boeckh M, Hirsch HH, et al. Definitions of cytomegalovirus infection and disease in transplant patients for Use in clinical trials. Clin Infect Dis 2017;64(1):87–91.

33. Kang EY, Patz EF Jr, Muller NL. Cytomegalovirus pneumonia in transplant patients: CT findings. J Comput Assist Tomogr 1996;20(2):295–9.

34. Kotton CN, Kumar D, Caliendo AM, et al. The third international Consensus guidelines on the management of cytomegalovirus in solid-organ transplantation. Transplantation 2018;102(6):900–31.

35. Nakhleh RE, Bolman RM 3rd, Henke CA, et al. Lung transplant pathology. A comparative study of pulmonary acute rejection and cytomegalovirus infection. Am J Surg Pathol 1991;15(12):1197–201.

36. Chemaly RF, Yen-Lieberman B, Castilla EA, et al. Correlation between viral loads of cytomegalovirus in blood and bronchoalveolar lavage specimens from lung transplant recipients determined by histology and immunohistochemistry. J Clin Microbiol 2004 May;42(5):2168–72.

37. Riise GC, Andersson R, Bergstrom T, et al. Quantification of cytomegalovirus DNA in BAL fluid: a longitudinal study in lung transplant recipients. Chest 2000;118(6):1653–60.

38. Westall GP, Michaelidies A, Williams TJ, et al. Human cytomegalovirus load in plasma and bronchoalveolar lavage fluid: a longitudinal study of lung transplant recipeints. J Infect Dis 2004; 190(6):1076–83.

39. Lodding IP, Schultz HH, Jensen JU, et al. Cytomegalovirus viral load in bronchoalveolar lavage to diagnose lung transplant associated CMV pneumonia. Transplantation 2018;102(2):326–32.

40. Manuel O, Kralidis G, Mueller NJ, et al. Impact of antiviral preventive strategies on the incidence and outcomes of cytomegalovirus disease in solid organ transplant recipients. Am J Transpl 2013; 13(9):2402–10.

41. Palmer SM, Limaye AP, Banks M, et al. Extended valganciclovir prophylaxis to prevent cytomegalovirus after lung transplantation: a randomized, controlled trial. Ann Intern Med 2010;152(12):761–9.

42. Paya C, Humar A, Dominguez E, et al. Efficacy and safety of valganciclovir vs. oral ganciclovir for prevention of cytomegalovirus disease in solid organ transplant recipients. Am J Transpl 2004;4(4):611–20.

43. Veit T, Pan M, Munker D, et al. Association of CMV-specific T-cell immunity and risk of CMV infection in lung transplant recipients. Clin Transpl Jun 2021; 35(6):e14294.

44. Sester U, Gärtner BC, Wilkens H, et al. Differences in CMV-specific T-cell levels and long-term susceptibility to CMV infection after kidney, heart and lung

transplantation. Am J Transpl Jun 2005;5(6): 1483–9.

45. Paez-Vega A, Cantisan S, Vaquero JM, et al. Efficacy and safety of the combination of reduced duration prophylaxis followed by immuno-guided prophylaxis to prevent cytomegalovirus disease in lung transplant recipients (CYTOCOR STUDY): an open-label, randomised, non-inferiority clinical trial. BMJ Open 2019;9(8):e030648.

46. Rogers R, Saharia K, Chandorkar A, et al. Clinical experience with a novel assay measuring cytomegalovirus (CMV)-specific CD4+ and CD8+ T-cell immunity by flow cytometry and intracellular cytokine staining to predict clinically significant CMV events. BMC Infect Dis 2020;20(1):58.

47. Frange P, Leruez-Ville M. Maribavir, brincidofovir, and letermovir: efficacy and safety of new antiviral drugs for treating cytomegalovirus infections. Med Mal Infect 2018;48(8):495–502.

48. Cherrier L, Nasar A, Goodlet KJ, et al. Emergence of letermovir resistance in a lung transplant recipient with ganciclovir-resistant cytomegalovirus infection. Am J Transpl 2018;18(12):3060–4.

49. Aryal S, Katugaha SB, Cochrane A, et al. Single-center experience with use of letermovir for CMV prophylaxis or treatment in thoracic organ transplant recipients. Transpl Infect Dis 2019;21(6): e13166.

50. Veit T, Munker D, Kauke T, et al. Letermovir for difficult to treat cytomegalovirus infection in lung transplant recipeints. Transplantation 2020;104(2): 410–4.

51. Asberg A, Humar A, Rollag H, et al. Oral valganciclovir is noninferior to intravenous ganciclovir for the treatment of cytomegalovirus disease in solid organ transplant recipients. Am J Transpl 2007; 7(9):2106–13.

52. Asberg A, Humar A, Jardine AG, et al. Long-term outcomes of CMV disease treatment with valganciclovir versus IV ganciclovir in solid organ transplant recipients. Am J Transpl 2009;9(5):1205–13.

53. Fisher CE, Knudsen JL, Lease ED, et al. Risk factors and outcomes of ganciclovir-resistant cytomegalovirus infection in solid organ transplant recipients. Clin Infect Dis 2017;65(1):57–63.

54. Khurana MP, Lodding IP, Mocroft A, et al. Risk factors for failure of primary valganciclovir prophylaxis against cytomegalovirus infection and disease in solid organ transplant recipients. Open Forum Infect Dis 2019;6(6):ofz215.

55. Le Page AK, Jager MM, Iwasenko JM, et al. Clinical aspects of cytomegalovirus antiviral resistance in solid organ transplant recipients. Clin Infect Dis 2013;56(7):1018.

56. Pierce B, Richaedson CL, Lacloche L, et al. Safety and efficacy of foscarnet for the management of ganciclovir-resistant or refractory cytomegalovirus

infections: a single-center study. Transpl Infect Dis 2018;20(2):e12852.

57. Chou S. Cytomegalovirus UL97 mutations in the era of ganciclovir and maribavir. Rev Med Virol 2008;18(4):233–46.

58. Papanicoloau GA, Silveira FP, Langston AA, et al. Maribavir for refractory or resistant cytomegalovirus infections in hematopoietic-cell or solid-organ transplant recipients: a randomized, dose-ranging, double-blind phase 2 study. Clin Infect Dis 2019;68(8):1255–64.

59. Fishman JA. Overview: cytomegalovirus and the herpesviruses in transplantation. Am J Transpl 2013;13(Suppl 3):1–8. quiz 8.

60. Martin-Gandul C, Stampf S, Hequet D, et al. Preventive strategies against cytomegalovirus and incidence of alpha-herpesvirus infections in solid organ transplant recipients: a nationwide cohort study. Am J Transpl 2017;17(7):1813–22.

61. Zuckerman RA, Limaye AP. Varicella zoster virus and herpes simplex virus in solid organ transplant patients. AM J Transpl 2013;13(Suppl 3):55–66. quiz 66.

62. Gourishankar S, McDermid JC, Jhangri GS, et al. Herpes zoster infection following solid organ transplantation: incidence, risk factors and outcomes in the current immunosuppressive era. Am J Transpl 2004;4(1):108–15.

63. Manuel O, Kumar D, Singer LG, et al. Incidence and clinical characteristics of herpes zoster after lung transplantation. J Jeart Lung Transpl 2008;27(1):11–6.

64. Kumar D, Husain S, Chen MH, et al. A prospective molecular surveillance study evaluating the clinical impact of community-acquired respiratory viruses in lung transplant recipients. Transplantation 2010;89(8):1028–33.

65. Vu DL, Bridevaux PO, Aubert JD, et al. Respiratory viruses in lung transplant recipients: a critical review and pooled analysis of clinical studies. Am J Transpl 2011;11(5):1071–8.

66. Palmer SM Jr, Henshaw NG, Howell DN, et al. Community acquired respiratory viral infection in adult lung transplant recipients. Chest 1998;113(4):944–50.

67. Milstone AP, Brumble LM, Barnes J, et al. A single-season prospective study of respiratory viral infections in lung transplant recipients. Eur Respir J 2006;28(1):131–7.

68. Garbino J, Soccal PM, Aubert JD, et al. Respiratory virus in bronchoalveolar lavage: a hospital based cohort study in adults. Thorax 2009;64(5):399–404.

69. Couch RB, Englund JA, Whimbey E. Respiratory viral infections in immunocompetent and immunocompromised persons. Am J Med 1997;102(3A):2–9. discussion 25-6.

70. Franquet T. Imaging of pulmonary viral pneumonia. Radiology 2011;260(1):18–39.

71. Ison MG. Respiratory viral infections in transplant recipients. Antivir Ther 2007;12(4 Pt B):627–38.

72. Lieberman D, Lieberman D, Shimoni A, et al. Identification of respiratory viruses in adults: nasopharyngeal versus oropharyngeal sampling. J Clin Microbiol 2009;47(11):3439–43.

73. Kumar D, Michaels MG, Morris MI, et al. Outcomes from pandemic influenza A H1N1 infection in recipients of solid organ transplants: a multicenter cohort study. Lancet Infect Dis 2010;10:521–6.

74. Kumar D, Ferreira VH, Blumberg E, et al. A 5-year prospective multicenter evaluation of influenza infection in transplant recipients. Clin Infect Dis 2018;67(9):1322–9.

75. Bridevaux PO, Aubert JD, Soccal PM, et al. Incidence and outcomes of respiratory viral infections in lung transplant recipients: a prospective study. Thorax 2014;69(1):32–8.

76. Mahony JB. Nucleic acid amplification-based diagnosis of respiratory virus infections. Expert Rev Anti Infect Ther 2010 Nov;8(11):1273–92.

77. Weinberg A, Zamora MR, Li S, et al. The value of polymerase chain reaction for the diagnosis of viral respiratory tract infections in lung transplant recipients. J Clin Virol 2002;25:171–5.

78. Englund JA, Piedra PA, Jewell A, et al. Rapid diagnosis of respiratory syncytial virus infections in immunocompromised adults. J Clin Microbiol 1996 Jul;34(7):1649–53.

79. Manuel O, Estabrook M, AST Infectious Diseases Community of Practice. RNA respiratory viruses in solid organ transplantation. Am J Transpl 2013;13(Suppl 4):212–9.

80. Colvin BL, Thomson AW. Chemokines, their receptors, and transplant outcome. Transplantation 2002;74(2):149–55.

81. Skoner DP, Gentile DA, Patel A, et al. Evidence for cytokine mediation of disease expression in adults experimentally infected with influenza A virus. J Infect Dis 1999;180(1):10–4.

82. Arnold R, Humbert B, Werchau H, et al. Interleukin-8, interleukin-6, and soluble tumor necrosis factor receptor type 1 release from a human pulmonary epithelial cell line (A549) exposed to respiratory syncytial virus. Immunology 1994;82(1):126–33.

83. Matsukura S, Kokobu F, Noda H, et al. Expression of IL-6, IL-8, and RANTES on human bronchial epithelial cells, NCI-H292, indueced by influenza virus A. J Allergy Clin Immunol 1996;98(6, Pt 1):1080–7.

84. Belperio JA, Keane MP, Burdick MD, et al. Critical role for CXCR3 chemokine biology in the pathogenesis of bronchiolitis obliterans syndrome. J Immunol 2002;169(2):1037–49.

85. Belperio JA, Keane MP, Burdick MD, et al. Role of CXCL9/CXCR3 chemokine biology during

pathogenesis of acute lung allograft rejection. J Immunol 2003;171(9):4844–52.

86. Weigt SS, Derhovanessian A, Liao E, et al. CXCR3 chemokine ligands during respiratory viral infections predict lung allograft dysfunction. Am J Transpl 2012 Feb;12(2):477–84.

87. Soccal PM, Aubert JD, Bridevaux PO, et al. Upper and lower respiratory tract viral infections and acute graft rejection in lung transplant recipients. Clin Infect Dis 2010;51:163–70.

88. Peghin M, Hirsch HH, Len O, et al. Epidemiology and immediate indirect effects of respiratory viruses in lung transplant recipients: a 5-year prospective study. Am J Trnasplant 2017;17(5): 1304–12.

89. Peghin M, Los-Arcos I, Hirsch HH, et al. Community-acquired respiratory viruses are a risk factor for chronic lung allograft dysfunction. Clin Infect Dis 2019;69(7):1192–7.

90. Allyn PR, Duffy EL, Humphires RM, et al. Graft loss and CLAD-onset is hastened by viral pneumonia after lung transplantation. Transplantation 2016; 100(11):2424–31.

91. Magnussen J, Westin J, Andersson LM, et al. Viral respiratory tract infection during the first postoperative year is a risk factor for chronic rejection after lung transplantation. Transpl Direct 2018;4(8): e370.

92. Khalifah AP, Hachem RR, Chakinala MM, et al. Respiratory viral infections are a distinct risk for bronchiolitis obliterans syndrome and death. Am J Respir Crit Care Med 2004;170(02):181–7.

93. Fisher CE, Preiksaitis CM, Lease ED, et al. Symptomatic respiratory virus infection and chronic lung allograft dysfunction. Clin Infect Dis 2016; 62(3):313–9.

94. Billings JL, Hertz MI, Savik K, et al. Respiratory viruses and chronic rejection in lung transplant recipeints. J Heart Lung Transpl 2002;21(5):559–66.

95. Vilchez RA, Dauber J, Kusne S. Infectious etiology of bronchiolitis obliterans: the respiratory viruses connection- myth or reality? Am J Transpl 2003;3: 245–9.

96. Sweet SC. Community-acquired respiratory viruses post-lung transplant. Semin Respir Crit Care Med 2021;42(3):449–59.

97. Vilchez RA, McCurry K, Dauber J, et al. Influenza virus infection in adult solid organ transplant recipients. Am J Transpl 2002 Mar;2(3):287–91.

98. Ison MG. Anti-influenza therapy: the emerging challenge of resistance. Therapy 2009;6:883.

99. Ison MG. Adenovirus infections in transplant recipients. Clin Infect Dis 2006;43(3):331–9.

100. Florescu DF, Schaenman JM. AST infectious diseases community of practice. Adenovirus in solid organ transplant recipients. Guidelines from the American Society of transplantation infectious

diseases community of practice. Clin Transpl 2019;33(9):e13527.

101. McCurdy LH, Milstone A, Dummer S. Clinical features and outcomes of paramyxoviral infection in lung transplant recipients treated with ribavirin. J Heart Lung Transpl 2003;22(7):745–53.

102. Hopkins P, McNeil K, Kermeen F, et al. Human metapneumovirus in lung transplant recipients and comparison to respiratory syncytial virus. Am J Respir Crit Care Med 2008;178(8):876–81.

103. Peleaz A, Lyon GM, Force SD, et al. Efficacy of oral ribavirin in lung transplant patients with respiratory syncytial virus lower respiratory tract infection. J Heart Lung Trasnplant 2009;28(1):67–71.

104. Burrows FS, Carlos LM, Benzimra M, et al. Oral ribavirin for respiratory syncytial virus infection after lung transplantation: efficacy and cost-efficiency. J Heart Lung Transpl 2015;34(7):958–62.

105. Raza K, Ismailjee SB, Crespo M, et al. Successful outcome of human metapneumovirus (hMPV) pneumonia in a lung transplant recipient treated with intravenous ribavirin. J Heart Lung Transpl 2007;26(8):862–4.

106. Vilchez R, McCurry K, Dauber J, et al. Influenza and parainfluenza respiratory viral infection requiring admission in adult lung transplant recipients. Transplantation 2002;73(7):1075–8.

107. Hall CB. Respiratory syncytial virus and parainfluenza virus. N Engl J Med 2001;344(25):1917–28.

108. Liu V, Dhillon GS, Weill D. A multi-drug regimen for respiratory syncytial virus and parainfluenza virus infections in adult lung and heart-lung transplant recipients. Transpl Infect Dis 2010;12(1):38–44.

109. Kennedy CC, Pennington KM, Beam E, et al. Fungal infection in lung transplantation. Semin Respir Crit Care Med 2021;42(3):471–82.

110. Vasquez R, Vasquez-Guillamet MC, Suarez J, et al. Invasive mold infections in lung and heart-lung transplant recipients: Stanford University Experience. Transpl Infect Dis 2015;17(2):259–66.

111. Weigt SS, Elashoff RM, Huang C, et al. Aspergillus colonization of the lung allograft is a risk factor for bronchiolitis obliterans syndrome. Am J Transpl 2009;9(8):1903–11.

112. Geltner C, Lass-Florl C. Invasive pulmonary Aspergillosis in organ transplants- Focus on lung transplants. Respir Investig 2016;54(2):76–84.

113. Lass-Florl C, Aigner M, Nachbaur D, et al. Diagnosing filamentous fungal infections in immunocompromised patients applying computed tomography-guided percutaneous lung biopsies: as 12-year experience. Infection 2017;45(6): 867–75.

114. Pfeiffer CD, Fine JP, Safdar N. Diagnosis of invasive aspergillosis using a galactomannan assay: a meta-analysis. Clin Infect Dis 2006;42(10): 1417–27.

115. Husain S, Carmago JF. Invasive aspergillosis in solid-organ transplant recipients: guidelines from the American Society of transplantation infectious disease community of practice. Clin Transpl 2019; 33(9):e13544.

116. Bergeron A, Belle A, Sulahian A, et al. Contribution of galactomannan antigen detection in BAL to the diagnosis of invasive pulmonary assspergillosis in patients with hematologic malignancies. Chest 2010;137(2):410–5.

117. Guo YL, Chen YQ, Wang K, et al. Accuracy of BAL galactomannan in diagnosing invasive aspergillosis: a bivariate metaanlysis and systematic review. Chest 2010;138(4):817–24.

118. Racil Z, Kocmanova I, Toskova M, et al. Galactomannan detection in bronchoalveolar lavage fluid for the diagnosis of invasive aspergillosis in patients with hematological diseases- the role of factors affecting assay performance. Int J Infect Dis 2011;15(12):e874–81.

119. Tran T, Beal SG. Application of the 1,3-B-D-Glucan (Fungitell) assay in the diagnosis of invasive fungal infections. Arch Pathol Lab Med 2016;140(2):181–5.

120. Patel TS, Eschenauer GA, Stuckey LJ, et al. Antifungal prophylaxis in lung transplant recipients. Transplantation 2016 Sep;100(9):1815–26.

121. Baker AW, Maziarz EK, Arnold CJ, et al. Invasive fungal infection after lung transplantation: epidemiology in the setting of antigunfal prophylaxis. Clin Infect Dis 2020;70(1):30–9.

122. Husain S, Zaldonis D, Kusne S, et al. Variation in antifungal prophylaxis strategies in lung transplantation. Transpl Infect Dis 2006;8(4):213–8.

123. He SY, Makhzoumi ZH, Singer JP, et al. Practice variation in Aspergillus prophylaxis and treatment among lung transplant centers: a national survey. Transpl Infect Dis 2015;17(1):14–20.

124. Hsu JL, Khan MA, Sobel RA, et al. Aspergillus fumigatus invasion increases with progressive airway ischemia. PLOS One 2013;8(10):e77136.

125. Verleden GM, Vos R, van Raemodonck D, et al. Pulmonary infection defense after lung transplantation: does airway ischemia play a role? Curr Opin Organ Transpl 2010;15(5):568–71.

126. Phoompoung P, Villalobos AP-C, Jain S, et al. Risk factors of invasive fungal infections in lung transplant recipients: a systematic review and meta-analysis. J Heart Lung Transpl 2022;41(2):255–62.

127. Bitterman R, Marinelli T, Husain S. Strategies for the prevention of invasive fungal infections after lung transplant. J Fungi (Basel) 2021;7(2):122.

128. Villalobos AP-C, Husain S. Infection prophylaxis and management of fungal infections in lung transplant. Ann Transl Med 2020;8(6):414.

129. Linder KA, Kauffman CA, Patel TS, et al. Evaluation of targeted versus universal prophylaxis for the prevention of invasive fungal infection following lung transplantation. Transpl Infect Dis 2021; 23(1):e13448.

130. Samanta P, Clancy CJ, Marini RV, et al. Isavuconazole is as effective as and better Tolerated than voriconazole for antifungal prophylaxis in lung transplant recipients. Clin Infect Dis 2021;73(3):416–26.

131. Marinelli T, Rotstein C. Comment: invasive fungal infections in lung transplant recipients. Clin Infect Dis 2021;72(2):365–6.

132. Marinelli T, Davoudi S, Foroutan F, et al. Antifungal prophylaxis in adult lung transplant recipients: Uncertainty despite 30 years of experience. A systematic review of the literature and network meta-analysis. Transpl Infect Dis 2022;24(3):e13832.

133. Singh N, Husain S. Aspergillus infections after lung transplantation: clinical differences in type of transplant and implications for management. J Heart Lung Transpl 2003;22(3):258–66.

134. Gordon SM, Avery RK. Aspergillosis in lung transplantation: incidence, risk factors, and prophylactic strategies. Transpl Infect Dis 2001;3(3):161–7.

135. Aguilar CA, Hamandi B, Fegbeutel C, et al. Clinical risk factors for invasive aspergillosis in lung transplant recipients: results of an international cohort study. J Heart Lung Transpl 2018;37(10):1226–34.

136. Helmi M, Love RB, Welter D, et al. Aspergillus infection in lung transplant recipients with cystic fibrosis: risk factors and outcomes comparison to other types of transplant recipients. Chest 2003; 123(3):800–8.

137. Paterson TF, Thompson GR 3rd, Denning DW, et al. Practice guidelines for the diagnosis and management of aspergillosis: 2016 update by the infectious diseases Society of America. Clin Infect Dis 2016;63(4):e1–60.

138. Marinelli T, Pennington KM, Hamandi B, et al. Epidemiology of candidemia in lung transplant recipeints and risk factors for candidemia in the early posttransplant period in the absence of universal antifungal prophylaxis. Transpl Infect Dis 2022; 24(2):e13812.

139. Roden MM, Zaoutis TE, Buchanan WL, et al. Epidemiology and Outcome of Zygomycosis: a review of 929 reported cases. Clin Infect Dis 2005;41(5): 634–53.

140. George IA, Santos CAQ, Olsen MA, et al. Epidemiology of Cryptococcosis and Cryptococcal meningitis in a large retrospective cohort of patients after solid organ transplantation. Open Forum Infect Dis 2017;4(1):ofx004.

141. Singh N, Lortholary Q, Alexander BD, et al. An immune reconstitution syndrome-like illness associated with Cryptococcus neoformans infection in organ transplant recipients. Clin Infect Dis 2005; 40(12):1756–61.

142. Carneiro HA, Coleman JJ, Restrep A, et al. Fusarium infection in lung ttransplant patients: report

of 6 cases and review of the literature. Medicine (Baltimore) 2011;90(01):69–80.

143. Sepkowitz KA. Opportunistic infections in patients with and patients without acquired immunodeficiency syndrome. Clin Infect Dis 2002;34:1098–107.

144. Gordon SM, LaRose SP, Kalmadi S, et al. Should prophylaxis for Pneuocystis carinii pneumonia in solid organ transplant recipients ever be discontinued? Clin Infect Dis 1999;28(2):240–6.

145. Thomas CF Jr, Limper AH. Pneumocystis pneumonia. N Engl J Med 2004;350(24):2487–98.

146. Miller R, Assi M. AST infectious diseases community of practice. Endemic fungal infections in solid organ transplant recipients- guidelines from the American Society of transplantation infectious diseases community of practice. Clin Transpl 2019;33(9):e13553.

147. Friedman DZP, Doucette K. Mycobacteria: selection of transplant candidates and post-lung transplant outcomes. Semin Respir Crit Care Med 2021 Jun;42(3):460–70.

148. Forbes BA, Hall GS, Miller MB, et al. Practical guidance for clinical microbiology laboratories: mycobacteria. Clin Microbiol Rev 2018;31(02):e00038.

149. Abad CLR, Razonable RR. Donor derived Mycobacterial tuberculosis infection after solid-organ transplantation: a comprehensive review. Transpl Infect Dis 2018;20(05):e12971.

150. Abad CLR, Razonable RR. Mycobacterium tuberculosis after solid organ transplantation: a review of more than 2000 cases. Clin Transpl 2018;32(06):e13259.

151. Subramanian AK, Theodoropoulos NM. Infectious Diseases Community of Practice of the American Society of Transplantation. Mycobacterium tuberculosis infections in solid organ transplantation: guidelines from the infectious diseases community of practice of the American Society of Transplantation. Clin Transpl 2019;33(09):e13513.

152. Subramanian AK. Tuberculosis in solid organ transplant candidates and recipients: current and future challenges. Curr Opin Infect Dis 2014 Aug;27(04):316–21.

153. Leard LE, Holm AM, Valapour M, et al. Consensus document for the selection of lung transplant candidates: an update from the International Society for Heart and Lung Transplantation. J Heart Lung Transpl 2021;40(11):1349–79.

154. Torre-Cisneros J, Doblas A, Aguado JM, et al. Spanish Network for Research in Infectious Diseases. Tuberculosis after solid-organ transplant: incidence, risk factors, and clinical characteristics in the RESITRA (Spanish Network of Infection in Transplantation) cohort. Clin Infect Dis 2009;48(12):1657–65.

155. Nahid P, Dorman SE, Alipanah N, et al. Official American thoracic Society/centers for disease control and prevention/infectious diseases Society of

America clinical practice guidelines: treatment of drug-susceptible tuberculosis. Clin Infect Dis 2016;63(7):e147–95.

156. Longworth SA, Daly JS. AST infectious diseases community of practice. Management of infections due to nontuberculous mycobacteria in solid organ transplant recipients- guidelines from the American Society of transplantation infectious diseases community of practice. Clin Transpl 2019;33(9):e13588.

157. Malouf MA, Glanville AR. The spectrum of mycobacterial infection after lung transplantation. Am J Respir Crit Care Med 1999;160(5 Pt 1):1611–6.

158. Keating MR, Daly JS, AST Infectious Diseases Community of Practice. Nontuberculous mycobacterial infections in solid organ transplantation. Am J Transpl 2013;13(Suppl 4):77–82.

159. Daley CL, Iaccarino JM, Lange C, et al. Treatment of nontuberculous mycobacterial pulmonary disease: an official ATS/ERS/SCMID/IDSA clinical practice guideline. Clin Infect Dis 2020;71(4):e1–36.

160. Hamad Y, Pilewski JM, Morrell M, et al. Outcomes in lung transplant recipeints with Mycobacterium abscessus infection: a 15-year experience from a large tertiary care center. Transpl Proc 2019;51(6):2035–42.

161. Perez AA, Singer JP, Schwartz BS, et al. Management and clinical outcomes after lung transplantation in patients with pre-transplant Mycobacterium abscessus infection: a single center experience. Transpl Infect Dis 2019;21(3):e13084.

162. Degiacomi G, Sammartino JC, Chiarelli LR, et al. Mycobacterium abscessus, an emerging and worrisome pathogen among cystic fibrosis patients. Int J Mol Sci 2019;20(23):E5868.

163. Furukawa BS, Flume PA. Nontuberculous mycobacteria in cystic fibrosis. Semin Respir Crit Care Med 2018;39(03):383–91.

164. Knoll BM, Kappagoda S, Gill RR, et al. Non-tuberculous mycobacterial infection among lung transplant recipients: a 15-year cohort study. Transpl Infect Dis 2012;14(5):452–60.

165. Chalermskulrat W, Sood N, Neuringer IP, et al. Nontuberculous mycobacteria in end stage cystic fibrosis: implications for lung transplantation. Thorax 2006;61(6):507–13.

166. Doucette K, Fishman JA. Nontuberculous mycobacterial infection in hematopoietic stem cell and solid organ transplant recipients. Clin Infect Dis 2004;38(10):1428–39.

167. Griffith DE, Aksamit T, Brown-Elliott BA, et al. ATS Mycobacterial Disease Society of America. An official ATS/IDSA statement: diagnosis, treatment, and prevention of nontuberculous mycobacterial diseases. Am J Respir Crit Care Med 2007;175(04):367–416.

168. Aslam S. Bacteriophage therapy as a treatment option for transplant infections. Curr Opin Infect Dis 2020;33(4):298–303.

Common Noninfectious Complications Following Lung Transplantation

Harpreet Singh Grewal, MD[a],[*],[1], Tany Thaniyavarn, MD[b],[1],
Selim M. Arcasoy, MD, MPH[a],[2], Hilary J. Goldberg, MD, MPH[b],[2]

KEYWORDS

- Lung transplantation • Thoracic complications • Extrathoracic complications • Immunosuppression

KEY POINTS

- Common noninfectious complications after lung transplantation can be both thoracic and/or extrathoracic.
- Common noninfectious complications after lung transplantation can have a significant impact on short-term and long-term outcomes.
- Long-term exposure to post-transplant immunosuppressive medications can lead to progression of preexisting chronic medical diseases or lead to development of new medical complications.
- Prevention, early detection, and evidence-based multidisciplinary management should remain the focus in management of both common noninfectious thoracic and extrathoracic complications.

According to the Scientific Registry of Transplant Recipients (SRTR), both transplant volume and survival among lung transplant recipients are improving over time.[1],[2] However, the outcomes of lung transplantation remain challenged by multiple thoracic (**Table 1**) and extrathoracic complications. With improving lung transplant survival, patients experience prolonged exposure to chronic immunosuppressive agents that can lead to multiple infectious and noninfectious complications. This article focuses on most common noninfectious complications with significant clinical impact.

THORACIC COMPLICATIONS FOLLOWING LUNG TRANSPLANTATION
Airway Complications

The airway anastomosis, either bronchial or tracheal, is considered the most vulnerable anastomotic site for operative complications due to compromised blood supply. Bronchial artery revascularization is not routinely performed, and therefore until 2 to 4 weeks posttransplant, when neovascularization from collateral circulation is established,[3] the perfusion of the airway anastomosis and proximal donor bronchus is retrograde from the low-pressure pulmonary circulation.

The incidence of airway complications varies depending on the case definition, but ranges between 7% and 18%.[4],[5] Compromise of the blood supply and infection are believed to be the cause of most airway complications. Risk factors that have been reported are longer donor bronchus, airway infections and colonization, severe primary graft dysfunction, prolonged mechanical ventilation (both donor and/or recipient), hemodynamic instability, early rejection, and use of mammalian target of rapamycin inhibitor before complete anastomosis healing.[4],[5] End-to-end anastomosis

[a] Lung Transplant Program, Columbia University, Irving Medical Center, 622 West 168th Street, PH 14E, Suite 104, New York, NY 10032, USA; [b] Lung Transplant Program, Brigham and Women's Hospital, 75 Francis Street, PBB Clinic 3, Boston, MA 02115, USA
[1] Co-first authors.
[2] Co-senior authors.
* Corresponding author.
E-mail address: hsg2138@cumc.columbia.edu

Clin Chest Med 44 (2023) 179–190
https://doi.org/10.1016/j.ccm.2022.11.001

Table 1 Noninfectious thoracic complications after lung transplantation	
Airway Complications	Anastomotic stenosis/ stricture Anastomotic dehiscence Anastomotic granulation Anastomotic fistula Bronchomalacia Distal bronchial stenosis Airway torsion
Native Lung	Native lung hyperinflation (NLH) Progression of pulmonary fibrosis Pneumothorax Malignancy
Vascular	Pulmonary embolism Pulmonary artery stenosis Pulmonary artery kinking Pulmonary vein obstruction Vascular torsion
Pleural/Diaphragm	Diaphragm dysfunction Pleural effusion (hemothorax, empyema, chylothorax) Pneumothorax Trapped lung (fibrothorax)
Allograft	Primary graft dysfunction Rejection Primary disease recurrence Malignancy Drug induced lung injury

seems protective unless there is donor-to-recipient airway size mismatch when telescoping anastomosis is preferred.

Computed tomography may reveal signs of airway complications; however, direct visualization with bronchoscopy is essential for diagnosis and management.

Anastomotic Ischemia, Necrosis, Dehiscence, and Fistula Formation

A Consensus Statement by the International Society for Heart and Lung Transplantation (ISHLT) classifies airway complications as ischemia/necrosis, dehiscence, stenosis, and malacia.[6] The severity of each category is based on location and extent (**Table 2**). The incidence of anastomotic dehiscence, which usually occurs within the first 6 weeks of transplantation, ranges between 1% and 10%.[6] Symptoms of anastomotic complications can range from none to severe. Those with significant dehiscence may present with persistent air leak, pneumothorax, pneumomediastinum, subcutaneous emphysema, sepsis, and fistula formation, such as bronchopleural, bronchoesophageal, bronchovascular, and bronchomediastinal fistulas. Complete anastomotic dehiscence is rare but can cause fatal hemorrhage.[4] Airway necrosis or dehiscence without persistent air leak can be managed conservatively (**Fig. 1**). Drainage and antimicrobial therapy are the main treatments for fistula formation. Frequent bronchoscopy and/or radiological follow-up to assess progression should be entertained based on the severity of necrosis. One study reported 84% success rate with conservative management alone.[4] Successful treatment of dehiscence has been reported with the use of uncovered self-expanding metallic stents that promote granulation platforms for healing[7]; this is preferred over silicone stenting, as it does not block the airway and allows for secretion drainage. Metallic stents are typically removed after 4 to 6 weeks to avoid excessive granulation (**Fig. 2**). Surgery ranging from simple anastomotic repair to transplant pneumonectomy is required in those with severe dehiscence.[4] Bronchovascular fistula is usually fatal due to abrupt massive hemoptysis but has been successfully treated with pneumonectomy.[8]

Exophytic Granulation Tissue

Significant airway obstruction from exophytic granulation tissue occurs in up to 20% of transplant recipients.[9] Cryodebridement and mechanical debridement with forceps offers a benefit of recanalization without inflammation as opposed to intervention with neodymium-yttrium-aluminum-garnet laser, argon plasma, or electrocautery that may cause inflammation but are useful in controlling bleeding following cryotherapy.[7]

Bronchial Stenosis

Bronchial stenosis (**Fig. 3**) is the most common airway complication, occurring in up to 24% of recipients within the first year.[7] It usually affects the anastomosis but occasionally airways distal to the anastomosis, especially the bronchus intermedius, known as vanishing bronchus intermedius syndrome. Serial balloon bronchoplasty repeated every few weeks (2–3 times) is often successful, especially if performed in conjunction with radial

Table 2
ISHLT adult airway complications after lung transplant[6]

Ischemia and Necrosis (I)		
Location	a.	Within 1 cm of anastomosis
	b.	>1 cm from anastomosis extending to major airways (BI/distal mainstem)
	c.	>1 cm from anastomosis extending to lobar or segmental airways
Extent	a.	<50% circumferential ischemia
	b.	>50% circumferential ischemia
	c.	<50% circumferential necrosis
	d.	>50% circumferential necrosis
Dehiscence (D)		
Location	a.	Cartilaginous
	b.	Membranous
	c.	Both
Extent	a.	0%−25% of circumference
	b.	>25%–50% of circumference
	c.	>50%–75% of circumference
	d.	>75% of circumference
Stenosis (S)		
Location	a.	Anastomotic
	b.	Anastomotic plus lobar/segmental
	c.	Lobar/segmental only
Extent	a.	0%–25% reduction in cross-sectional area
	b.	>25%–50% reduction in cross-sectional area
	c.	>50% but <100% reduction in cross-sectional area
	d.	100% obstruction
Malacia (M)		
Location	a.	Within 1 cm of anastomosis
	b.	Diffuse involving anastomosis and extending beyond 1 cm

Crespo MM, McCarthy DP, Hopkins PM, et al. ISHLT Consensus Statement on adult and pediatric airway complications after lung transplantation: Definitions, grading system, and therapeutics. J Heart Lung Transplant 2018;37(5):548-563.

incision, cryotherapy, and local steroid injection.[10] In patients with critically narrow anastomosis and symptomatic, especially on single lung transplant recipients, failing multiple dilations, the use of stents may be indicated. Silicone stents are preferred over metallic stents in those with refractory stenosis, as they can be customized and easily deployed and removed. Those with bronchial diameter less than 12 mm may require self-expanding metallic stent placement until a silicone stent can be placed.[7] The optimal duration for the stent is unknown but has been reported in the range of 6 to 12 months.[4,7] On rare occasions, surgical intervention such as anastomotic reconstruction, sleeve resection, or even retransplantation may be required.[7,11]

Bronchomalacia

Bronchomalacia may be defined as expiratory luminal collapse of greater than 70% in diameter.[12] Malacia can be localized to the anastomosis or can be diffuse, affecting more commonly the longer native left-side bronchus. Pulmonary hygiene and nocturnal noninvasive positive pressure ventilation are essential for those who are symptomatic. In refractory cases with feasible anatomy, silicone stenting is preferred over metallic stenting to promote airway remodeling. The duration for therapeutic stenting has been proposed as 9 to 12 months.[7] If a metallic stent is used, it should be removed in 4 to 6 weeks to avoid excessive granulation. Surgical treatments are typically not recommended.[7]

Native Lung and Thoracic Complications in Single Lung Transplant Recipients

Limited data exist regarding native lung complications after single lung transplantation. The most common complications include hyperinflation of a native lung with emphysema or chronic obstructive pulmonary disease, development of malignancy (discussed later), progression of pulmonary fibrosis in the native lung, and diaphragm dysfunction.[13,14]

Native Lung Hyperinflation

After lung transplantation for chronic obstructive pulmonary disease (COPD)/emphysema, native lung hyperinflation (NLH) can occur in up to one-third of those receiving a SLTxp.[15] Native lung compliance in patients with COPD is much higher when compared with the newly transplanted allograft, a differential that can worsen ventilation perfusion mismatch. The risk of NLH increases with development of primary graft dysfunction (PGD), underlying severe pretransplant airflow obstruction with hyperinflation and pretransplant pulmonary hypertension (**Fig. 4**). NLH can manifest with posttransplant hemodynamic instability from decreased preload, radiographic diaphragm flattening, and mediastinal shift toward the new

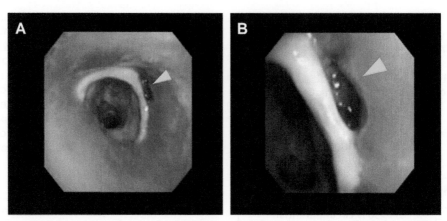

Fig. 1. Airway dehiscence: (*A*) A small defect is observed on the anterior aspect of the left anastomosis (*green arrowhead*); (*B*) closer photograph reveals suture material inside the defect. (This was managed conservatively with complete healing).

allograft, resulting in restriction of the allograft and worsening respiratory failure.[15] Lung volume reduction peritransplant has been associated with longer hospitalization, longer operative times, and higher rate of perioperative and postoperative complications (bleeding, renal failure, phrenic nerve injury, diminished peak lung function, and 6-minute walk distance posttransplant) without survival benefit.[16,17] Management of NLH should focus on prevention. Effective measures include lung protective ventilation, minimizing positive end expiratory pressure, early extubation, bronchodilation, chest physiotherapy, and early mobilization. Therapeutic bronchoscopy can be used to clear secretions and mucous plugs, and placement of endobronchial coils, valves, or bronchial

blockers in select cases helps decrease hyperinflation.[18–20] Donor allograft sizing in a hyperinflated chest should be optimized.[15] In cases of severe PGD following single lung transplantation for COPD, early utilization of veno-venous extracorporeal membrane oxygenation support with low pressure ventilator settings or rarely independent lung ventilation may be necessary.

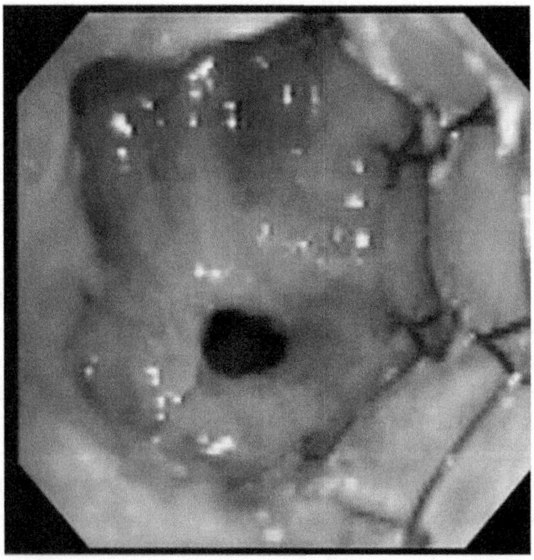

Progression of Native Lung Pulmonary Fibrosis

The data on progression of pulmonary fibrosis are limited to single-center case studies. Pulmonary fibrosis can rapidly progress or be exacerbated by a new insult after SLTxp. Gas exchange does not seem affected by progression of native lung fibrosis.[21,22] In a study of 21 patients, the rate of disease progression was estimated at 11% per year based on radiographic assessments.[21]

Diaphragm Dysfunction

The incidence of diaphragm dysfunction in lung transplant recipients ranges from 2.8% to 40%.[23–25] Multiple mechanisms of injury are at play, including ischemic, thermal, stretch, or transection type injuries to the phrenic nerve during lung transplant surgery. Critical illness–related polyneuropathy, myopathy, and disuse atrophy from prolonged ventilation can also result in a weak diaphragm.[26,27] Other risk factors include use of cardiopulmonary bypass and extracorporeal life support.[24,26] The diaphragmatic dysfunction or paralysis related to the surgical procedure is more commonly unilateral versus the dysfunction related to myopathy, critical illness, or prolonged mechanical ventilation that is often bilateral. Diagnosis rests on clinical suspicion, particularly in

Fig. 2. Excessive granulation tissue complicating metallic bronchial stent.

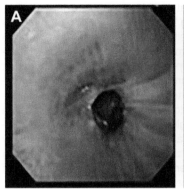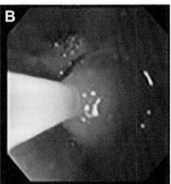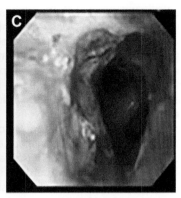

Fig. 3. Bronchial anastomotic stenosis. (*A*) Severe stenosis of left bronchial anastomosis; (*B*) balloon dilatation in process; (*C*) major improvement in anastomotic caliber with visible suture material after balloon dilatation.

patients who have unexplained ventilator dependence. The diagnosis can typically be established with bedside ultrasonography or fluoroscopy during spontaneous breathing (which can be routinely done during the initial surveillance bronchoscopies). Other complementary tests include upright and supine pulmonary function testing, measurement of transdiaphragmatic pressures, and nerve conduction studies with diaphragmatic electromyographic evaluation.[26]

Lung transplant recipients with bilateral diaphragm dysfunction may require prolonged mechanical ventilatory support and have decreased

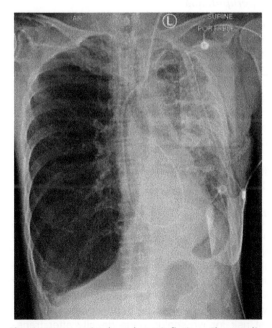

Fig. 4. Acute native lung hyperinflation. Chest radiograph discloses right-sided native lung hyperinflation with mediastinal displacement to the left in a patient who received left single lung transplantation for advanced bullous emphysema and developed primary graft dysfunction.

survival.[24,26,27] The impact on quality of life and survival is more significant in patients with single lung transplantation. Diaphragmatic dysfunction can take up to a year to recover; noninvasive ventilation can be used to help provide respiratory support for those liberated from invasive mechanical ventilation.[26,27] Surgical intervention with plication or diaphragmatic pacing strategies have a limited role with possible benefit in carefully selected patients.[28,29]

Pleural Complications

Pleural complications occur in up to half of all lung transplant recipients.[30–32] Those with pleural complications have worse long-term outcomes.[32] Such complications include pneumothorax, hemothorax, chylothorax, infection, inflammation/rejection, malignancy, or vascular pleural complications.[32–34] Pleural effusion can occur early or late after transplantation.[32,33] Early postoperative pleural effusions are related to poor drainage mechanisms and usually resolve within 2 weeks of transplantation.[30,34,35] Early perioperative management includes chest tube placement in all lung transplant recipients. Other interventions include thoracentesis and chronic pleural drainage catheters.[32] Late pleural effusions (effusions after the immediate postoperative period) with a lymphocytic predominance, as high as 90%, are often associated with acute cellular rejection in the correct clinical setting. Chylothorax has also been described in the lung transplant population.

Pneumothorax is extremely common in the early postoperative period and may be accompanied by prolonged air leak and subcutaneous emphysema. A feared complication early posttransplant remains development of bronchopleural fistula and anastomotic dehiscence.[30,31,34,35] However, most pneumothoraces resolve with expectant management and chest tube drainage in the perioperative period.[34] Rarely, some require further bronchoscopic or surgical intervention.

Hemothorax can occur early after surgery and can lead to hemodynamic derangement requiring medical support and surgical reexploration in up to half of these patients.[36] Patients with hemodynamic instability, multiple transfusions, and evidence of active bleeding often require early surgical exploration for local control of the bleeding source and to avoid the deleterious effects of multiple blood transfusions and vasopressor; this can lead to prolonged intensive care unit stay, ventilator dependence, and can affect both short-term and long-term graft and survival outcomes.[36]

Chylous effusions can occur in a small number of lung transplant recipients (<2%) from injury to the thoracic duct or its tributaries.[37] Diagnostic studies will reveal pleural fluid triglycerides greater than 110 mg/dL. Definitive management is lymphoscintigraphy and ductal embolization.[38] Medical management includes a very low-fat diet, or support with total parenteral nutrition and elimination of enteral nutrition, and octreotide. Surgical options are pleurodesis and shunting of chyle to the peritoneal space or into the venous system.[37,39,40] Sirolimus can be helpful after healing of the anastomosis in patients with underlying lymphangioleiomyomatosis.[39,41]

EXTRATHORACIC COMPLICATIONS IN LUNG TRANSPLANTATION
Diabetes Mellitus

Posttransplant diabetes mellitus (PTDM) is common after lung transplantation with prevalence of 19.1% and 33.3% at 1 and 5 years, respectively.[2] The diagnostic criteria are similar to that of the general population. Transient hyperglycemia is common due to high-dose steroid therapy in the early transplant phase and for treatment of rejection and should be distinguished from PTDM. PTDM diagnosis should be made as an outpatient when the patient is on maintenance dose of immunosuppression.[42] Hemoglobin A1C may have reduced sensitivity especially early after transplant due to medication-induced hyperglycemia or anemia related to blood loss. Early initiation of insulin for transient hyperglycemia may prevent the development of PTDM.[43] Once insulin requirements decrease, oral hypoglycemic agents can be used to control PTDM. Tacrolimus can be associated with worsening glycemic control, with few patients needing transition to cyclosporine.

Hypertension

Fifty percent of patients develop hypertension by the first year after lung transplantation.[44] The suggested goal for blood pressure is less than 130/80 mm Hg.[45] The treatment choice depends on the clinical situation in distinct phases of transplant. For example, β-blockers are useful in patients with hypertension and atrial arrhythmia, which occurs in 30% to 50% in the early posttransplant setting.[46] Inhibition of the renin-angiotensin-aldosterone system may contribute to decreasing glomerular filtration rate, hyperkalemia as well as anemia, all of which are commonly encountered in the posttransplant setting. Calcium channel blockers (CCB) are, therefore, preferred over angiotensin-converting enzyme inhibitor, angiotensin receptor blocker, or renin inhibitor therapies.[47] In addition, CCB may counteract renal vasoconstriction caused by calcineurin inhibitors (CNI).[48] CCB therapy, especially nondihydropyridine such as diltiazem, may result in increased CNI levels, which warrants close monitoring. Other classes of antihypertensives such as α-blockers, central alpha-2 agonists, direct vasodilators, and diuretics may be considered or added in cases of refractory hypertension or if dictated by other clinical situations. Secondary hypertension, especially that due to posterior reversible leukoencephalopathy syndrome caused by CNI, should be considered in those with refractory or severe hypertension.

Hyperlipidemia

More than half of the patients develop hyperlipidemia at 5 years posttransplantation.[44] Treatment of hyperlipidemia would benefit long-term cardiovascular outcomes. However, given a median survival of lung transplant recipients of 10.2 years (conditional to survival for 1 year),[2] the benefit of treating hyperlipidemia remains debatable. Nonetheless, management guidelines used for the nontransplant population are usually used. If tolerated, treatment before transplantation is continued but drug-drug interactions especially with CCB and CNI deserve special attention.

Bone Disease

Because of advanced age, medication use, especially steroids, and comorbidities such as chronic obstructive pulmonary disease, osteopenia and osteoporosis are found in one-third of those who are referred for lung transplantation.[49] Those with low bone density pretransplant are at greatest risk for worsening bone density after transplantation.[49] Risk factors include CNI use, which increases bone resorption. Steroids reduce bone formation and intestinal calcium absorption while increasing bone resorption and renal calcium wasting. Azathioprine and mycophenolate have no effect on bone health, whereas sirolimus and everolimus reduce bone resorption. In addition, CNI-related chronic kidney disease could complicate bone health. Rates of bone loss and fractures are highest in the first year after transplantation related to immobilization and higher steroid dose requirements.[49] Hence, prevention and treatment should be used early. Management mimics that of postmenopausal osteoporosis.[50] Prophylactic calcium and vitamin D as well as regular exercise are encouraged. Further treatment with antiresorptive and bone anabolic agents is often necessary, but hypocalcemia and hypovitaminosis D should be corrected before initiation of those agents. Both oral and intravenous bisphosphonates are effective in preventing bone loss,[49] although their use may be limited in those with renal dysfunction, where denosumab or bone anabolic agents are more appropriate. Treatment should be individualized. For instance, oral bisphosphonate is irritative to the mucosa and should be avoided in those with gastroesophageal reflux disease or gastric bypass. Intravenous antiresorptive bisphosphonate and denosumab have the advantage of longer intervals between doses. Bone anabolic agents teriparatide, abaloparatide, and romosozumab are given subcutaneously to those with severe osteoporosis and extremely high risk of fracture.[50] Abaloparatide may cause severe hyperuricemia. Romosozumab, a sclerostin inhibitor, is the newest and most potent bone anabolic agent; however, due to association with increased cardiovascular death, it should not be used in those with myocardial ischemia/infarction or stroke in the previous year.[50] Other treatments such as estrogen, raloxifene, tibolone, or calcitonin have been used in the transplant population, but the evidence is limited.[51–53] Bone density with dual radiograph absorptiometry is recommended every 1 to 3 years.[50]

Acute Kidney Injury

The incidence of acute kidney injury (AKI) perioperatively/postoperatively can be as high as 80% and varies widely among studies depending on the diagnostic criteria used.[54–59] AKI in the immediate posttransplant period is associated with increased hospital length of stay, longer duration of mechanical ventilation, risk of developing chronic kidney disease (CKD), and increased mortality.[1,60–62] Renal replacement therapy is needed in 5% to 8% of recipients after developing perioperative AKI, and this cohort has a nearly 10-fold increased risk of 30-day and greater than 5-fold increased risk of 1-year mortality.[61] It is important

to reassess renal function and transplant candidacy regularly for candidates at risk of developing AKI and CKD.[55,61] Glomerular filtration rate (GFR) can be overestimated in those with poor nutritional status or muscle wasting.[63] Early involvement of nephrology consultants for accurate diagnosis and classification of renal dysfunction should be entertained.[64]

A modified surgical approach avoiding the use of intraoperative cardiopulmonary bypass, if possible, should be considered. Multidisciplinary engagement with surgery, anesthesiology, and perfusion teams can help optimize renal perfusion during surgery. Appropriate fluid and hemodynamic resuscitation strategies in all phases of care are essential. Alteration of immunosuppressive regimens may allow delay in the initiation of nephrotoxic CNI therapy in at-risk lung transplant recipients. Appropriate selection and dosing of medications should be used with involvement of transplant pharmacy.[56]

Chronic Kidney Disease

CKD is a well-established complication after lung transplantation. CKD is defined as structural abnormalities on imaging or decreased function for more than 3 months according to Kidney Disease Improving Global Outcomes (KDIGO) guidelines. The most recent SRTR report showed the incidence of CKD, defined as creatinine greater than >2.5 mg/dL or need for renal replacement therapy or renal transplant, to be 6.2% at 1 year and 17.3% at 5 years.[1] The incidence of doubling of serum creatinine as a marker for CKD is 34% at 1 year and 53% at 5 years after transplantation in the SRTR report.[58,59] AKI remains the most important risk factor for CKD.[54,65] Early decline in GFR in the first month after lung transplantation can predict CKD.[65]

CKD management rests on prevention of postoperative AKI and targeted management of risk factors after transplant. Both preoperative and postoperative hypertension and calcineurin use are important contributors to CKD.[59,66,67] Avoidance of nephrotoxic medications, preventing CNI-induced insults, and transition to alternative immunosuppression strategies while balancing the adverse effects and risk of rejection with this strategy are important in mitigating the risk of CKD (these alternatives and medications are discussed in more detail in the immunosuppression article in this issue).[68,69] BK polyomavirus nephropathy remains an underdiagnosed cause of native kidney disease.[70] It is increasingly being recognized as a potential culprit for worsening renal function in lung transplant recipients.[70]

Involving a nephrologist in management of these patients may be helpful, and in select cases with advanced CKD, renal transplantation may be considered.

Malignancy

Among lung transplant recipients who survive more than 5 years, malignancy is the second most common cause of death after bronchiolitis obliterans syndrome, accounting for approximately 17% of deaths.[2] This section focuses on the most common malignancies in this population, including posttransplant lymphoproliferative disorder (PTLD), cutaneous squamous cell carcinoma (SCC) and lung cancer.[71,72]

POSTTRANSPLANT LYMPHOPROLIFERATIVE DISORDER

PTLD affects 1.8% to 9.4% of lung transplant recipients. The incidence may be as high as 20% to 30% in Epstein-Barr virus (EBV)-seronegative recipients who receive lungs from EBV-seropositive donors (EBV D+/R−).[72,73] About 60.8% of those with EBV D+/R− serostatus who develop PTLD do so within the first posttransplant year.[73] Most of these early PTLDs originate from B lymphocytes of the recipient, are EBV-related, often involve the lung allograft, and respond to reduction in immunosuppression.[72,74] Late PTLDs occurring beyond the first year of lung transplantation are typically T-cell and natural killer–cell derived. Late PTLD is more likely to be EBV-negative, extrapulmonary, and may be disseminated at the time of diagnosis.[72]

PTLD can be found incidentally or present with symptoms specific to organ involved and with type B symptoms. Nodular (single or multiple) findings on radiologic images with or without effusion may be seen with intrathoracic PTLD.[75] Patients may also present with secondary symptoms including strokelike presentation with central nervous system involvement, urinary infection with sepsis in case of bladder outlet obstruction, and new-onset cough in case of lung involvement or abdominal symptoms with gastrointestinal PTLD.[75,76] The initial steps in management of PTLD involve reduction in immunosuppression and obtaining oncology consultation.[75] Anti-B-cell therapy, chemotherapy, and radiation have demonstrated significant treatment benefit.[77,78]

Skin Cancer

Skin cancer is the most common malignancy after lung transplantation. The cumulative incidence of skin cancer is 31% at 5 years and 47% at 10 years.[79] The most common skin cancers include SCC and basal cell carcinoma (BCC), accounting for 95% of all skin cancers.[75,80] Cutaneous SCC and BCC primarily affect the sun exposed areas. BCC favors face and upper torso, and SCC tends to involve arms along with upper torso and face.[75] Cutaneous SCC in lung transplant recipients can be poorly differentiated and invasive.[81] The risk of recurrence and metastatic disease in lung transplant recipients after treatment of cutaneous SCC at 1.5 years can be as high as 14% and 8%, respectively.[81]

In those with a diagnosis of skin cancer, reduction in the intensity of immunosuppression is commonly considered.[75] Prolonged fungal prophylaxis or treatment with voriconazole has been associated with an increased risk of SCC.[82] In skin cancers, resection or destructive techniques, such as Mohs procedure, are available for treatment.[75] Other therapies include topical treatments and systemic therapies. A multidisciplinary approach with early involvement of dermatology, oncology, and surgery specialists when indicated and close monitoring should be used to ensure optimal outcomes.

Lung Cancer

After lung transplant lung cancers may develop as a recurrence of the recipient's primary lung cancer, can occur in the allograft as donor transmitted or de novo malignancy, or develop de novo in the native lung. Lung cancer may also be seen as an incidental finding in the explanted lung with later metastatic recurrence in the recipient. In a study by Triplette and colleagues, the incidence of lung cancer was 5-fold higher in lung transplant recipients compared with general population.[83] In the same study, SLTxp recipients had a 13-fold higher lung cancer incidence, with most occurring in the native lung.[83] The median time to diagnosis was 3.9 years posttransplant.[83] Patients aged 50 to 80 years, who had a 20 or more pack-year history of smoking and had quit less than 15 years before listing for transplantation, are considered at high risk for developing malignancy. The additional risk of immunosuppression contributing to risk of lung cancer in the native lung should be a consideration in the listing decision for a bilateral lung transplant.

Both small cell and non–small cell carcinoma can present with constitutional symptoms such as anorexia, fatigue, and weight loss or with pulmonary symptoms including new-onset cough, dyspnea, chest pain, or rarely hemoptysis. The presentation may also be asymptomatic with incidental finding of lung nodule or lymphadenopathy on routine chest imaging.[75] Lung cancer can progress rapidly due to immunosuppression, and this presentation can mimic infection.[84,85] Diagnostic and staging strategies remain similar to the non-transplant population but may be limited due to nodal resection at the time of transplantation.[75] Curative resection should be attempted when possible.[75] Therapeutic options are limited by recipient comorbidities such as CKD or cytopenia and in the case of immune checkpoint inhibitors, increased risk of rejection.[72,75] Reduction in immunosuppression, as with PTLD and skin cancers, is commonly undertaken, although benefits remain unclear.[72,75]

SUMMARY

Lung transplant outcomes continue to be affected by common noninfectious thoracic and extrathoracic complications. Common thoracic complications include airway, native lung disease–specific complications, diaphragm dysfunction, and pleural complications. Common extrathoracic complications include diabetes mellitus, lipid disorders, bone disease, hypertension, both acute and chronic kidney disease, and malignancy. Prevention, early detection, and evidence-based disease-specific management strategies with ongoing close follow-up remain key to survival.

CLINICS CARE POINTS

- The incidence of airway complications ranges between 7% and 18%, and direct visualization with bronchoscopy is essential for diagnosis and management planning.
- Native lung hyperinflation in patients receiving lung transplantation for COPD occurs in up to a third of the patients. Effective management measures include lung protective ventilation, minimizing positive end expiratory pressure, early extubation, bronchodilators and chest physiotherapy, therapeutic bronchoscopy, and liberal use of extracorporeal membrane oxygenation (ECMO) and independent lung ventilation.
- Diaphragm dysfunction can occur from multiple mechanisms of injury including thermal, stretch, ischemia or nerve transection. The impact on quality of life and survival is more significant in single lung transplant recipients. It can take up to one year for the diaphragm to recover in those with preserved phrenic nerve function.

- Pleural complications occur in up to half of all lung transplant recipients and include pneumothorax, hemothorax, empyema, effusion due to rejection, malignancy and chylothorax and are associated with worse long-term outcomes.
- Common extra thoracic complications include post-transplant diabetes mellitus (19.1% in the first year), hypertension (between 30 to 50% within the first year), hyperlipidemia (26.7% in the first year), and bone disease (already present in up to a third of pre lung transplant patients at time of transplantation).
- Acute Kidney Injury (AKI) is observed frequently in patients receiving lung transplantation with 5% to 8% requiring renal replacement therapy after developing perioperative AKI.
- Chronic Kidney disease (CKD) is a common complication after lung transplantation and is usually caused by chronic exposure to calcineurin inhibitors. Its management rests on prevention of post-operative AKI, therapeutic drug monitoring and targeted management of risk factors.
- Malignancy is the second most common cause of death after chronic rejection in recipients who survive more than 5 years after lung transplantation and accounts for 17.1% of all mortality.

DISCLOSURES

None of the authors have any commercial or financial conflicts of interest or funding associated with this project.

REFERENCES

1. Valapour M, Lehr CJ, Skeans MA, et al. OPTN/SRTR 2019 annual data report: lung. Am J Transpl 2021; 21(S2):441–520.
2. Chambers DC, Cherikh WS, Harhay MO. The international thoracic organ transplant registry of the international society for heart and lung transplantation: thirty-sixth adult lung and heart-lung transplantation report – 2019; focus theme: donor and recipient size match. J Heart Lung Transpl 2019;38(10):1042–55.
3. Guthaner DF, Wexler L, Sadeghi AM, et al. Revascularization of tracheal anastomosis following heart—lung transplantation. Invest Radiol 1983;18(6): 500–3.
4. Yserbyt J, Dooms C, Vos R, et al. Anastomotic airway complications after lung transplantation: risk factors, treatment modalities and outcome—a

single-centre experience. Eur J Cardiothorac Surg 2016;49(1):e1–8.

5. Santacruz JF, Mehta AC. Airway complications and management after lung transplantation: ischemia, dehiscence, and stenosis. Proc Am Thorac Soc 2009;6(1):79–93.

6. Crespo MM, McCarthy DP, Hopkins PM, et al. ISHLT consensus statement on adult and pediatric airway complications after lung transplantation: Definitions, grading system, and therapeutics. J Heart Lung Transplant 2018;37(5):548–63.

7. Mahajan AK, Folch E, Khandhar SJ, et al. The diagnosis and management of airway complications following lung transplantation. Chest 2017;152(3): 627–38.

8. Rea F, Marulli G, Loy M, et al. Salvage right pneumonectomy in a patient with bronchial–pulmonary artery fistula after bilateral sequential lung transplantation. J Heart Lung Transplant 2006; 25(11):1383–6.

9. Tendulkar RD, Fleming PA, Reddy CA, et al. High-dose-rate endobronchial brachytherapy for recurrent airway obstruction from hyperplastic granulation tissue. Int J Radiat Oncology*Biology*Physics 2008; 70(3):701–6.

10. Tremblay A, Coulter TD, Mehta AC. Modification of a mucosal-sparing technique using electrocautery and balloon dilatation in the endoscopic management of web-like benign airway stenosis. J Bronchology Interv Pulmonology 2003;10(4):268–71.

11. Marulli G, Loy M, Rizzardi G, et al. Surgical treatment of posttransplant bronchial stenoses: case reports. Transplant Proc 2007;39(6):1973–5.

12. Ridge CA, O'Donnell CR, Lee EY, et al. Tracheobronchomalacia: current concepts and controversies. J Thorac Imaging 2011;26(4):278–89.

13. Gonzalez FJ, Alvarez E, Moreno P, et al. The influence of the native lung on early outcomes and survival after single lung transplantation. PLOS ONE 2021;16(4):e0249758.

14. Sekulovski M, Simonska B, Peruhova M, et al. Factors affecting complications development and mortality after single lung transplant. WJT 2021;11(8): 320–34.

15. Siddiqui FM, Diamond JM. Lung transplantation for chronic obstructive pulmonary disease: past, present, and future directions. Curr Opin Pulm Med 2018;24(2):199–204.

16. Backhus L, Sargent J, Cheng A, et al. Outcomes in lung transplantation after previous lung volume reduction surgery in a contemporary cohort. J Thorac Cardiovasc Surg 2014;147(5):1678–83.e1.

17. Shigemura N, Gilbert S, Bhama JK, et al. Lung transplantation after lung volume reduction surgery. Transplantation 2013;96(4):421–5.

18. Perch M, Riise GC, Hogarth K, et al. Endoscopic treatment of native lung hyperinflation using endobronchial valves in single-lung transplant patients: a multinational experience: endobronchial valves in lung transplants. Clin Respir J 2015;9(1): 104–10.

19. Shehata IM, Elhassan A, Urits I, et al. Postoperative management of hyperinflated native lung in single-lung transplant recipients with chronic obstructive pulmonary disease: a review article. Pulm Ther 2021;7(1):37–46.

20. Grewal HS, Mehta AC. Emphysema management: from investigational endobronchial coils to lung transplantation. Am J Respir Crit Care Med 2018; 198(3):e14.

21. Elicker BM, Golden JA, Ordovas KG, et al. Progression of native lung fibrosis in lung transplant recipients with idiopathic pulmonary fibrosis. Respir Med 2010;104(3):426–33.

22. Grgic A, Lausberg H, Heinrich M, et al. Progression of fibrosis in usual interstitial pneumonia: serial evaluation of the native lung after single lung transplantation. Respiration 2008;76(2):139–45.

23. Hernández-Hernández MA, Sánchez-Moreno L, Orizaola P, et al. A prospective evaluation of phrenic nerve injury after lung transplantation: incidence, risk factors, and analysis of the surgical procedure. J Heart Lung Transplant 2022;41(1):50–60.

24. Shigemura N, D'Cunha J, Bhama J, et al. Diaphragm dysfunction following lung transplantation: the largest single-center experience. Chest 2013; 144(4):1009A.

25. Soetanto V, Grewal US, Mehta AC, et al. Early postoperative complications in lung transplant recipients. Indian J Thorac Cardiovasc Surg 2021. https://doi.org/10.1007/s12055-021-01178-1.

26. McCool FD, Tzelepis GE. Dysfunction of the diaphragm. N Engl J Med 2012;366(10):932–42.

27. LoMauro A, Righi I, Privitera E, et al. The impaired diaphragmatic function after bilateral lung transplantation: a multifactorial longitudinal study. J Heart Lung Transplant 2020;39(8):795–804.

28. Rappaport JM, Tang A, Siddiqui HU, et al. Diaphragm plication helps salvage allograft function in lung transplant patients with diaphragm dysfunction. J Am Coll Surgeons 2021;233(5):e188.

29. Onders R, Elgudin Y, Abu-Omar Y, et al. Diaphragm pacing in lung transplant patients: to identify and treat diaphragm function abnormalities. J Heart Lung Transplant 2021;40(4):S316–7.

30. Ferrer J, Roldan J, Roman A, et al. Acute and chronic pleural complications in lung transplantation. J Heart Lung Transplant 2003;22(11):1217–25.

31. Herridge MS, de Hoyos AL, Chaparro C, et al. Pleural complications in lung transplant recipients. J Thorac Cardiovasc Surg 1995;110(1):22–6.

32. Tang A, Siddiqui HU, Thuita L, et al. Natural history of pleural complications after lung transplantation. Ann Thorac Surg 2021;111(2):407–15.

33. Rappaport JM, Siddiqui HU, Tang A, et al. Pleural space management after lung transplant: early and late outcomes of pleural decortication. J Heart Lung Transplant 2021;40(7):623–30.

34. Garrido G, Dhillon GS. Medical course and complications after lung transplantation. In: Sher Y, Maldonado JR, editors. Psychosocial care of end-stage organ disease and transplant patients. Cham: Springer; 2019. p. 279–88.

35. Arndt A, Boffa DJ. Pleural space complications associated with lung transplantation. Thorac Surg Clin 2015;25(1):87–95.

36. Hong A, King CS, Brown AWW, et al. Hemothorax following lung transplantation: incidence, risk factors, and effect on morbidity and mortality. Multidiscip Respir Med 2016;11:40.

37. Jacob S, Meneses A, Landolfo K, et al. Incidence, management, and outcomes of chylothorax after lung transplantation: a single-center experience. Cureus 2019. https://doi.org/10.7759/cureus.5190.

38. Jacob S, Ali M, El-Sayed Ahmed MM, et al. Refractory chylous effusions in lymphangioleiomyomatosis patient post lung transplant. SAGE Open Med Case Rep 2020;8. 2050313X2092133.

39. Nakagiri T, Shintani Y, Minami M, et al. Lung transplantation for lymphangioleiomyomatosis in a single Japanese institute, with a focus on late-onset complications. Transplant Proc 2015;47(6):1977–82.

40. Fremont RD, Milstone AP, Light RW, et al. Chylothoraces after lung transplantation for lymphangioleiomyomatosis: review of the literature and utilization of a pleurovenous shunt. J Heart Lung Transpl 2007;26(9):953–5.

41. Ohara T, Oto T, Miyoshi K, et al. Sirolimus ameliorated post lung transplant chylothorax in lymphangioleiomyomatosis. Ann Thorac Surg 2008;86(6): e7–8.

42. American Diabetes Association. 7. Diabetes technology: standards of medical care in diabetes—2021. Diabetes Care 2021;44(Supplement_1): S85–99.

43. Hecking M, Haidinger M, Döller D. Early basal insulin therapy decreases new-onset diabetes after renal transplantation. J Am Soc Nephrol 2012;23(4): 739–49.

44. Yusen RD, Edwards LB, Dipchand AI. The registry of the international society for heart and lung transplantation: thirty-third adult lung and heart-lung transplant report – 2016; focus theme: primary diagnostic indications for transplant. J Heart Lung Transpl 2016;35(10):1170–84.

45. Whelton PK, Carey RM, Aronow WS. ACC/AHA/AAPA/ABC/ACPM/AGS/APhA/ASH/ASPC/NMA/PCNA guideline for the prevention, detection, evaluation, and management of high blood pressure in adults: executive summary: a report of the american college of cardiology/american heart association task force on clinical practice guidelines. Hypertension 2017;71(6):1269–324.

46. Fan J KZ, S L. Incidence, risk factors and prognosis of postoperative atrial arrhythmias after lung transplantation: a systematic review and meta-analysis. Interact Cardiovasc Thorac Surg 2016;23(5):790–9.

47. Cross NB, Webster AC, Masson P. Antihypertensives for kidney transplant recipients: systematic review and meta-analysis of randomized controlled trials. Transplantation 2009;Jul;88(1):7–18.

48. Grześk G. Calcium blockers inhibit cyclosporine A-induced hyperreactivity of vascular smooth muscle cells. Mol Med Rep 2012. https://doi.org/10.3892/mmr.2012.847.

49. Wang TKM, O'Sullivan S, Gamble GD, et al. Bone density in heart or lung transplant recipients-a longitudinal study. Transplant Proc 2013;45(6):2357–65.

50. Shoback D, Rosen CJ, Black DM, et al. Pharmacological management of osteoporosis in postmenopausal women: an endocrine society guideline update. J Clin Endocrinol Metab 2020;105(3): 587–94.

51. Kulak CAM, Borba VZC, Kulak Júnior J, et al. Bone disease after transplantation: osteoporosis and fractures risk. Arq Bras Endocrinol Metab 2014;58(5): 484–92.

52. Lan GB, Xie XB, Peng LK, et al. Long. current status of research on osteoporosis after solid organ transplantation: pathogenesis and management. Biomed Res Int 2015;2015:1–10.

53. Kapetanakis EI, Antonopoulos AS, Antoniou TA, et al. Effect of long-term calcitonin administration on steroid-induced osteoporosis after cardiac transplantation. J Heart Lung Transplant 2005;24(5):526–32.

54. Lertjitbanjong P, Thongprayoon C, Cheungpasitporn W, et al. Acute kidney injury after lung transplantation: a systematic review and meta-analysis. JCM 2019;8(10):1713.

55. Puttarajappa CM, Bernardo JF, Kellum JA. Renal complications following lung transplantation and heart transplantation. Crit Care Clin 2019;35(1): 61–73.

56. Du WW, Wang XX, Zhang D, et al. Retrospective analysis on incidence and risk factors of early onset acute kidney injury after lung transplantation and its association with mortality. Ren Fail 2021;43(1): 535–42.

57. Chaudhry R, Wanderer JP, Mubashir T, et al. Incidence and predictive factors of acute kidney injury after off-pump lung transplantation. J Cardiothorac Vasc Anesth 2022;36(1):93–9.

58. Hingorani S. Chronic kidney disease after liver, cardiac, lung, heart–lung, and hematopoietic stem cell transplant. Pediatr Nephrol 2008;23(6):879–88.

59. Ishani A, Erturk S, Hertz MI, et al. Predictors of renal function following lung or heart-lung transplantation. Kidney Int 2002;61(6):2228–34.

60. Fidalgo P, Ahmed M, Meyer SR, et al. Incidence and outcomes of acute kidney injury following orthotopic lung transplantation: a population-based cohort study. Nephrol Dial Transplant 2014;29(9):1702–9.

61. Banga A, Mohanka M, Mullins J, et al. Characteristics and outcomes among patients with need for early dialysis after lung transplantation surgery. Clin Transpl 2017;31(11):e13106.

62. Osho AA, Castleberry AW, Snyder LD, et al. Assessment of different threshold preoperative glomerular filtration rates as markers of outcomes in lung transplantation. Ann Thorac Surg 2014;98(1):283–90.

63. Barraclough K, Menahem S, Bailey M, et al. Predictors of decline in renal function after lung transplantation. J Heart Lung Transplant 2006;25(12):1431–5.

64. Yerokun BA, Mulvihill MS, Osho AA, et al. Simultaneous or sequential lung-kidney transplantation confer superior survival in renal-failure patients undergoing lung transplantation: a national analysis. J Heart Lung Transplant 2017;36(4):S95.

65. Wehbe E, Brock R, Budev M, et al. Short-term and long-term outcomes of acute kidney injury after lung transplantation. J Heart Lung Transplant 2012; 31(3):244–51.

66. Kunst H, Thompson D, Hodson M. Hypertension as a marker for later development of end-stage renal failure after lung and heart-lung transplantation: a cohort study. J Heart Lung Transplant 2004;23(10): 1182–8.

67. Esposito C, De Mauri A, Vitulo P, et al. Risk factors for chronic renal dysfunction in lung transplant recipients. Transplantation 2007;84(12):1701–3.

68. Naesens M, Kuypers DRJ, Sarwal M. Calcineurin inhibitor nephrotoxicity. CJASN 2009;4(2):481–508.

69. Ivulich S, Westall G, Dooley M, et al. The evolution of lung transplant immunosuppression. Drugs 2018; 78(10):965–82.

70. Albasha W, Vahdani G, Ashoka A, et al. Native BK virus nephropathy in lung transplant: a case report and literature review. Clin Kidney J 2022;15(4): 808–11.

71. Engels EA, Pfeiffer RM, Fraumeni JF. Spectrum of cancer risk among U.S. solid organ transplant recipients: the transplant cancer match study. JAMA 2011;306(17):1891–901.

72. Shtraichman O, Ahya VN. Malignancy after lung transplantation. Ann Transl Med 2020;8(6):416.

73. Courtwright AM, Burkett P, Divo M. Posttransplant lymphoproliferative disorders in epstein-barr virus donor positive/recipient negative lung transplant recipients. Ann Thorac Surg 2018;105(2):441–7.

74. Neuringer IP. Posttransplant lymphoproliferative disease after lung transplantation. Clin Developmental Immunol 2013;2013:1–11.

75. Benvenuto L, Aversa M, Arcasoy SM. Malignancy following lung transplantation. In: Reference module in biomedical sciences. Elsevier; 2021. https://doi.org/10.1016/B978-0-08-102723-3.00120-7. B9780081027233001000.

76. Grewal HS, Lane C, Highland KB, et al. Post-transplant lymphoproliferative disorder of the bladder in a lung transplant recipient. Oxford Med Case Rep 2018;2018(3). https://doi.org/10.1093/omcr/omx093.

77. Trappe R, Oertel S, Leblond V, et al. Sequential treatment with rituximab followed by CHOP chemotherapy in adult B-cell post-transplant lymphoproliferative disorder (PTLD): the prospective international multicentre phase 2 PTLD-1 trial. Lancet Oncol 2012;13(2):196–206.

78. Choquet S. Efficacy and safety of rituximab in B-cell post-transplantation lymphoproliferative disorders: results of a prospective multicenter phase 2 study. Blood 2006;107(8):3053–7.

79. Rashtak S, Dierkhising RA, Kremers WK. Incidence and risk factors for skin cancer following lung transplantation. J Am Acad Dermatol 2015;72(1):92–8.

80. Tejwani V, Deshwal H, Ho B, et al. Cutaneous complications in recipients of lung transplants. Chest 2019;155(1):178–93.

81. Mittal A, Colegio OR. Skin cancers in organ transplant recipients. Am J Transpl 2017;17(10):2509–30.

82. Clancy CJ, Nguyen MH. Long-term voriconazole and skin cancer: is there cause for concern? Curr Infect Dis Rep 2011;13(6):536–43.

83. Triplette M, Crothers K, Mahale P. Risk of lung cancer in lung transplant recipients in the United States. Am J Transpl 2019;19(5):1478–90.

84. Arcasoy SM, Hersh C, Christie JD, et al. Bronchogenic carcinoma complicating lung transplantation. J Heart Lung Transpl 2001;20(10):1044–53.

85. Grewal AS, Padera RF, Boukedes S, et al. Prevalence and outcome of lung cancer in lung transplant recipients. Respir Med 2015;109(3):427–33.

Lung Transplantation for Coronavirus Disease-2019 Patients and Coronavirus Disease-2019 in Lung Transplant Recipients

Diego Avella, MD[a], Henry Neumann, MD[b], Ankit Bharat, MD[a],*

KEYWORDS

- Lung • Transplant • COVID-19 • ARDS • ECMO

KEY POINTS

- Respiratory failure.
- Coronavirus disease-2019 infection.
- Acute respiratory distress syndrome.
- Extracorporeal membrane oxygenation.
- Lung transplantation.

BACKGROUND

Coronavirus disease-2019 (COVID-19) infection has affected millions of people, resulting in a wide spectrum of manifestations ranging from self-limited disease to severe acute respiratory distress syndrome (ARDS) requiring hospitalization and respiratory support, which, in some cases, can progress into lung fibrosis. For the most severe forms of the severe acute respiratory syndrome coronavirus 2 (SARS-CoV-2) infection resulting in ARDS, modalities of respiratory support include mechanical ventilation (MV) and extracorporeal membrane oxygenation (ECMO). After initiation of respiratory support, a certain percentage of patients will not recover sufficient lung function to remain free from mechanical respiratory support. In addition, certain patients infected with COVID-19 will develop long-lasting deterioration in their respiratory function, oxygen dependence, and overall deterioration in their performance due to the development of pulmonary fibrosis. Although these patients remain free from respiratory support, their quality of life is significantly affected, similar to patients with chronic respiratory diseases. In addition, they may be at risk for the development of secondary pulmonary hypertension and cardiac dysfunction.[1,2] Lung transplantation for respiratory complications secondary to COVID-19 infection has been performed in over 200 patients in the United States with outcomes comparable to transplants performed for the traditional indications of chronic lung diseases.[3] **Table 1** summarizes the relevant literature related to the lung transplantation in patients with respiratory failure secondary to COVID-19 infection.

Determination of the transplant candidacy for patients with respiratory failure secondary to COVID-19 requires careful consideration. Prior reports have used lung transplantation for COVID-19 in patients who are younger and with less

a Thoracic Surgery, Department of Surgery, Feinberg School of Medicine Northwestern University, 676 North St. Clair Street Suite 650, Chicago, IL 60611, USA; b Transplant Infectious Diseases, Division of Infectious Diseases, Department of Medicine, NYU School of Medicine, New York, NY, USA
* Corresponding author. Northwestern Medicine, 676 North Saint Clair Street, Suite 650, Chicago, IL 60611.
E-mail address: ankit.bharat@nm.org

Clin Chest Med 44 (2023) 191–199
https://doi.org/10.1016/j.ccm.2022.11.002
0272-5231/23/© 2022 Elsevier Inc. All rights reserved.

chestmed.theclinics.com

Table 1	
Relevant published articles on lung transplantation for severe coronavirus disease-2019 infection	
Demonstration of need and feasibility of lung transplantation for severe COVID-19 infection	Lung transplantation for patients with severe COVID-19. Bharat, A. et al. *Sci Transl Med.* 2020.[16]
Early recommendations of criteria for lung transplantation in patients with COVID-19 infection	When to consider lung transplantation for COVID-19. Cypel, M. *Lancet Respir Med.* 2020.[14]
Multi-institutional international early experience and outcomes of lung transplantation for severe COVID-19 infection	Early outcomes after lung transplantation for severe COVID19: a series of the first consecutive cases from four countries. Bharat, A. et al. *Lancet Respir Med.* 2021.[15]
Larger, single institutional experience with lung transplantation for COVID-19-associated ARDS	Clinical Characteristics and Outcomes of Patients With COVID-19–Associated Acute Respiratory Distress Syndrome Who Underwent Lung Transplant. Kurihara, C et al. *JAMA.* 2022.[17]
Experts' opinions on approaching lung transplantation for patients with COVID-19 infection	Lung transplantation for patients with COVID-19. King, C., et al. *Chest,* 2022.[29]
Reported national outcomes for patients that underwent lung transplantation for respiratory failure secondary to COVID-19; analysis of the UNOS data	Lung transplantation for COVID-19 related respiratory failure in the United States. Roach, A., et al. *NEJM.* 2022.[3]

comorbidities, and have had excellent performance status before the onset of COVID-19. However, prolonged hospitalizations, dependence on the ventilator, recurrent infections, malnutrition, physical deconditioning, and other respiratory complications, such as hemothorax and pneumothorax, make the transplant evaluation and the procedure quite challenging. It is imperative that the patients and their caregivers be provided with a clear understanding of the potential complications associated with changes in lifestyle and the need for lifelong immunosuppressive medications following transplantation.

SELECTION OF CANDIDATES FOR LUNG TRANSPLANTATION

Approximately 5% of patients infected with COVID-19 develop a severe form of the disease[4] although this is expected to reduce with the vaccination and is now less common with the most prevalent Omicron variants (BA.2, BA.4, and BA.5). The mortality of patients with severe disease is close to 30%[5,6] despite optimized medical care. The number of patients with severe disease or long-term sequelae after a COVID-19 infection is substantial when considering the number of patients infected with COVID-19. However, there is still a lack of strong data demonstrating the long-term course of the disease. The course of the disease differs significantly between patients that remain free of MV since the development of

symptoms or after a period of mechanical respiratory support and the patients that cannot be weaned from ventilator support or ECMO.

In a Spanish study that investigated the incidence of COVID-19 infection in Catalonia, 1.83% of the patients had an outpatient COVID-19 diagnosis and mortality was 3.01%. In the same study, the patients that required hospitalization for COVID-19 represented 0.3% of the population but the mortality in this group was 19.16%.[7] Other studies have reported a decrease in the functional respiratory reserve shown by a reduction in the pulmonary function testing and exercise tolerance as well as radiographic evidence of lung fibrosis after 3 to 4 months of initial symptoms of COVID-19 infection.[8,9] However, there is a lack of understanding of the implications of these findings in the long term.

Radiographic findings after COVID-19 infection include ground glass opacities (GGO), frank lung consolidation, and atelectasis. These findings are considered early manifestations and do not necessarily represent signs of irreversible damage. However, the GGOs can represent fibrosis, particularly when they present late in the course of the disease and other signs of lung fibrosis are present simultaneously. Traction bronchiectasis, honey combing, and subpleural fibrosis are more definitive signs of lung fibrosis and irreversible changes[9,10]; however, anecdotally some patients have shown resolution of similar radiographic findings. The development of pleural effusions represents a unique challenge, particularly in coagulopathic patients and patients receiving therapeutic anticoagulation and ECMO support due to spontaneous bleeding in the pleural cavity and bleeding associated with placement of chest tubes. Spontaneous pneumothorax is another frequent complication of COVID-19 infection more frequently seen in patients who are receiving MV likely related to the effects of positive pressure ventilation on a fibrotic, stiff lung parenchyma. Lung expansion after placement of thoracostomy tubes is frequently incomplete with persistent air in the pleural spaces and prolonged air leaks. However, the development of lung fibrosis after COVID-19 infection is not uniform in all hospitalized or ventilated patients and has been associated with advanced age, history of chronic obstructive pulmonary disease and idiopathic pulmonary fibrosis, alcoholism, smoking, prolonged mechanic ventilation, and length of intensive care unit (ICU) stay.[11]

The COVID-19 findings closely resemble the course of the disease seen in patients with other coronavirus infections such as Middle East acute respiratory syndrome (MERS) and severe acute respiratory syndrome (SARS). In patients with SARS and MERS, the majority recovered from their symptoms after two weeks, but about one-third of the patients developed severe respiratory complications, including pneumonia and ARDS, and a subgroup of patients developed chronic lung fibrosis.[12,13]

Waiting a reasonable period of time for the lungs to recover coupled with optimal respiratory care to maximize the chances of lung recovery is recommended before considering a patient for a lung transplant. Patients should be referred for a lung transplant evaluation after a multidisciplinary team with experience in the management of ARDS and lung transplant patients determines if there is: (i) no recovery after 4 to 6 weeks from the onset of symptoms of COVID-19, (ii) significant respiratory deterioration from base line and (iii) the need for oxygen supplementation, MV or extracorporeal life support. Contraindications for a lung transplant, such as an active or recent malignancy, severe chest wall deformities, irreversible bleeding disorders, compromise of other major organ systems, active substance abuse, inability to comply with a complex medical regimen, lack of adequate financial, or social support, should be ruled out first. Based on initial reports from our center and others, it is recommended that patients who undergo lung transplantation for COVID-19 include those younger than 70 years old, have been cleared of COVID-19 infection, single organ failure, no permanent neurologic damage, and a body mass index below 35.[14–17]

Once a patient has been deemed a suitable candidate for transplantation, any decision related to timing of the transplant should include several factors. The ideal time to perform a lung transplant in patients with lung disease after COVID-19 is determined by a combination of reasonable evidence indicating that the lung changes are irreversible, the physiologic reserve of the patient is adequate, and the physical deconditioning and complications associated with the disease have not placed the patient at too high a risk of death and complications–thus, reducing the benefit of a transplantation. For patients with significant functional limitations due to the COVID-19 infection or who require mechanical respiratory support, the risk of developing further complications affecting other organ systems, increasing physical deconditioning, and malnutrition should be considered. In such patients, there should be an emphasis on decreasing sedation, increasing the patients' involvement in their care, optimizing nutritional support, and minimizing threats to other systems. Judicious management of fluids is critical to improve the respiratory function without compromising other organ systems.

Approximately one-third of the patients admitted to the hospital for COVID-19 infection developed acute kidney injury and approximately 15% required renal replacement therapy.[18,19] Hospitalized patients requiring high ventilator support for a prolonged period have a low likelihood of recovery. In our series, without a lung transplant, there was a near 100% mortality rate for patients who required more than seven days of MV for COVID-19 ARDS.[20] Therefore, an early preliminary evaluation for lung transplantation candidacy of these patients before starting mechanical life support is recommended to help tailor individual therapy.

For patients who are not admitted to the hospital, a standard evaluation for lung transplantation should be performed. A sufficient time for recovery of 4 weeks, or ideally 8 weeks, from the beginning of COVID-19 symptoms is recommended before considering lung transplantation. Recently published high-quality studies support the use of ECMO for ARDS, and large multicenter studies have reported good outcomes with the use of ECMO for COVID-19-associated ARDS. Considering this evidence, prolonged ECMO support, extending past 28 days, may be necessary to bridge some patients with COVID-19-associated ARDS to recovery, instead of bridging to lung transplant.[21] A complete standard evaluation is recommended, including all the physiologic and socioeconomic factors used for the evaluation of all patients considered for lung transplantation.

To date, in the United States, patients who have received lung transplants for COVID-19 are younger than patients receiving lung transplants for other indications[3,17]

Demonstration of eradication of the COVID-19 infection is critical before performing a lung transplantation. Strong immunosuppression, needed immediately after the lung transplant, can be detrimental in patients with a persistent COVID-19 infection. We recommend that patients receive two negative polymerase chain reaction (PCR) tests 24 h apart performed using samples obtained from the distal airways with a bronchoalveolar lavage, as those areas have a higher viral load and have a lower false negative rate in comparison to the upper airway. When the patient is not intubated, we recommend two negative PCR tests from samples obtained from the upper airway at least 24 h apart.[15,17]

INTRAOPERATIVE CONSIDERATIONS DURING TRANSPLANT

To date, most transplanted patients for COVID-19 ARDS have received a double lung transplant as the most common procedure for any lung transplant recipient with acute respiratory failure requiring MV or ECMO support, and also in part due to the high prevalence of severe pulmonary hypertension.[3,17] However, a few single lung transplants in patients with respiratory disease secondary to COVID-19 infection have been performed successfully.[3] Many COVID-19 patients develop structural abnormalities such as cavitary lesions and recurrent pleural infections with recurrent bacterial infections. The presence of persistent infections or structural abnormalities, such as large cavities that could be potential sources of infection in the postoperative period, pose a high risk for patients' undergoing a single lung transplant for respiratory disease secondary to COVID-19 infection. As such, single lung transplantation should be considered on a case-by-case basis and mostly reserved for patients with long-term COVID-19 fibrosis rather than ARDS.

Owing to the high incidence of pulmonary hypertension and right ventricular dysfunction, in addition to the higher incidence of severe pleural adhesions, the use of intraoperative venoarterial (VA) ECMO support is highly recommended. As many of these patients are already on peripheral venous-venous (VV) ECMO support, it is important to consider conversion to VA ECMO for a better hemodynamic support. Pneumonectomies also pose significant challenges because of the presence of adhesions between the lungs and the pleura and mediastinum. In these patients, the dissection planes are frequently altered, and bleeding is often significant. Surgical teams, as well as perfusion and anesthesia teams, should be aware of this and prepare to transfuse and support the patient. The chest cavities are often small, requiring caudad retraction of the diaphragm to facilitate the operation. As expected, the operative time and organ cold ischemic time is longer in COVID-19 patients, as is the requirement for transfusion of blood products in comparison with other pathologies.[17]

A unique challenge in COVID-19 ARDS patients is the presence of diaphragmatic dysfunction. In a recent study, 76% of patients discharged to rehabilitation after severe COVID-19 ARDS had sonographic evidence of diaphragm dysfunction.[22] The mechanisms associated with the diaphragmatic dysfunction in these patients include critical illness myopathy, ventilator-induced diaphragmatic dysfunction, iatrogenic injury of the phrenic nerve during placement of central lines, postinfectious inflammatory neuropathy of the phrenic nerve, and direct neuromuscular involvement of the COVID-19 virus. Peripheral nerves and muscles express angiotensin-converting enzyme 2 (ACE2) receptor to which viral structural proteins bind. Autopsy studies have shown diaphragmatic fibrosis and a unique myopathic phenotype compared with other ICU patients.[23–25]

The prevalence and impact of these findings in transplanted patients is unknown, but they play a role in the increased number of complications, need for ventilator support, and ICU stay. A diaphragmatic and phrenic nerve evaluation with bedside ultrasound is a useful tool in ventilated patients to assess the function of the diaphragm longitudinally and detect improvement or deterioration of the diaphragmatic function. Although to date there are no studies evaluating the effect of any therapeutic intervention for diaphragmatic dysfunction after lung transplants for respiratory disease after COVID-19 infection, some transplant centers advocate for the early use of diaphragmatic pacing in a selected group of patients. However, the short and long-term results of this intervention are unknown. Nonetheless, these findings stress the importance of protecting the phrenic nerve during the conduction of the operation minimizing trauma or traction of the nerves.

POSTOPERATIVE CARE OF THE TRANSPLANTED PATIENTS

Postoperative care in the ICU involves respiratory support with MV and extracorporeal life support with VV and VA ECMO. The length of stay in the hospital and in the ICU after a lung transplant for

COVID-19 has been reported to be almost twice as long for patients receiving lung transplants for other reasons. In our series, the median length of stay for COVID-19 transplant patients versus other lung transplant patients was 28.5 versus 16 days in the hospital and 6.5 versus 2 days in the ICU. The need for care in the ICU was largely determined by the need for MV. Analysis of the United Network for Organ Sharing (UNOS) database for patients receiving transplants related to COVID-19, indicate that over 70% of such patients have needed MV for at least 48 h after the transplant.[3] In our series, the median time on a ventilator was 6.5 days.[17] In addition, according to the UNOS database, approximately 12.3% of patients needed postoperative ECMO,[3] and there was a 30-day mortality of 2.2% (4 of 183 patients analyzed) and a 6-month survival rate of 92%.

In our series, 1-year survival rate after transplantation of 30 patients for COVID-19 was 100% after a median follow-up of 351 days in comparison with 83.3% survival of patients that received transplants for a different pathology. Thirty percent of the patients needed ECMO support after transplant.[17] The difference in the need for ECMO support posttransplant is likely explained by institutional preferences in the postoperative management of these patients and the heterogeneity in patient complexity. The causes of early, postoperative deaths include respiratory failure, rejection after transplant, gastrointestinal infection, hyperammonemia, and COVID-19 infection. Other frequent postoperative complications after lung transplant for COVID-19 include primary graft dysfunction (PGD), stroke, acute renal failure, and transplant rejection, and pleural effusions.

Renal dysfunction occurs more frequently in patients with COVID-19. This is true also for patients after lung transplants due to COVID-19 in comparison with patients undergoing lung transplants for other reasons. Approximately 30% of patients hospitalized with COVID-19 develop kidney injury, and 50% of COVID-19 patients in the ICU with kidney injury require dialysis. Vascular endothelial injury associated with COVID-19 infection, hemodynamic instability, tissue inflammation, and immune infiltration may play a role in the origin of kidney injury.[26] Even though the long-term outcomes are unknown, patients with COVID-19 infection and renal failure have higher mortality and worse outcomes. Approximately 5% of COVID-19 patients who have received a lung transplant needed dialysis before transplantation.[3] In comparison with non-COVID-19 patients, the rate of permanent hemodialysis after lung transplant is significantly higher in COVID-19 patients (13.3% vs 5.5%). Of note, a similar percentage of COVID-19 patients that received a lung transplant (10%) required only temporary postoperative dialysis.[20] However, it is unclear what percentage of patients that had renal failure before transplant required permanent dialysis after lung transplant. Some centers have performed simultaneous lung and kidney transplants when the potential of recovery of kidney function was deemed low.

The degree of PGD after transplant is not clearly understood. In our series, 70% of the patients had some degree of PGD. However, their rate of acute rejection or development of donor specific antibodies was zero in comparison with a 12% in non-COVID-19 patients. A potential explanation for the low rate is the dilution of human leukocyte antigen titers due to a higher rate of bleeding and transfusions.[17] The impact of these findings in the development of chronic allograft dysfunction in these patients is unknown. Despite the higher frequency of PGD, the patients that received a lung transplant for respiratory diseases after COVID-19 infection had more significant improvement in their performance in comparison with the non-COVID-19 patients.[20] This is not surprising considering the more critical condition of the COVID-19 patients at the time of the transplant relative to the non-COVID-19 patients as well as the younger age and healthier base line of such patients before COVID-19 infection.

With the high prevalence of COVID-19 infection, a particular subject with impactful implications for the future is the selection of lungs from donors that could have had infection for COVID-19. The current recommendation from the UNOS is to obtain samples from the lower respiratory tract from donors and analyze those by PCR for COVID-19, due to the higher frequency of the viral receptor ACE2 in the lower respiratory tract and because the viral testing in samples obtained from bronchoalveolar lavage remains positive for a longer period in comparison to samples obtained from the upper respiratory tract.[27] However, to maximize the use of the organs and decrease the false positive rates of COVID-19 tests, if a positive test is found and the clinical probability of a positive infection is low, it is recommended to repeat the test in samples obtained from the distal airways. In donors with a history of infection of COVID-19 more than 21 days before the lung procurement, the likelihood of active COVID-19 infection and transmissibility is extremely low. The assessment of the organ at the time of procurement also provides valuable information about the condition of the organ. Evaluation of the donor lungs with a computed tomography scan looking for fibrotic changes, persistent hypoxia in central and selective arterial gases sampling, thick and rigid lungs at in situ palpation of the organs, and reduced lung compliance in the ventilator are all indicators of fibrotic changes in the lung. **Fig. 1** shows an algorithm for evaluating the donor lungs in the setting of a potential history of COVID-19.[28]

In conclusion, lung transplant is a life-saving treatment for carefully selected patients with COVID-19-associated respiratory failure. Despite a complex pretransplant medical course, the post-transplant outcomes are excellent when performed by experienced centers.

PREVENTION AND SPECIFIC POST EXPOSURE PROPHYLAXIS

General measures that include avoiding close contact with sick individuals, frequent hand sanitation, social distancing, and mask wearing in public are important for the prevention of SARS-CoV-2 infection. There are multiple COVID-19 vaccines available worldwide; four are used in the United States. Pfizer/BioNTech® and Moderna® COVID-19 are FDA approved for two doses and two booster doses are approved including a bivalent booster. For up-to-date recommendations, please check www.cdc.gov/coronavirus/2019-ncov/vaccines/recommendations/immuno.html. Novavax® subunit vaccine and J&J/Janssen® adenovirus vaccine are only recommended as alternatives for patients who are hesitant about or have a contraindication for mRNA vaccines. Tixagevimab/cilgavimab (EVUSHELD®) has been administered as pre-exposure prophylaxis in lung transplant recipients beginning two weeks after completion of COVID-19 immunization or in cases where vaccination is contraindicated or deferred. It is important to note that Evusheld® lacks activity

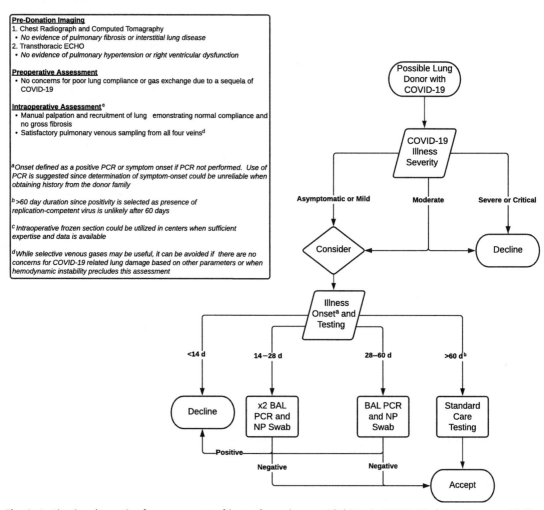

Fig. 1. Institutional practice for assessment of lungs from donor with historic COVID-19. (*From* Querrey M, Kurihara C, Manerikar A, et al. Lung donation following SARS-CoV-2 infection. Am J Transplant. 2021;21(12):4073-4078.[27])

against BA4.6 and other emerging variants such as BQ.1 and BQ.1.1. Post-exposure prophylaxis with monoclonal antibodies included Casirivimab/Imdevimab (REGEN-COV®) and Bamlanivimab/etesevimab, are no longer recommended as they lack sufficient activity against the omicron variants.

TREATMENT FOR POST LUNG TRANSPLANT PATIENTS WITH COVID 19 NOT REQUIRING HOSPITALIZATION

Monoclonal antibody therapy has been a mainstay for COVID-19 treatment for immunocompromised transplant recipients since late 2020. However, the most recently available monoclonal antibody treatment, Bebtelovimab, is no longer recommended due to lack of efficacy against omicron subvariants BQ.1 & BQ1.1, which are now the dominant subvariants circulating. Therefore, currently there are no monoclonal antibody options for treatment.

For patients with mild to moderate symptoms not requiring hospitalization, we recommend an antiviral within 5 days of symptom onset. The preferred antiviral treatment for outpatients at this time based on the available data of clinical efficacy is nirmatrelvir/ritonavir (Paxlovid®). However, its use is limited by renal function and drug-drug interactions, particularly with calcineurin inhibitors (CNIs). Molnupiravir is also an option for outpatient antiviral treatment, but data on the efficacy of molnupiravir in immunocompromised hosts is limited. Medications should be reviewed, if possible, with the help of a clinical ID and transplant pharmacist.

A 3-day course of Remdesivir to prevent progression of disease and hospitalization is recommended but is limited at this time logistically due to the need for daily infusion.

Molnupiravir (Lagevrio®) 800 mg PO twice daily for 5 days is the preferred antiviral therapy if the patient is on extended-release tacrolimus, or if Paxlovid® is contraindicated due to other drug-drug interactions, pregnancy or CrCl <30.

TREATMENT FOR POST LUNG TRANSPLANT PATIENTS WITH COVID 19 REQUIRING HOSPITALIZATION

Patients with no oxygen requirement have limited options. The most common antiviral used is Remdesivir for 3 days of therapy. It can be given to patients with severe renal failure/ESRD based on CATCO data [2]. Monitoring of AST/ALT is recommended, and remdesivir is not recommended if the ALT is 10 times the upper limit of normal. One should also monitor for bradycardia. Prophylactic anticoagulation (AC) is recommended while hospitalized. In patients requiring low flow supplemental oxygen: Remdesivir 5-10 days duration, plus dexamethasone 6 mg daily for 10 days (Oral or IV) is recommended. Therapeutic AC is recommended irrespective of D-dimer value, while hospitalized. If disease severity progresses to severe illness during the hospital admission and there is no evidence of thrombosis, the AC strategy should be modified to prophylactic doses of AC.

For patients requiring high flow oxygen, or non-invasive or invasive ventilation: Remdesivir for 5-10 days, and dexamethasone 6 mg daily for 10 days (Oral or IV) is recommended. Baricitinib, a JAK inhibitor, is the preferred agent if inflammatory markers are increased, for ARDS, and if there are no contraindications such as ESRD, severe neutropenia or leukopenia. The Baricitinib dose is 4 mg PO daily for 14 days, and the dose will need to be adjusted if the eGFR <60 mL/min/1.73m2.

When Baricitinib is contraindicated, tocilizumab, an IL-6 inhibitor, is recommended for patients with severe COVID-19, and if the patient has not already received more than 2 doses of baricitinib. The patient must have already received at least 1 dose of dexamethasone, have increased inflammatory markers (C-Reactive Protein > 75mg/L), and abnormal chest imaging with bilateral consolidation and ground glass opacities. Tocilizumab is given as a single dose that is weight based <40kg: 8mg/kg, 41-65kg: 400mg, 66kg-90kg: 600mg and > 90kg: 800mg.

Tocilizumab should be used with caution when the patient has elevated procalcitonin due to concern for secondary bacterial infection, and if there is a current uncontrolled serious bacterial, fungal, or non-COVID-19 viral infection, this agent should be avoided. Tocilizumab should also be avoided if alanine transaminase is >5 times the upper limit of normal, if there is a high risk for gastrointestinal perforation, neutropenia (Neutrophil count <500 cells/μL) or thrombocytopenia (Platelet count <50,000 cells/μL).[30–34]

CLINICS CARE POINTS

- Patients undergoing lung transplant for Coronavirus 2019 infection ARDS have a more complicated perioperative course than non-Coronavirus 2019 patients undergoing lung transplant.

- The long term results after lung transplantation for Coronavirus 2019 infection ARDS are comparable to outcomes in non-Coronavirus 2019 patients.

DISCLOSURE

D. Avella and A. Bharat have no commercial or financial conflicts.

REFERENCES

1. Tudoran C, Tudoran M, Lazureanu VE, et al. Evidence of pulmonary hypertension after SARS-CoV-2 infection in subjects without previous significant cardiovascular pathology. J Clin Med 2021;10(2). https://doi.org/10.3390/jcm10020199.
2. Nishiga M, Wang DW, Han Y, et al. COVID-19 and cardiovascular disease: from basic mechanisms to clinical perspectives. Nat Rev Cardiol 2020;17(9): 543–58.
3. Roach A, Chikwe J, Catarino P, et al. Lung transplantation for covid-19-related respiratory failure in the United States. N Engl J Med 2022;386(12): 1187–8.
4. Richardson S, Hirsch JS, Narasimhan M, et al. Presenting characteristics, comorbidities, and outcomes among 5700 patients hospitalized with COVID-19 in the New York city area. JAMA 2020;323(20):2052–9.
5. Group RC, Horby P, Lim WS, et al. Dexamethasone in hospitalized patients with covid-19. N Engl J Med 2021;384(8):693–704.
6. Beigel JH, Tomashek KM, Dodd LE, et al. Remdesivir for the treatment of covid-19 - final report. N Engl J Med 2020;383(19):1813–26.
7. Burn E, Tebe C, Fernandez-Bertolin S, et al. The natural history of symptomatic COVID-19 during the first wave in Catalonia. Nat Commun 2021;12(1):777.
8. Guler SA, Ebner L, Aubry-Beigelman C, et al. Pulmonary function and radiological features 4 months after COVID-19: first results from the national prospective observational Swiss COVID-19 lung study. Eur Respir J 2021;57(4). https://doi.org/10.1183/13993003.03690-2020.
9. Han X, Fan Y, Alwalid O, et al. Six-month follow-up chest CT findings after severe COVID-19 pneumonia. Radiology 2021;299(1):E177–86.
10. Solomon JJ, Heyman B, Ko JP, et al. CT of post-acute lung complications of COVID-19. Radiology 2021;301(2):E383–95.
11. Ojo AS, Balogun SA, Williams OT, et al. Pulmonary fibrosis in COVID-19 survivors: predictive factors and risk reduction strategies. Pulm Med 2020;2020: 6175964.
12. Luyt CE, Combes A, Becquemin MH, et al. Long-term outcomes of pandemic 2009 influenza A(H1N1)-associated severe ARDS. Chest 2012;142(3):583–92.
13. Hosseiny M, Kooraki S, Gholamrezanezhad A, et al. Radiology perspective of coronavirus disease 2019 (COVID-19): lessons from severe acute respiratory syndrome and Middle East respiratory syndrome. AJR Am J Roentgenol 2020;214(5):1078–82.
14. Cypel M, Keshavjee S. When to consider lung transplantation for COVID-19. Lancet Respir Med 2020; 8(10):944–6.
15. Bharat A, Machuca TN, Querrey M, et al. Early outcomes after lung transplantation for severe COVID-19: a series of the first consecutive cases from four countries. Lancet Respir Med 2021;9(5):487–97.
16. Bharat A, Querrey M, Markov NS, et al. Lung transplantation for patients with severe COVID-19. Sci Transl Med Dec 16 2020;12(574). https://doi.org/10.1126/scitranslmed.abe4282.
17. Kurihara C, Manerikar A, Querrey M, et al. Clinical characteristics and outcomes of patients with COVID-19-associated acute respiratory distress syndrome who underwent lung transplant. JAMA 2022;327(7):652–61.
18. Bowe B, Cai M, Xie Y, et al. Acute kidney injury in a national cohort of hospitalized US veterans with COVID-19. Clin J Am Soc Nephrol 2020;16(1):14–25.
19. Hirsch JS, Ng JH, Ross DW, et al. Acute kidney injury in patients hospitalized with COVID-19. Kidney Int 2020;98(1):209–18.
20. Kurihara C, Manerikar A, Gao CA, et al. Outcomes after extracorporeal membrane oxygenation support in COVID-19 and non-COVID-19 patients. Artif Organs 2022;46(4):688–96.
21. Rudym D, Chang SH, Angel LF. Characteristics and outcomes of patients with COVID-19-associated ARDS who underwent lung transplant. JAMA 2022;327(24):2454.
22. Farr E, Wolfe AR, Deshmukh S, et al. Diaphragm dysfunction in severe COVID-19 as determined by neuromuscular ultrasound. Ann Clin Transl Neurol 2021;8(8):1745–9.
23. Shi Z, de Vries HJ, Vlaar APJ, et al. Diaphragm pathology in critically ill patients with COVID-19 and postmortem findings from 3 medical centers. JAMA Intern Med 2021;181(1):122–4.
24. Patel Z, Franz CK, Bharat A, et al. Diaphragm and phrenic nerve ultrasound in COVID-19 patients and beyond: imaging technique, findings, and clinical applications. J Ultrasound Med 2022;41(2):285–99.
25. Liotta EM, Batra A, Clark JR, et al. Frequent neurologic manifestations and encephalopathy-associated morbidity in Covid-19 patients. Ann Clin Transl Neurol 2020;7(11):2221–30.
26. Legrand M, Bell S, Forni L, et al. Pathophysiology of COVID-19-associated acute kidney injury. Nat Rev Nephrol 2021;17(11):751–64.
27. Kaul DR, Valesano AL, Petrie JG, et al. Donor to recipient transmission of SARS-CoV-2 by lung transplantation despite negative donor upper respiratory tract testing. Am J Transplant 2021;21(8):2885–9.
28. Querrey M, Kurihara C, Manerikar A, et al. Lung donation following SARS-CoV-2 infection. Am J Transplant 2021;21(12):4073–8.
29. King CS, Mannem H, Kukreja J, et al. Lung transplantation for patients with COVID-19. Chest 2022; 161(1):169–78.

30. Gottlieb RL, Vaca CE, Paredes R, et al. Early remdesivir to prevent progression to severe Covid-19 in outpatients. N Engl J Med 2022;386:305–15.

31. Jayk Bernal A, Gomes da Silva MM, Musungaie DB, et al. Molnupiravir for oral treatment of covid-19 in nonhospitalized patients. N Engl J Med 2021; 386(6):509–20.

32. AST statement on oral antiviral therapy for COVID-19 for organ transplant recipients. Available at: https://www.myast.org/sites/default/files/AST%20Statement %20on%20Oral%20Antiviral%20Therapy%20for% 20COVID%20Jan%204%20%282%29.pdf.

33. Cheng M, Fowler R, Murthy S, et al. Remdesivir in patients with severe kidney dysfunction: a secondary analysis of the CATCO randomized trial. JAMA Netw Open 2022;5(8):e2229236.

34. The ATTACC, ACTIV-4a, and REMAP-CAP Investigators. Therapeutic anticoagulation with heparin in noncritically Ill patients with Covid-19. N Engl J Med 2021;385:790–802.

Future of Lung Transplantation
Xenotransplantation and Bioengineering Lungs

Justin C.Y. Chan, MD, MPhil[a],*, Ryan Chaban, MD[b,c],
Stephanie H. Chang, MD[a], Luis F. Angel, MD[a],
Robert A. Montgomery, MD, DPhil[a], Richard N. Pierson III, MD[b]

KEYWORDS

• Lung transplant • Xenotransplantation • Bioengineering • Ex vivo lung perfusion
• Tissue engineering

KEY POINTS

• Significant progress is being made in xenotransplantation, and lessons from other solid organ xenotransplants can be adapted to advance lung xenotransplantation.
• The use of genetically modified pigs with knockout of known xeno-antigens and addition of human complement and coagulation pathway regulating proteins have extended lung xenotransplant survival in a pig-to-baboon model for up to 31 days.
• The theoretic risk of zoonosis can be mitigated through animal husbandry techniques to maintain designated pathogen-free herds and by donor screening or genetic modification.
• The ongoing research into tissue engineering techniques may also provide an alternative source of lungs in the future.

BACKGROUND

Recent accomplishments in human xenotransplantation, including the first pig-to-human kidney transplants[1,2] into three brain-dead human recipients and a transiently successful life-supporting pig-to-human heart transplant,[3] have reinvigorated interest in xenotransplantation.

With approximately three patients per week dying on the lung transplant waiting list in the United States,[4] the use of animal organs for transplantation promises to alleviate or even eliminate the issue of the lung donor organ shortage and revolutionize the practice of transplant medicine.

However, despite considerable progress in solid organ xenotransplantation, lung xenotransplantation presents unique challenges and still requires significant advancements in the laboratory before being applied to clinical use. In this article, we outline the current state-of-the-art in lung xenotransplantation, highlighting recent advances and remaining obstacles to be overcome.

History of Lung Xenotransplantation

For heart and kidney xenografts, survival of months and years has been reported in nonhuman primates carrying life-supporting pig organs. In contrast, lung xenotransplantation had relatively

[a] NYU Transplant Institute, New York University, 530 1st Avenue, Suite 7R, New York, NY 10016, USA; [b] Department of Surgery, Center for Transplantation Sciences, Massachusetts General Hospital and Harvard Medical School, 55 Fruit Street, Boston, MA 02114, USA; [c] Department of Cardiovascular Surgery, University Hospital of Johannes Gutenberg University, Langenbeckstr. 1, Bau 505, 5. OG55131 Mainz, Germany
* Corresponding author. Department of Cardiothoracic Surgery, New York University, 530 1st Avenue, Suite 7R, New York, NY 10016.
E-mail address: justin.chan2@nyulangone.org

Clin Chest Med 44 (2023) 201–214
https://doi.org/10.1016/j.ccm.2022.11.003
0272-5231/23/© 2022 Elsevier Inc. All rights reserved.

limited success, with recipient survival limited to days or weeks.[5] Lung xenotransplantation has not yet been tested in vivo in a human. Anatomically, the lung contains a large surface area of vascular endothelium which is exposed to the full cardiac output multiple times per minute. In addition, the lung contains an innate immune system that surveils the environment and is overly sensitive to perceived pathogens arriving through the airways or in circulation. The resulting inflammation is often associated with localized loss of alveolocapillary barrier function which, because of the highly interconnected anatomy of the bronchial tree, renders the lung especially sensitive to the loss of alveolocapillary barrier function that is associated with lung xenograft failure.

Experimental Models in Lung Xenotransplantation

The phenotype of lung xenograft rejection has been characterized primarily in ex vivo experiments, where pig lungs were perfused with human blood and in various in vivo transplant models.[6] Ex vivo experiments with xenogeneic lungs were first reported in 1968 by Bryant and colleagues who perfused swine lungs with human blood and ventilated them simultaneously.[7] The Pierson laboratory modified this model, using fresh rather than stored human blood to evaluate the contribution of leukocytes and platelets, and developed a side-by-side 'paired' model,[8] to facilitate mechanistic studies and evaluate therapeutic interventions. Ex vivo xenogeneic perfusion of swine lung (performed with both wild-type and genetically modified pigs) with human blood seems to accurately model 'hyperacute rejection' changes that occur within the range of 6 to 8 hours during in vivo pig-to-baboon lung xenotransplantation.[9] (Although a mouse model of lung xenotransplantation was developed,[10] its value is limited by ill-defined interspecies differences in immune and other physiologic pathways, and the clinical irrelevance of even 'successful' genetic modifications to the donor.)

Particularly important for lung xenotransplantation research is the pig-to-baboon experimental model. Baboons have been used intensively in xenotransplantation research as a nonhuman primate host that is presumed to simulate the human response to a pig organ xenograft because of their relative anatomic and presumed immunologic similarity. Relative to cynomolgus or rhesus monkeys, baboons are preferred among non human primates (NHPs) because of their larger size.[11] Baboons have been used to cross-circulate pig lungs in ex vivo models that allow mechanistic studies and evaluate the interaction with pig tissues without sacrificing them.[12] Orthotopic left-sided lung xenotransplantation with flow and pressure measurements in the pulmonary artery coupled with a right pulmonary artery snare to intermittently direct the full cardiac output to the transplanted lung allows evaluation of life-supporting function of xeno-lung transplant and yields several valuable data.[9]

Selection of a Lung Xenograft Donor for Clinical Use

On the donor side, pigs have become the main source for xeno-organs because of (1) ready availability as a commercially farmed domesticated species, (2) size matching, fast maturity at 9 months, allowing rapid propagation of pigs with desirable traits, (3) relatively large litter size (typically 4–10) compared with other domesticated species' number of offspring, (4) short gestation period of 115 days (about 4 months), which enables rapid propagation due to shorter and multiple pregnancies. Those factors together make the propagation of pigs with desirable genetic modifications more feasible as it shortens the development cycle and lowers the cost. There is an improved public perception of pigs over primates as xenograft donors to save human lives with most studies showing that people view pigs to be a more acceptable source of xenografts.[13–15]

Several developments have allowed for the recent progress in lung xenotransplantation. Genetic engineering technologies, such as zinc finger nucleases and transcription activator-like effector nucleases, and more recently and most prominently, clustered regularly interspaced short palindromic repeats, associated protein 9 (CRISPR-Cas9)[16] were pioneered in mice. This technique has been applied to swine,[17] the initial report of modification of genes coding for myostatin, and mutations resulting in increased muscle growth. Since then, CRISPR-Cas9 technology has been applied successfully to nonhuman primates[18] and (controversially), to human embryos.[19–21] CRISPR-Cas9 technology is the main technique now used to develop the transgenic pigs used in pig-to-human xenotransplantation experiments.[22]

Another important technology is that of somatic cell nuclear transfer (cloning). This technique was first reported through a clone of a Finnish Dorset sheep (Dolly the sheep)[23] by the use of transfer of nucleic material from the mammary gland of a ewe to an unfertilized oocyte and subsequent transfer of the embryo into a recipient which subsequently birthed the clone. This technique builds on work performed in in vitro fertilization (IVF) which was successfully reported in a human in 1978 with the birth of baby Louise Brown in the United Kingdom.[24]

Without all three of these technologies, genetic engineering for the development and propagation of the multiply gene-edited 'transgenic' pig as potential organ 'donors' for clinical use would not be possible. Gene editing of the pig has contributed fundamentally to the recent progress in xenotransplantation.

Notably, survival of up to 31 days was recorded in a baboon recipient of a left lung transplant from a pig engineered to lack two carbohydrate antigens and to additionally express multiple human proteins.[25]

Immunologic and Physiologic Challenges

When wild-type pig lungs are perfused with human blood, a rapid elevation in pulmonary vascular resistance, loss of alveolocapillary barrier function, development of lung edema, increased ventilation resistance, and eventually, complete loss of graft function happens in a matter of minutes.[26] This 'hyperacute rejection' is driven by pre-formed natural antibodies found in human and primate blood, against pig tissues.[27] Most of these antibodies target the galactolse-a1.3-galactose (alpha-Gal), a carbohydrate which is expressed ubiquitously in almost all mammals, except for humans and old-world primates who carry millions of years old loss-of-function mutations in the producing enzyme.[28] N-glycolylneuraminic acid[29] and the Sid blood group (sd[a]) antigen[30] are further targets of the 5% to 15% and 1% to 5% of the natural anti-pig antibodies, respectively. Humans develop those natural antibodies early in their life because contact with various gastrointestinal microorganisms that express the same antigens.[31]

Hyperacute acute rejection still happens in lungs from double and triple-knockout swine which do not express the above-mentioned carbohydrate pig antigens, driven mainly by complement system activation, coagulation dysregulation, and likely pre-formed antibodies against unknown epitopes.[25,32,33] Under physiologic conditions, the complement system is kept deactivated with the help of regulatory proteins that are collectively known as complement-pathway-regulatory proteins (CPRPs). But interspecies incompatibilities make pig CPRPs less effective in preventing destructive overactivation of the human complement system. Early approaches focus on neutralizing the complement system by administration of agents, such as cobra venom factor, and were partially successful.[34] Especially important in this regard are the membrane cofactor protein

(MCP_CD46), decay accelerating factor (DAF_CD55) and the membrane-attack-complex-inhibitory protein (MAC-IP_CD59).

Diffuse microvascular thrombosis and consumptive coagulopathy are characteristic of early lung xenotransplantation.[35,36] The problem had been largely mitigated by introducing knockout pigs and transgenic human CPRPs. However, much like pig CPRPs, pig coagulation-regulatory proteins are inefficient in exhibiting an anticoagulative regulatory role when in contact with human blood. For example, pig aortic endothelial cells were found to activate human prothrombin and to trigger human platelets to express the procoagulant tissue factor (TF) on contact with them.[37,38] Pig thrombomodulin (TBM), and its cofactor, endothelial protein C receptor, are both less potent in activating protein C with only 1% to 10% of the human analogs activity.[39–41] Pig TF pathway inhibitor (TFPI) is also suspected to be inefficient in regulating the human tissue factor-initiated coagulation.[42] Pig von Willebrand factor, a large multimer protein that is found in the endothelium, platelets, and megakaryocytes, and is involved in initiating platelet adhesion to the endothelium, seems to aggregate and activate human platelets spontaneously through aberrant interaction with their glycoprotein receptor GPIb.[43,44]

A cluster of differentiation antigen 47 (CD47) acts as a self-recognition marker that is ubiquitously expressed on endothelial, epithelial, and hematopoietic cells.[45] Its interaction with signal-regulatory proteins (SIRP-a) on macrophages is recognized as an inhibitory signal against phagocytosis.[46] CD39 is expressed by endothelial cells and a variety of immunocytes[47] and acts as an anti-inflammatory mediator by converting the extracellular pro-inflammatory and vasoconstrictive adenosine triphosphate (ATP) into adenosine monophosphate (AMP).[48] CD73 is found in a variety of tissues and augments the effect of CD39 by further converting AMP in adenosine.[49] All the above-listed regulatory proteins and others suffer from similar interspecies incompatibility, and it makes biological sense to consider introducing the human analogues in future xenografts. Further, natural killer (NK) cells recognize major histocompatibility complex (MHC) class I (HLA) molecules as an inhibitory signal.[50] Pig MHC class I (also termed swine leukocyte antigen, SLA) binds poorly to the inhibitory receptor expressed by human NK cells, resulting in NK-mediated pig cell killing in vitro.[51] Introducing transgenic expression of human leukocyte antigen E (HLA-E) to pig grafts protects against pig cell injury by human NK cells.[52] Although antibodies in patients who are highly sensitized to human HLA may in theory cross-react with the swine leukocyte antigen, a literature review of xeno-studies suggests that such a scenario is unlikely.[28]

Ex Vivo and in Vivo Results

Early ex vivo lung perfusion with human blood experiments was less successful because of antibody-mediated hyperacute rejection, marked by severe pulmonary hypertension and pulmonary edema[53] with survival of less than 60 minutes.[54] Eliminating anti-pig antibody by absorption[55] and inhibiting complement activity by heat treatment enabled the survival of more than 90 minutes in the late nineties.[56,57] Complement system inhibitors alone did not improve survival.[58] Macchiarini and colleagues[59] used an ex vivo pig heart–lung perfusion model to adsorb (immunodeplete) xenoantibodies and subsequently perform pig-to-goat lung xenotransplantation. Although they were able to overcome hyperacute rejection by this approach, xenoantibody titers rebounded within 2 to 4 days, associated with xenograft necrosis and recipient death.

In the pig-to-primate model, removing the alpha-Gal-antigen prolonged survival of the alpha-Gal knockout (GalTKO) swine lungs beyond 2 hours in both ex vivo experiments,[8,60] and in vivo pig-to baboon model.[61] Introducing human transgenic pig organs using genetic modification techniques has also extended the survival of pig lungs.[26] The expression of human decay accelerating factor (CD55) partially protected pig lung from hyperacute rejection.[62,63] Ex vivo perfusion experiments have shown improvement in rejection resistance for lungs that both lack the alpha-Gal and express the human hCD46 by down-modulation of the complement system, reducing platelet and coagulation cascade activation, neutrophil sequestration, and histamine release, with a median survival of almost 3 hours.[64]

Survival has been further improved through inhibiting the interaction between platelet-GPIb and von Willebrand factor (vWF),[65] or using GPIb, GPIIb/IIIa depleting treatment[66] or with thromboxane and histamine inhibitors.[67] GalTKO.hCD46 pig lungs perfused with human blood survived up to 4 hours with the help of the aforementioned pharmacologic methods.

Transgenic pigs that express "humanized vWF" were made and they demonstrated reduced platelet sequestration during lung ex vivo perfusion experiments and after pig-to-baboon lung transplantation by reducing the non-physiological human platelet aggregation, without influencing the in vitro platelet activation by collagen.[68] Transgenic GalTKO.hCD46 pig lungs that further express HLA-E were associated with significant decrease in antibody-dependent and independent NK-mediated cytotoxicity and neutrophil sequestration in the ex vivo organ perfusion model.[69]

Yamada and colleagues have achieved survival of more than 7 days in pig-to-baboon by using GalTKO lungs that additionally express hCD47.[70] Miura and colleagues achieved regular survival of more than 8 hours in ex vivo perfusion of GalT-KO.hCD46 lungs that also express both human TFPI and CD47.[71] Burdorf and colleagues have achieved survival of more than 7 days in pig-to-baboon in vivo transplantation of GalTKO.hCD46 that further express HO-1, hEPCR, and hTBM.[25] As noted above, they achieved recipient survival of 31 days in one baboon after transplanting a GalTKO-.β4GalT-KO.hCF46.-hEPCR.hTBM.hCF47.HO-1 lung.[25]

Anatomic Differences Between Pig and Human Lungs

Significant differences exist in the anatomy of the pigs compared with that of humans. Pig lungs have seven lobes (**Fig. 1**) compared with human five, with four lobes on the right (cranial, middle, accessory, and caudal lobes) and three on the left (cranial, middle, and caudal).[72] The right cranial lobe is of particular interest for human transplantation as the bronchus for this lobe arises directly from the trachea (the so-called "pig bronchus"), a significant distance from the carinal bifurcation. This anatomy complicates the normal end-to-end bronchial anastomosis technique of right lung transplantation unless the right porcine cranial lobe is surgically excluded. Therefore, most porcine-to-primate transplantation experiments have used the left single lung transplant as the experimental model.[9] In human lung transplantation, donor tracheal bronchus abnormalities have been reported, with various techniques of implantation including the incorporation of the tracheal bronchus into the right bronchial anastomosis,[73] implantation of the tracheal bronchus using an island of trachea,[74] or resection of the affected segments or lobes.[75] For the porcine cranial lobe bronchus, the distance between the carina and the lobar takeoff typically exceeds 1 cm. A long patch tracheoplasty might be vulnerable to healing problems, rendering resection of the right cranial lobe a logical consideration. Gallifant and colleagues.[76] conducted a study of lobar gas exchange in pigs using whole lung computed tomography (CT) and demonstrated that the right cranial lobe contributed approximately 13% to total lung tidal ventilation, and 9% of proportional oxygen uptake of the lung. Thus, resection of the

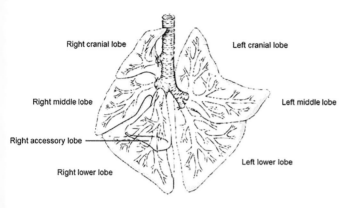

Fig. 1. Lobar anatomy of the porcine lung, ventral view.

cranial lobe (especially if appropriately sized pigs are selected to allow for the difference) would be a feasible technique to overcome this technical challenge. Implantation of both lungs *en bloc*, with a primary tracheal anastomosis, would also be a potential technique to avoid this issue.

One further anatomic difference between porcine lungs and human lungs is the branching pattern of the airways (**Fig. 2**). Porcine lungs tend to have a monopodial branching pattern,[77] where the main bronchus tends to continue in the same direction and the segmental bronchi branch off at obtuse angles.[78] This is in contrast to the bipodial branching pattern seen in human lungs. However, other than bronchoscopic differences[72] and the need to adapt nomenclature for the porcine lung, the clinical implications of this variant branching pattern remain unclear.

Infectious Challenges

Transmission of infectious diseases from the animal population (zoonosis) to immunosuppressed human recipients is a significant concern for xenotransplantation. The types of pathogens vary depending on the species of the animal; however, most research and clinical work have now focused on swine as the source animal for transplant organs. Diseases that can be carried by feral swine include brucellosis, tuberculosis, and leptospirosis as well as microorganisms such as *Salmonella* spp., Shiga toxin-producing *Escherichia coli,* and hepatitis E. These diseases and microorganisms have been known to transmit between humans and feral swine and mixing of feral and domestic swine populations have also been documented in the United States.[79]

The risk of these zoonotic infections can be minimized through careful breeding practices, maintaining clean and disinfected animal housing, and screening of the pig herd.[80] Due to the inherent characteristics of pigs, having early

sexual maturity, short gestational period, and large litter size, the development of designated pathogen-free (DPF) herds is feasible,[81] and will be required by regulatory agencies to minimize the risk of transmission of zoonotic disease to potential recipients.[80,82]

Porcine endogenous retroviruses

Of particular concern when considering porcine xenotransplantation is the potential transmission of porcine endogenous retroviruses (PERV). All pigs carry PERV in their genome,[83] and therefore, this made the eradication of PERV through traditional animal husbandry methods infeasible. Subtypes PERV-A and PERV-B are capable of infecting human cells[84,85] in vitro, with PERV-C being less capable, although possible through phenotypic mixing.[86]

PERV infection of humans has never been observed in clinical circumstances following transplantation of living tissues (skin) or cells (splenocytes, islets) from pigs.[87] Theoretic concerns exist as PERV has been shown to infect human embryonic kidney cell lines (HEK-293 cells) in vitro,[88,89] and human-to-human in vitro infectivity has been demonstrated by Niu and colleagues[90] in co-cultures of infected HEK293 T cells. It is important to note, however, that neither pig-to-human nor human-to-human transmission of PERV has ever been shown to occur in vivo.

Additionally, pre-clinical studies of 101 nonhuman primates (monkey and baboon) transplant recipients, have not revealed transmission of PERVs.[91] Additionally, porcine-to-human pancreatic islet cell xenotransplantation has been carried out without evidence of PERV infection in the recipients.[92,93] However, it should be noted that in these clinical islet xenograft cases, either no or low-dose immunosuppression was used. Additionally, there is some evidence that pig islet cells do not release PERV,[94] thus, the applicability

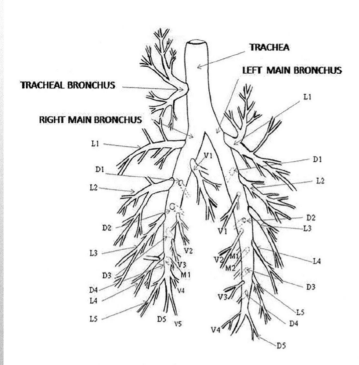

Fig. 2. Monopodial branching pattern of the bronchial tree in the pig.[134] (*From Monteiro A, Smith RL. Bronchial tree Architecture in Mammals of Diverse Body Mass. International Journal of Morphology. 2014;32:312-316.*)

of these findings to lung xenotransplantation is uncertain.

The clinical effect of PERV infection remains unknown; however, all retroviruses are potentially oncogenic and immunosuppressive. PERVs have been isolated from porcine leukemic cells[95] as well as radiation-induced leukemic cells.[96] Similar endogenous retroviruses in humans (HERV-K) have been found expressed in human breast cancer, prostate cancer, lymphoma melanoma, and other cancers.[97] It is unclear, however, whether there is a direct role in HERV activation and oncogenesis or whether it is expressed due to transcriptional activation in tumor cells.

There is also concern that PERV infection could induce immunosuppression. PERV, a type 3 retrovirus, is closely related to the murine leukemia virus, feline leukemia virus, and koala retrovirus. These viruses have been linked to immunodeficiency in their infected hosts.[98] In experiments using purified PERVs on human peripheral blood mononuclear cells, inhibition of cell proliferation of PERV in a viral-load-dependent manner was observed, suggesting that PERV infection in the human could induce an immunosuppressive state.[99]

Finally, concerns regarding the potential risk of human-to-human PERV transmission as well as the incorporation of PERV into the human genome exist. Additionally, potential recombination of the PERV with closely related HERV could theoretically give rise to a new virus with unknown pathologic potential.[100]

Strategies to minimize the prevalence of PERV include animal selection, although as mentioned earlier, it is impossible to eliminate the ubiquitous PERV-A and PERV-B. However, the selection of low-titer pigs and pigs screened to be free of PERV-C (to reduce the risk of PERV recombination) play a role in risk reduction and mitigation. Anti-retroviral drugs are effective against PERV in vitro,[101] however, concern regarding resistance would suggest that combination therapy would be required.

The most definitive strategy for eliminating the risk of PERV transmission is genomic editing of the pig. Yang and colleagues developed a method to inactivate all 62 copies of PERVs in porcine cell lines.[102] To do this, they used CRISPR-Cas9 RNA-guided nuclease to inactivate all copies of the PERV *pol* gene, a strategy designed to prevent infectivity for human cells. Subsequently, the group was able to similarly modify a porcine fibroblast cell line, and, using somatic cell nuclear transfer (cloning), developed viable pig embryos which were then successfully transferred into surrogate sows. The resulting PERV-inactivated pig strain, with at least 1000-fold less transmission to human cells, is proposed as a foundation for genetically engineered pigs intended for human use.[90] However, implications of potential off-target effects of such extensive gene editing must be considered in risk-benefit calculations.

The current clinical work with pig-to-human kidney transplantation has used pig donors which have been screened to be free of PERV-C but are positive for PERV-A and PERV-B. Similar to previous work in pancreatic islet cell transplant, the transmission of PERV-A and PERV-B was not detected in the kidney recipients for up to 53 hours.[1,2] PERV was similarly not detected in the most recent pig-to-human heart transplant.[3]

PORCINE CYTOMEGALOVIRUS

Recently, the report of porcine cytomegalovirus (PCMV) infection of the 2022 pig-to-human heart transplant performed at the University of Maryland has raised concern regarding the screening process for this virus and its role in the eventual failure of the organ.[3]

The role of human CMV (human herpesvirus 5) infection in lung transplant recipients is well understood, with a significant negative effect on both early survival[103] as well as potentiating chronic effects, leading to chronic lung allograft disease. Therefore, a period of antiviral prophylaxis is routinely prescribed to CMV-negative recipients undergoing transplant with CMV-positive organ (CMV mismatch transplant).[104] Despite the name, however, PCMV is more closely related to human herpesvirus (HHV) 6 and HHV-7. HHV-6 is significant, in that, it can accelerate the course of acquired immunodeficiency syndrome immunosuppression[105] as well as being potentially oncogenic, potentially associated with Hodgkins's lymphoma, gastrointestinal cancer, glial tumors, and oral cancers.[106]

Porcine CMV is endemic to the worldwide pig population and is transmitted through nasal secretions and in utero. Clark and colleagues[107] demonstrated 50% detection of porcine CMV in lung tissue in adult pigs and 66% in piglets raised conventionally for research in the United Kingdom. Prevention of CMV transmission to piglets was demonstrated using a combination of cesarean section and barrier rearing, although splenic samples from these piglets demonstrated PCMV DNA, although at lower concentrations than in farm-raised animals. Through early weaning of piglets and screening removal of PCMV-positive animals from the breeding herd, PCMV can be eliminated in animal herds used for xenotransplantion.[108]

The effect of PCMV on lung xenotransplantation has been demonstrated in experiments on nonhuman primates. PCMV transmitted by cardiac xenotransplantation has been shown to have high viral loads in the recipient baboon lung[109] and is associated with poorer cardiac graft survival. Comparable results have been seen with pig-to-baboon kidney xenotransplantation.[110] PCMV when transmitted by xenotransplantation, is potentially associated with consumptive coagulopathy[111] as well as graft edema (in cardiac xenografts[109]), both of which would have deleterious impacts on lung xenotransplantation.

Despite theoretic concerns regarding zoonosis, clinical experience to date using pancreatic islet cells, kidney and heart transplants from pig-to-human has not demonstrated significant infectious concerns. The concerning infectious entities including PERV and porcine CMV have effective techniques for surveillance and eradication in the host herds, and mitigation through pharmacologic treatment of the recipient is also an option. Maintaining herds of DPF animals,[112] screening for pathogens both known and potential, as well as novel techniques in gene editing allowing for endogenous retroviruses to be eliminated from donor animals, could allow for safe lung xenotransplantation concerning zoonosis.

Alternatives to Xenotransplantation and Lung Bioengineering

Although lung allotransplantation is the standard care for end-stage lung failure, it still suffers from fundamental limitations that do not have solutions in the near future, like donor scarcity, waiting time, less-than-optimal graft quality (due to donor age, donor co-morbidity, and so on) and technical issues regarding the limitation imposed by the restricted time window of the procurement and transplantation process.[113] Mechanical devices to supplement or replace lung function—extra- or intra-corporeal membrane oxygenator 'artificial lung' technologies, with or without an integrated pump—have witnessed considerable advances recently, but no durable mechanical lung replacement system has yet been developed. Alternative approaches to lung transplantation (both allotransplantation and xenotransplantation) include bioengineering and regenerative medicine. The general approach for bioengineering is to use some form of scaffold or matrix which is then populated by one or more phenotypes of cells, usually generated from human stem cells, to create the desired tissue properties.[114] If the intended recipient's cells can be used, the bioengineered organ would be expected to function without the need for immunosuppression medication. Alternatively, 'universal donor' cells, not susceptible to conventional rejection mechanisms, would offer the promise of replacing the lung with biocompatible tissue on demand. To date, tissue engineering (**Fig 3**) approaches have been applied to human skin substitutes,[115] vascular grafts,[116] and bladder tissue.[117] However, tissue engineering for primarily vascularized solid organs is more

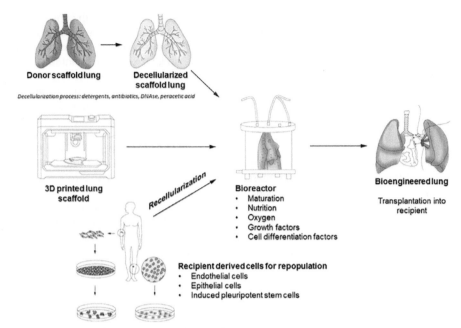

Fig. 3. Decellularization/recellularization process used in tissue engineering.

challenging given the multiple cell types involved (over 40 different cell types in the lung[118]) as well as the need not just for structural integrity, but, in the case of lung, alveolocapillary barrier and gas exchange functions.

In terms of animal transplants performed with bioengineered lungs, the current experiments are summarized in **Table 1**. In large animals compared to humans, the longest survival report to date is from Nichols and colleagues,[119] who performed transplantation of porcine lungs using a decellularized pig scaffold with the survival of one animal to 2 months. Of note, only the airway was anastomosed in this experiment, but vascularization of the airway was observed. Animal transplantation experiments with bioengineered lungs 3D-printed artificial scaffolds are ongoing, however, peer-reviewed data have yet to be published.[120]

Lung Xenotransplantation: Future and Remaining Challenges

Despite the considerable number of remaining challenges, xenotransplantation in general and lung, in particular, have made great advances and discoveries in the last decades. Recently, pigs have been produced that have up to 16 genetic modifications (Revivicor, Blacksburg, Virginia, USA; Quhan Bio Inc, Hangyhou, China; eGenesis Inc, Cambridge, MA, USA; to name a few). Survival is now measured by years for nonhuman primates carrying life-supporting pig kidneys and by months for pig hearts. Lung

xenotransplantation still must achieve similar in vivo results before moving to clinical studies. Further genetic modifications may not be necessary, and we may work better on optimizing the ones we know. Removing the three main pig carbohydrates and introducing 7 to 10 human regulatory proteins may be sufficient to develop a 'xeno-lung' for human use as long as gene expression is sufficient in the correct anatomic locations. Additional optimization of lung xenotransplantation may require novel immunosuppressive treatments distinct from the classical triple treatment (antimetabolite, anti-calcineurin, and steroid), as shown for other organs.[121,122]

Xenotransplantation carries the potential to revolutionize transplantation medicine by providing unlimited supplies of high-quality organs. Ideally, the future transplantation centers will routinely have access to a supply of consistent donor pigs who are maintained under DPF conditions. Organ procurement can be conducted under planned conditions as dictated by the intended recipient's situation, eliminating the need for long waiting times and clinical deterioration. In theory, bred pigs with consistent gene editing and expression of transgenes would permit the availability of pigs of all ages for precision donor-recipient size matching and compatibility testing.

In conclusion, based on the accelerated pace of advancements in xenotransplantation, we are optimistic that lung xenotransplantation will be a reality in the future.

Table 1
Summary of bioengineered animal transplantation experiments and survival

Author	Animal	n	Bioreactor Culture Time	Recellularization Cell Line	Survival	Anastomosis
Ott[123]	Rat	3	9 d	Human umbilical cord endothelial cells and human alveolar basal epithelial cells	6 h	Airway and vascular anastomosis
Doi[124]	Rat	3	8 d	eGFP-labeled vascular endothelial cells, QDs655-labeled adipose-derived stromal cells	3 h	Airway and vascular anastomosis
Petersen[125]	Rat	4	8 d	Neonatal rat lung epithelial cells and microvascular lung endothelial cells	2 h	Airway and vascular anastomosis
Song[126]	Rat	12	7 d	Human umbilical cord endothelial cells	14 d	Airway and vascular anastomosis
Gilpin[127]	Rat	5	10 d	Human ventralized iPSC-derived endothelial cells	60 min	Airway and vascular anastomosis
Ren[128]	Rat	6	8 d	Human umbilical vein endothelial cells and human mesenchymal stromal cells (n = 3) Human-induced pluripotent stem cells (n = 3)	3 d	Airway and vascular anastomosis
Obata[129]	Rat	16	3 d	Rat adipose-derived stromal cells and rat lung microvascular endothelial cells	30 min	Vascular anastomosis
Jensen[130]	Mouse	Unknown	24 h	Predifferentiated murine embryonic stem cells	14 d	Implanted subcutaneously
Nichols[119]	Pig	5	30 d	Adult pig-derived lung cells from pneumonectomy	2 mo	Airway anastomosis only
Yanagiya[131]	Pig	3	3 wk	Autologous airway epithelial cells and vascular endothelial cells obtained by wedge resection 3 wk before transplantation	2 h	Airway and vascular anastomosis
Zhou[132]	Pig	3	6 d	Human umbilical vein endothelial cells and human airway epithelial progenitor cells	6 d	Airway and vascular anastomosis
Kitano[133]	Pig	3	6 d	Human umbilical vein endothelial cells and basal endothelial stem cells	24 h	Airway and vascular anastomosis

CLINICS CARE POINTS

- Successful lung xenotransplantation will require development of an animal lung that is resistant to hyperacute rejection, compliment mediated rejection and coagulation dysregulation. The use of CRISPR-Cas9 gene editing technology has significantly advanced progress in developing these organs.

- Strict attention to the raising of animals to prevent zoonosis as well as humane and ethical practices must be adhered to ensure public acceptability of xenotransplantation.

- Lung xenotransplantation faces unique challenges that has limited progress in comparison to heart and kidney xenotransplantation, in which experimental and clinical pig-to-human transplant trials have met with early success.

DISCLOSURE

R. Chaban is supported by the Benjamin Research Fellowship from the German Research Foundation, United States (DFG). R.A. Montgomery receives research funding from Lung Biotechnologies, a wholly owned subsidiary of United Therapeutics, United States. No other author declares a conflict of interest.

REFERENCES

1. Montgomery RA, Stern JM, Lonze BE, et al. Results of two cases of pig-to-human kidney xenotransplantation. N Engl J Med 2022;386(20): 1889–98.
2. Porrett PM, Orandi BJ, Kumar V, et al. First clinical-grade porcine kidney xenotransplant using a human decedent model. Am J Transplant 2022; 22(4):1037–53.
3. Griffith BP, Goerlich CE, Singh AK, et al. Genetically modified porcine-to-human cardiac xenotransplantation. N Engl J Med 2022;387(1):35–44.
4. Valapour M, Lehr CJ, Skeans MA, et al. OPTN/ SRTR 2020 annual data report: lung. Am J Transplant 2022;22(S2):438–518.
5. Cooper DK. A brief history of cross-species organ transplantation. Proc (Bayl Univ Med Cent) 2012; 25:49–57.
6. Laird C, Burdorf L, Pierson RN 3rd. Lung xenotransplantation: a review. Curr Opin Organ Transplant 2016;21(3):272–8.
7. Bryant LR, Eiseman B, Avery A. Studies of the porcine lung as an oxygenator for human blood. J Thorac Cardiovasc Surg 1968;55(2):255–63.
8. Schroeder C, Allan JS, Nguyen BN, et al. Hyperacute rejection is attenuated in GalT knockout swine lungs perfused ex vivo with human blood. Transpl Proc 2005;37(1):512–3.
9. Burdorf L, Azimzadeh AM, Pierson RN 3rd. Xenogeneic lung transplantation models. Methods Mol Biol 2012;885:169–89.
10. Schroeder C, Guosheng GS, Price E, et al. Hyperacute rejection of mouse lung by human blood: characterization of the model and the role of complement. Transplantation 2003;76:755–60.
11. Sadeghi AM, Laks H, Drinkwater DC, et al. Heart-lung xenotransplantation in primates. J Heart Lung Transplant 1991;10(3):442–7.
12. Daggett CW, Yeatman M, Lodge AJ, et al. Total respiratory support from swine lungs in primate recipients. J Thorac Cardiovasc Surg 1998;115: 19–27.
13. Hurst DJ, Padilla LA, Cooper DKC, et al. Factors influencing attitudes toward xenotransplantation clinical trials: a report of focus group studies. Xenotransplantation 2021;28(4):e12684.
14. Hurst DJ, Padilla LA, Cooper DKC, et al. Scientific and psychosocial ethical considerations for initial clinical trials of kidney xenotransplantation. Xenotransplantation 2022;29(1):e12722.
15. Mitchell C, Lipps A, Padilla L, et al. Meta-analysis of public perception toward xenotransplantation. Xenotransplantation 2020;27(4):e12583.
16. Knott GJ, Doudna JA. CRISPR-Cas guides the future of genetic engineering. Science 2018; 361(6405):866–9.
17. Wang K, Ouyang H, Xie Z, et al. Efficient generation of myostatin mutations in pigs using the CRISPR/Cas9 system. Scientific Rep 2015;5(1): 16623.
18. Musunuru K, Chadwick AC, Mizoguchi T, et al. In vivo CRISPR base editing of PCSK9 durably lowers cholesterol in primates. Nature 2021; 593(7859):429–34.
19. Zuccaro MV, Xu J, Mitchell C, et al. Allele-specific chromosome removal after Cas9 cleavage in human embryos. Cell 2020;183(6):1650–64. e15.
20. Liang P, Xu Y, Zhang X, et al. CRISPR/Cas9-mediated gene editing in human tripronuclear zygotes. Protein & Cell 2015;6(5):363–72.
21. Alanis-Lobato G, Zohren J, McCarthy A, et al. Frequent loss of heterozygosity in CRISPR-Cas9-edited early human embryos. Proc Natl Acad Sci 2021;118(22). e2004832117.
22. Ryczek N, Hryhorowicz M, Zeyland J, et al. CRISPR/Cas technology in pig-to-human xenotransplantation research. Int J Mol Sci 2021;22(6). https://doi.org/10.3390/ijms22063196.
23. Wilmut I, Schnieke AE, McWhir J, et al. Viable offspring derived from fetal and adult mammalian cells. Nature 1997;385(6619):810–3.
24. Steptoe PC, Edwards RG. Birth after the Reimplantation of a human embryo. Lancet 1978;312(8085): 366.
25. Burdorf L, Laird CT, Harris DG, et al. Pig-to-baboon lung xenotransplantation: extended survival with targeted genetic modifications and pharmacologic treatments. Am J Transpl 2022;22:28–45.
26. Burdorf L, Azimzadeh AM, Pierson RN 3rd. Progress and challenges in lung xenotransplantation: an update. Curr Opin Organ Transpl 2018;23: 621–7.
27. Pierson RN 3rd, Kaspar-König W, Tew DN, et al. Profound pulmonary hypertension characteristic of pig lung rejection by human blood is mediated

by xenoreactive antibody independent of complement. Transpl Proc 1995;27(1):274.

28. Cooper DK, Good AH, Koren E, et al. Identification of alpha-galactosyl and other carbohydrate epitopes that are bound by human anti-pig antibodies: relevance to discordant xenografting in man. Transpl Immunol 1993;1:198–205.

29. Basnet NB, Ide K, Tahara H, et al. Deficiency of N-glycolylneuraminic acid and Galalpha1-3Galbeta1-4GlcNAc epitopes in xenogeneic cells attenuates cytotoxicity of human natural antibodies. Xenotransplantation 2010;17(6):440–8.

30. Byrne GWDZ, Stalboerger P, Kogelberg H, et al. Cloning and expression of porcine β1,4 N-acetyl-galactosaminyl transferase encoding a new xenoreactive antigen. Xenotransplantation 2014;21:543–54.

31. Rood PPTH, Hara H, Long C, et al. Late onset of development of natural anti-nonGal antibodies in infant humans and baboons: implications for xenotransplantation in infants. Transpl Int 2007;20:1050–8.

32. Lutz AJLP, Estrada JL, et al. Double knockout pigs deficient in N-glycolylneuraminic acid and galactose α-1,3-galactose reduce the humoral barrier to xenotransplantation. Xenotransplantation 2013;20:27–35.

33. Estrada JLMG, Li P, Adams A, et al. Evaluation of human and non-human primate antibody binding to pig cells lacking GGTA1/CMAH/β4GalNT2 genes. Xenotransplantation 2015;22:194–202.

34. Leventhal JR, Dalmasso AP, Cromwell JW, et al. Prolongation of cardiac xenograft survival by depletion of complement. Transplantation 1993;55:857–65.

35. Lin CC, Cooper DK, Dorling A. Coagulation dysregulation as a barrier to xenotransplantation in the primate. Transpl Immunol 2009;21(2):75–80.

36. Robson SC, Cooper DK, d'Apice AJ. Disordered regulation of coagulation and platelet activation in xenotransplantation. Xenotransplantation 2000;7(3):166–76.

37. Siegel JB, Grey ST, Lesnikoski BA, et al. Xenogeneic endothelial cells activate human prothrombin. Transplantation 1997;64:888–96.

38. Lin CC, Chen D, McVey JH, et al. Expression of tissue factor and initiation of clotting by human platelets and monocytes after incubation with porcine endothelial cells. Transplantation 2008;86(5):702–9.

39. Kopp CW, Grey ST, Siegel JB, et al. Expression of human thrombomodulin cofactor activity in porcine endothelial cells. Transplantation 1998;66:244–51.

40. Roussel JC, Moran CJ, Salvaris EJ, et al. Pig thrombomodulin binds human thrombin but is a poor cofactor for activation of human protein C and TAFI. Am J Transpl 2008;8:1101–12.

41. Lawson JH, Daniels LJ, Platt JL. The evaluation of thrombomodulin activity in porcine to human xenotransplantation. Transplant Proc 1997;29(1-2):884–5.

42. Schulte am Esch J, Rogiers X, Robson SC. Molecular incompatibilities in hemostasis between swine and men–impact on xenografting. Ann Transplant 2001;6(3):12–6.

43. Schulte Am Esch J 2nd RS, Knoefel WT, Hosch SB, et al. O-linked glycosylation and functional incompatibility of porcine von Willebrand factor for human platelet GPIb receptors. Xenotransplantation 2005;12:30–7.

44. Mazzucato M, De Marco L, Pradella P, et al. Porcine von Willebrand factor binding to human platelet GPIb induces transmembrane calcium influx. Thrombosis and haemostasis 1996;75(4):655–60.

45. Kaur S, Isenberg JS, Roberts DD. CD47 (Cluster of Differentiation 47). Atlas Genet Cytogenet Oncol Haematol 2021;25(2):83–102.

46. Martínez-Sanz P, Hoogendijk AJ, Verkuijlen PJJH, et al. CD47-SIRPα checkpoint inhibition enhances neutrophil-mediated killing of dinutuximab-opsonized neuroblastoma cells. Cancers (Basel) 2021;13:4261.

47. Allard B, Longhi MS, Robson SC, et al. The ectonucleotidases CD39 and CD73: novel checkpoint inhibitor targets. Immunol Rev 2017;276(1):121–44.

48. Antonioli L, Pacher P, Vizi ES, et al. CD39 and CD73 in immunity and inflammation. Trends Mol Med 2013;19(6):355–67.

49. Knapp KZM, Zebisch M, Pippel J, et al. Crystal structure of the human ecto-5'-nucleotidase (CD73): insights into the regulation of purinergic signaling. Structure 2012;20:2161–73.

50. Watzl C. How to trigger a killer: modulation of natural killer cell reactivity on many levels. Adv Immunol 2014;124:137-170.

51. Puga Yung G, Bongoni AK, Pradier A, et al. Release of pig leukocytes and reduced human NK cell recruitment during ex vivo perfusion of HLA-E/human CD46 double-transgenic pig limbs with human blood. Xenotransplantation 2018;25(1).

52. Forte P, Baumann BC, Schneider MK, et al. HLA-Cw4 expression on porcine endothelial cells reduces cytotoxicity and adhesion mediated by CD158a+ human NK cells. Xenotransplantation 2009;16(1):19-26.

53. Macchiarini P, Mazmanian GM, Oriol R, et al. Ex vivo lung model of pig-to-human hyperacute xenograft rejection. J Thorac Cardiovasc Surg 1997;114(3):315–25.

54. Pierson RN 3rd, Tew DN, Konig WK, et al. Pig lungs are susceptible to hyperacute rejection by human blood in a working ex vivo heart-lung model. Transpl Proc 1994;26(3):1318.

55. Macchiarini P, Oriol R, Azimzadeh A, et al. Evidence of human non-alpha-galactosyl antibodies involved in the hyperacute rejection of pig lungs and their removal by pig organ perfusion. J Thorac Cardiovasc Surg 1998;116(5):831–43.

56. Pfeiffer S, Zorn GL 3rd, Kelishadi S, et al. Role of anti-Gal alpha13Gal and anti-platelet antibodies in hyperacute rejection of pig lung by human blood. Annals of thoracic surgery 2001;72(5): 1681–9. discussion 1690.

57. Pierson RN 3rd, Kasper-Konig W, Tew DN, et al. Hyperacute lung rejection in a pig-to-human transplant model: the role of anti-pig antibody and complement. Transplant 1997;63(4):594–603.

58. Blum MG, Collins BJ, Chang AC, et al. Complement inhibition by FUT-175 and K76-COOH in a pig-to-human lung xenotransplant model. Xenotransplantation 1998;5(1):35–43.

59. Macchiarini P, Oriol R, Azimzadeh A, et al. Characterization of a pig-to-goat orthotopic lung xenotransplantation model to study beyond hyperacute rejection. J Thorac Cardiovasc Surg 1999;118(5):805–14.

60. Nguyen BN, Azimzadeh AM, Schroeder C, et al. Absence of Gal epitope prolongs survival of swine lungs in an ex vivo model of hyperacute rejection. Xenotransplantation 2011;18(2):94–107.

61. Nguyen BN, Azimzadeh AM, Zhang T, et al. Life-supporting function of genetically modified swine lungs in baboons. J Thorac Cardiovasc Surg 2007;133(5):1354–63.

62. Pierson RN 3rd, Pino-Chavez G, Young VK, et al. Expression of human decay accelerating factor may protect pig lung from hyperacute rejection by human blood. J Heart Lung Transpl 1997; 16(2):231–9.

63. White DJG, Langford GA, Cozzi E, et al. Production of pigs transgenic for human DAF: a strategy for xenotransplantation. Xenotransplantation 1995;2: 213–7.

64. Burdorf L, Stoddard T, Zhang T, et al. Expression of human CD46 modulates inflammation associated with GalTKO lung xenograft injury. Am J Transpl 2014;14:1084–95.

65. Pfeiffer S, Zorn GL 3rd, Zhang JP, et al. Hyperacute lung rejection in the pig-to-human model. III. Platelet receptor inhibitors synergistically modulate complement activation and lung injury. Transplantation 2003;75(7):953–9.

66. Burdorf L, Riner A, Rybak E, et al. Platelet sequestration and activation during GalTKO.hCD46 pig lung perfusion by human blood is primarily mediated by GPIb, GPIIb/IIIa, and von Willebrand Factor. Xenotransplantation 2016;23(3):222–36.

67. Burdorf L, Harris D, Dahi S, et al. Thromboxane and histamine mediate PVR elevation during xenogeneic pig lung perfusion with human blood. Xenotransplantation 2019;26(2):e12458.

68. Connolly MR, Kuravi K, Burdorf L, et al. Humanized von Willebrand factor reduces platelet sequestration in ex vivo and in vivo xenotransplant models. Xenotransplantation 2021;28:e12712.

69. Laird CT, Burdorf L, French BM, et al. Transgenic expression of human leukocyte antigen-E attenuates GalKO.hCD46 porcine lung xenograft injury. Xenotransplantation 2017;24(2).

70. Watanabe H, Sahara H, Nomura S, et al. GalT-KO pig lungs are highly susceptible to acute vascular rejection in baboons, which may be mitigated by transgenic expression of hCD47 on porcine blood vessels. Xenotransplantation 2018;25(5):e12391.

71. Miura S, Habibabady ZA, Pollok F, et al. Effects of human TFPI and CD47 expression and selectin and integrin inhibition during GalTKO.hCD46 pig lung perfusion with human blood. Xenotransplantation 2022;29(2):e12725.

72. Judge EP, Hughes JML, Egan JJ, et al. Anatomy and bronchoscopy of the porcine lung. A model for translational respiratory medicine. Am J Respir Cell Mol Biol 2014;51(3):334–43.

73. Schmidt F, McGiffin DC, Zorn G, et al. Management of congenital abnormalities of the donor lung. Ann Thorac Surg 2001;72(3):935–7.

74. Hendriks JMH, Deblier I, Dieriks B, et al. Successful bilateral lung transplant from a donor with a tracheal right upper lobe bronchus. J Thorac Cardiovasc Surg 2009;137(3):771–3.

75. Mendogni P, Tosi D, Rosso L, et al. Lung transplant from donor with tracheal bronchus: case report and literature review. Transplant Proc 2019;51(1):239–41.

76. Gallifant J, Cronin JN, Formenti F. Quantification of lobar gas exchange: a proof-of-concept study in pigs. Br J Anaesth 2021;127(2):e55–8.

77. Azad MK, Mansy HA, Gamage PT. Geometric features of pig airways using computed tomography. Physiol Rep 2016;4(20). https://doi.org/10.14814/phy2.12995.

78. Noble PB, McLaughlin RA, West AR, et al. Distribution of airway narrowing responses across generations and at branching points, assessed in vitro by anatomical optical coherence tomography. Respir Res 2010;11(1):9.

79. Brown VR, Bowen RA, Bosco-Lauth AM. Zoonotic pathogens from feral swine that pose a significant threat to public health. Transboundary Emerging Dis 2018;65(3):649–59.

80. U.S. Department of Health and Human Services FaDA, Center for Biologics Evaluation and Research. Source animal, product, preclinical, and clinical issues concerning the use of xenotransplantation products in humans. https://www.fda.gov/regulatory-information/search-fda-guidance-documents/source-animal-product-preclinical-and-clinical-issues-concerning-use-xenotransplantation-products.

81. Boneva RS, Folks TM, Chapman LE. Infectious disease issues in xenotransplantation. Clin Microbiol Rev 2001;14(1):1–14.

82. PHS guideline on infectious disease issues in xenotransplantation.

83. Wilson CA. Endogenous retroviruses. Cell Mol Life Sci 2008/11/01 2008;65(21):3399–412.

84. Patience C, Takeuchi Y, Weiss RA. Infection of human cells by an endogenous retrovirus of pigs. Nat Med 1997;3(3):282–6.

85. Le Tissier P, Stoye JP, Takeuchi Y, et al. Two sets of human-tropic pig retrovirus. Nature 1997;389(6652):681–2.

86. Takeuchi Y, Patience C, Magre S, et al. Host range and interference studies of three classes of pig endogenous retrovirus. J Virol 1998;72(12):9986–91.

87. McGregor CGA, Takeuchi Y, Scobie L, et al. PERVading strategies and infectious risk for clinical xenotransplantation. Xenotransplantation 2018;25(4):e12402.

88. Martin U, Kiessig V, Blusch JH, et al. Expression of pig endogenous retrovirus by primary porcine endothelial cells and infection of human cells. Lancet 1998;352(9129):692–4.

89. Wilson CA, Wong S, Muller J, et al. Type C retrovirus released from porcine primary peripheral blood mononuclear cells infects human cells. J Virol 1998;72(4):3082–7.

90. Niu D, Wei H-J, Lin L, et al. Inactivation of porcine endogenous retrovirus in pigs using CRISPR-Cas9. Science 2017;357(6357):1303–7.

91. Denner J, Tönjes RR. Infection barriers to successful xenotransplantation focusing on porcine endogenous retroviruses. Clin Microbiol Rev 2012;25(2):318–43.

92. Heneine W, Tibell A, Switzer WM, et al. No evidence of infection with porcine endogenous retrovirus in recipients of porcine islet-cell xenografts. Lancet 1998;352(9129):695–9.

93. Garkavenko O, Croxson MC, Irgang M, et al. Monitoring for presence of potentially xenotic viruses in recipients of pig islet xenotransplantation. J Clin Microbiol 2004;42(11):5353–6.

94. Irgang M, Laue C, Velten F, et al. No evidence for PERV release by islet cells from German landrace pigs. Ann Transpl 2008;13(4):59–66.

95. Moennig V, Frank H, Hunsmann G, et al. C-type particles produced by a permanent cell line from a leukemic pig. II. Physical, chemical, and serological characterization of the particles. Virol 1974;57(1):179–88.

96. Frazier ME. Evidence for retrovirus in miniature swine with radiation-induced leukemia or metaplasia. Arch Virol 1985;83(1–2):83–97.

97. Salavatiha Z, Soleimani-Jelodar R, Jalilvand S. The role of endogenous retroviruses-K in human cancer. Rev Med Virol 2020;30(6):e2142.

98. Denner J, Young PR. Koala retroviruses: characterization and impact on the life of koalas. Retrovirology 2013;10:108.

99. Tacke SJ, Kurth R, Denner J. Porcine endogenous retroviruses inhibit human immune cell function: risk for xenotransplantation? Virology 2000;268(1):87–93.

100. Łopata K, Wojdas E, Nowak R, et al. Porcine Endogenous Retrovirus (PERV) – Molecular Structure and Replication Strategy in the Context of Retroviral Infection Risk of Human Cells. Review. Frontiers in Microbiology 2018;9.

101. Denner J. Can antiretroviral drugs Be used to treat porcine endogenous retrovirus (PERV) infection after xenotransplantation? Viruses 2017;9(8):213.

102. Yang L, Güell M, Niu D, et al. Genome-wide inactivation of porcine endogenous retroviruses (PERVs). Sci 2015;350(6264):1101–4.

103. Fishman JA, Rubin RH. Infection in organ-transplant recipients. N Engl J Med 1998;338(24):1741–51.

104. Herrera S, Khan B, Singer LG, et al. Extending cytomegalovirus prophylaxis in high-risk (D+/R−) lung transplant recipients from 6 to 9 months reduces cytomegalovirus disease: a retrospective study. Transpl Infect Dis 2020;22(4):e13277.

105. Emery VC, Atkins MC, Bowen EF, et al. Interactions between β-herpesviruses and human immunodeficiency virus in vivo: evidence for increased human immunodeficiency viral load in the presence of human herpesvirus 6. J Med Virol 1999;57(3):278–82.

106. Eliassen E, Lum E, Pritchett J, et al. Human herpesvirus 6 and malignancy: a review. Front Oncol 2018;8:512.

107. Clark DA, Fryer JFL, Tucker AW, et al. Porcine cytomegalovirus in pigs being bred for xenograft organs: progress towards control. Xenotransplantation 2003;10(2):142–8.

108. Egerer S, Fiebig U, Kessler B, et al. Early weaning completely eliminates porcine cytomegalovirus from a newly established pig donor facility for xenotransplantation. Xenotransplantation 2018;25(4):e12449.

109. Denner J, Längin M, Reichart B, et al. Impact of porcine cytomegalovirus on long-term orthotopic cardiac xenotransplant survival. Scientific Rep 2020;10(1):17531.

110. Yamada K, Tasaki M, Sekijima M, et al. Porcine cytomegalovirus infection is associated with early rejection of kidney grafts in a pig to baboon xenotransplantation model. Transplantation 2014;98(4):411–8.

111. Mueller NJ, Kuwaki K, Dor FJMF, et al. Reduction of consumptive coagulopathy using porcine cytomegalovirus-free cardiac porcine grafts in pig-to-primate xenotransplantation. Transplantation 2004;78(10):1449–53.

112. Fishman JA. Prevention of infection in xenotransplantation: designated pathogen-free swine in the safety equation. Xenotransplantation 2020;27(3): e12595.

113. US. Department Of health and human, services., organ transplantation:, OPTN., &, SRTR., Annual data report 2020.

114. Langer R, Vacanti JP. Tissue engineering. Science 1993;260(5110):920–6.

115. Cortez Ghio S, Larouche D, Doucet EJ, et al. The role of cultured autologous bilayered skin substitutes as epithelial stem cell niches after grafting: a systematic review of clinical studies. Burns Open 2021;5(2):56–66.

116. Matsuzaki Y, John K, Shoji T, et al. The evolution of tissue engineered vascular graft technologies: from preclinical trials to advancing patient care. Appl Sci (Basel) 2019;9(7). https://doi.org/10.3390/app9071274.

117. Atala A, Bauer SB, Soker S, et al. Tissue-engineered autologous bladders for patients needing cystoplasty. Lancet 2006;367(9518):1241–6.

118. Franks TJ, Colby TV, Travis WD, et al. Resident cellular components of the human lung. Proc Am Thorac Soc 2008;5(7):763–6.

119. Nichols JE, Francesca SL, Niles JA, et al. Production and transplantation of bioengineered lung into a large-animal model. Sci Translational Med 2018;10(452):eaao3926.

120. United therapeutics provides an update on its organ printing programs. https://ir.unither.com/news/press-releases/press-release-details/2022/United-Therapeutics-Provides-an-Update-on-Its-Organ-Printing-Programs/default.aspx. [Accessed 6 June 2022]. Accessed.

121. Pierson RN. Progress toward pig-to-human xenotransplantation. N Engl J Med 2022;386(20): 1871–3.

122. Pierson RN, Fishman JA, Lewis GD, et al. Progress toward cardiac xenotransplantation. Circulation 2020;142(14):1389–98.

123. Ott HC, Clippinger B, Conrad C, et al. Regeneration and orthotopic transplantation of a bioartificial lung. Nat Med 2010;16(8):927–33.

124. Doi R, Tsuchiya T, Mitsutake N, et al. Transplantation of bioengineered rat lungs recellularized with endothelial and adipose-derived stromal cells. Sci Rep 2017;7(1):8447.

125. Petersen TH, Calle EA, Zhao L, et al. Tissue-engineered lungs for in vivo implantation. Science 2010;329(5991):538–41.

126. Song JJ, Kim SS, Liu Z, et al. Enhanced in vivo function of bioartificial lungs in rats. Ann Thorac Surg 2011;92(3):998–1005 [discussion: 1005–6].

127. Gilpin SE, Ren X, Okamoto T, et al. Enhanced lung epithelial specification of human induced pluripotent stem cells on decellularized lung matrix. Ann Thorac Surg 2014;98(5):1721–9 [discussion: 1729].

128. Ren X, Moser PT, Gilpin SE, et al. Engineering pulmonary vasculature in decellularized rat and human lungs. Nat Biotechnol 2015;33(10):1097–102.

129. Obata T, Tsuchiya T, Akita S, et al. Utilization of natural detergent potassium laurate for decellularization in lung bioengineering. Tissue Eng Part C Methods 2019;25(8):459–71.

130. Jensen T, Roszell B, Zang F, et al. A rapid lung decellularization protocol supports embryonic stem cell differentiation in vitro and following implantation. Tissue Eng Part C Methods 2012;18(8): 632–46.

131. Yanagiya M, Kitano K, Yotsumoto T, et al. Transplantation of bioengineered lungs created from recipient-derived cells into a large animal model. Semin Thorac Cardiovasc Surg 2021;33(1):263–71.

132. Zhou H, Kitano K, Ren X, et al. Bioengineering human lung grafts on porcine matrix. Ann Surg 2018; 267(3):590–8.

133. Kitano K, Ohata K, Economopoulos KP, et al. Orthotopic transplantation of human bioartificial lung grafts in a porcine model: a feasibility study. Semin Thorac Cardiovasc Surg 2022;34(2):752–9.

134. Monteiro A, Smith RL. Bronchial tree architecture in mammals of diverse body mass. Int J Morphol 2014;32:312–6.

Moving?

Make sure your subscription moves with you!

To notify us of your new address, find your **Clinics Account Number** (located on your mailing label above your name), and contact customer service at:

Email: journalscustomerservice-usa@elsevier.com

800-654-2452 (subscribers in the U.S. & Canada)
314-447-8871 (subscribers outside of the U.S. & Canada)

Fax number: 314-447-8029

Elsevier Health Sciences Division
Subscription Customer Service
3251 Riverport Lane
Maryland Heights, MO 63043

*To ensure uninterrupted delivery of your subscription, please notify us at least 4 weeks in advance of move.

Printed and bound by CPI Group (UK) Ltd, Croydon, CR0 4YY

08/05/2025

01864719-0005